ADVANCES IN CHEMICAL ENGINEERING
Volume 29

Molecular and Cellular Foundations of Biomaterials

ADVANCES IN
CHEMICAL ENGINEERING

Editor-in-Chief

ARUP CHAKRABORTY
Department of Chemical Engineering
University of California at Berkeley
Berkeley, California

Editors

MORTON M. DENN
College of Chemistry
University of California at Berkeley
Berkeley, California

JOHN H. SEINFELD
Department of Chemical Engineering
California Institute of Technology
Pasadena, California

GEORGE STEPHANOPOULOS
Department of Chemical Engineering
Massachusetts Institute of Technology
Cambridge, Massachusetts

JACKIE Y. YING
Department of Chemical Engineering
Massachusetts Institute of Technology
Cambridge, Massachusetts

NICHOLAS PEPPAS
Department of Chemical and Biomedical Engineering,
and Division of Pharmaceutics,
University of Texas,
Austin, TX, USA

JAMES WEI
School of Engineering and Applied Science
Princeton University
Princeton, New Jersey

ADVANCES IN CHEMICAL ENGINEERING
Volume 29

Molecular and Cellular Foundations of Biomaterials

Edited by

NICHOLAS A. PEPPAS
*Department of Chemical and
Biomedical Engineering,
and Division of Pharmaceutics,
University of Texas,
Austin, TX, USA*

MICHAEL V. SEFTON
*Institute of Biomaterials
and Biomedical Engineering,
Department of Chemical Engineering
and Applied Chemistry,
University of Toronto,
Ontario, Canada*

2004

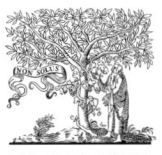

ELSEVIER
ACADEMIC
PRESS

AMSTERDAM - BOSTON - HEIDELBERG - LONDON - NEW YORK - OXFORD
PARIS - SAN DIEGO - SAN FRANCISCO - SINGAPORE - SYDNEY - TOKYO

ELSEVIER B.V.
Sara Burgerhartstraat 25
P.O.Box 211, 1000 AE
Amsterdam, The Netherlands

ELSEVIER Inc.
525 B Street, Suite 1900
San Diego, CA 92101-4495
USA

ELSEVIER Ltd
The Boulevard, Langford Lane
Kidlington, Oxford OX5 1GB
UK

ELSEVIER Ltd
84 Theobalds Road
London WC1X 8RR
UK

© 2004 Elsevier Inc. All rights reserved.

This work is protected under copyright by Elsevier Inc., and the following terms and conditions apply to its use:

Photocopying
Single photocopies of single chapters may be made for personal use as allowed by national copyright laws. Permission of the Publisher and payment of a fee is required for all other photocopying, including multiple or systematic copying, copying for advertising or promotional purposes, resale, and all forms of document delivery. Special rates are available for educational institutions that wish to make photocopies for non-profit educational classroom use.

Permissions may be sought directly from Elsevier's Rights Department in Oxford, UK: phone (+44) 1865 843830, fax (+44) 1865 853333, e-mail: permissions@elsevier.com. Requests may also be completed on-line via the Elsevier homepage (http://www.elsevier.com/locate/permissions).

In the USA, users may clear permissions and make payments through the Copyright Clearance Center, Inc., 222 Rosewood Drive, Danvers, MA 01923, USA; phone: (+1) (978) 7508400, fax: (+1) (978) 7504744, and in the UK through the Copyright Licensing Agency Rapid Clearance Service (CLARCS), 90 Tottenham Court Road, London W1P 0LP, UK; phone: (+44) 20 7631 5555; fax: (+44) 20 7631 5500. Other countries may have a local reprographic rights agency for payments.

Derivative Works
Tables of contents may be reproduced for internal circulation, but permission of the Publisher is required for external resale or distribution of such material. Permission of the Publisher is required for all other derivative works, including compilations and translations.

Electronic Storage or Usage
Permission of the Publisher is required to store or use electronically any material contained in this work, including any chapter or part of a chapter.

Except as outlined above, no part of this work may be reproduced, stored in a retrieval system or transmitted in any form or by any means, electronic, mechanical, photocopying, recording or otherwise, without prior written permission of the Publisher.
Address permissions requests to: Elsevier's Rights Department, at the fax and e-mail addresses noted above.

Notice
No responsibility is assumed by the Publisher for any injury and/or damage to persons or property as a matter of products liability, negligence or otherwise, or from any use or operation of any methods, products, instructions or ideas contained in the material herein. Because of rapid advances in the medical sciences, in particular, independent verification of diagnoses and drug dosages should be made.

First edition 2004

ISBN: 0-12-008529-1
ISSN: 0065-2377 (Series)

∞ The paper used in this publication meets the requirements of ANSI/NISO Z39.48-1992 (Permanence of Paper).
Printed in Great Britain.

CONTENTS

CONTRIBUTORS ix
PREFACE xi

The New New Biomaterials
MICHAEL V. SEFTON

I. What Happened to Inert Biomaterials? 1
II. Biocompatibility of Modern Biomaterials 2
References 5

Cell–Material Interactions
KRISTYN S. MASTERS AND KRISTI S. ANSETH

I. Introduction 7
II. Cell Surface Receptors and their Ligands 8
   A. Integrins 10
   B. Proteoglycans and Selectins 13
   C. Immunoglobulins 16
   D. Anti-adhesive Matrix Molecules 17
III. Integrin–Ligand Binding and Signal Transduction 18
   A. Focal Adhesions 19
   B. Effect of Cell Adhesion and Shape on Cell Function 21
IV. Nonspecific Interactions of Cells with Materials 25
   A. Dynamics of Protein Adsorption 26
   B. Surface Chemistry 28
   C. Surface Topography 31
V. Controlled Cell–Material Interactions 33
   A. Ideal Surfaces 34
   B. Adhesion Ligands 36
VI. Conclusion 41
References 42

Polymeric Biomaterials for Nerve Regeneration

SURYA K. MALLAPRAGADA AND JENNIFER B. RECKNOR

I. Introduction	47
II. Polymers for Regeneration in the Peripheral Nervous System	48
A. Nondegradable Polymers for Entubulization	50
B. Degradable Polymers for Entubulization	52
C. Comparative Studies	57
III. Polymers for Regeneration in the Central Nervous Systems	60
IV. Polymers for Controlled Release	64
V. Cell Encapsulation	66
VI. Conclusions	68
Acknowledgments	68
References	68

Structural and Dynamic Response of Neutral and Intelligent Networks in Biomedical Environments

ANTHONY M. LOWMAN, THOMAS D. DZIUBLA, PETR BURES, AND NICHOLAS A. PEPPAS

I. Introduction	75
II. Structure of Three-dimensional Polymeric Networks as Biomaterials	76
A. Hydrogel Classification	77
B. Network Structure of Hydrogels	77
C. Solute Transport in Hydrogels	83
D. Environmentally Responsive Hydrogels	88
E. Complexation in Polymers	92
F. Tissue Engineering Aspects of Neutral Networks	98
III. Applications of Hydrogels	105
A. Neutral Hydrogels	105
B. Responsive Networks	110
C. Oral Insulin Delivery Systems	119
D. Protein Based Hydrogels	120
E. Other Promising Applications	121
References	122

Biomaterials and Gene Therapy

F. KURTIS KASPER AND ANTONIOS G. MIKOS

I. Introduction	131
A. Gene Therapy and Protein Delivery	132
B. Methods of Gene Delivery	133
II. Biomaterials for Nonviral Gene Therapy	136
A. Cationic Lipids	136

	B. Cationic Polymers	138
	C. Polymers for Controlled Delivery	141
III.	Polymer Based Particles for Controlled DNA Release	141
	A. Genetic Immunization	142
	B. Advantages of Encapsulation Over Injection	143
	C. PLGA for Release of DNA in Vaccination Applications	143
IV.	Polymeric Scaffolds for Controlled DNA Delivery	157
	A. Gene Activated Matrices	157
	B. Wound Healing and Bone Regeneration	158
	C. Bone Tissue Engineering	159
	D. Release of DNA from Scaffolds	161
V.	Conclusion	162
VI.	Abbreviations	162
	Acknowledgments	163
	References	163

Surface-Erodible Biomaterials for Drug Delivery

Balaji Narasimhan and Matt J. Kipper

I.	Introduction	169
II.	Chemistry and Synthesis	172
	A. Early Synthesis of Polyanhydrides	172
	B. Synthesis of Polyanhydrides for Drug Delivery	173
	C. Chemistries of Polyanhydrides Used in Drug Delivery	176
III.	Polyanhydride Characterization	189
	A. Chemical Characterization of Polyanhydrides	189
	B. Characterization of Thermal Properties, Crystallinity, and Phase Behavior of Polyanhydrides	192
	C. Biocompatibility of Polyanhydrides	199
IV.	Degradation, Erosion, and Drug Release Kinetics	200
	A. Experiments	200
	B. Modeling Degradation, Erosion, and Drug Release Kinetics	207
V.	Design of Polyanhydride Carriers for Controlled Release	209
	A. Implantable Systems	210
	B. Injectable Systems	211
	C. Aerosols and Systems Designed for Mucosal Delivery	212
VI.	Conclusions and Future Opportunities	213
	References	214

Index	219
Contents of Volumes in This Serial	227

CONTRIBUTORS

Numbers in parentheses indicates the pages on which the authors' contribution begin.

KRISTI S. ANSETH, *Howard Hughes Medical Institute, Department of Chemical and Biological Engineering, University of Colorado, Boulder, CO 80309-0424, USA* (7)

PETR BURES, *Departments of Chemical and Biomedical Engineering, and Division of Pharmaceutics, CPE 3.466, The University of Texas at Austin, Austin, TX 78712-0231, USA* (75)

THOMAS D. DZIUBLA, *Institute for Environmental Medicine, University of Pennsylvania School of Medicine, Philadelphia, PA 19104, USA* (75)

F. KURTIS KASPER, *Department of Bioengineering, Rice University, Houston, TX 77005, USA* (131)

MATT J. KIPPER, *Department of Chemical Engineering, Iowa State University, Ames, IA 50011, USA* (169)

ANTHONY M. LOWMAN, *Department of Chemical Engineering, Drexel University, Philadelphia, PA 19104, USA* (75)

SURYA K. MALLAPRAGADA, *Department of Chemical Engineering, Iowa State University, Ames, IA 50011-2230, USA* (47)

KRISTYN S. MASTERS, *Howard Hughes Medical Institute, Department of Chemical and Biological Engineering, University of Colorado, Boulder, CO 80309, USA* (7)

ANTONIOS G. MIKOS, *Department of Bioengineering, Rice University, Houston, TX 77005, USA* (131)

BALAJI NARASIMHAN, *Department of Chemical Engineering, Iowa State University, Ames, IA 50011, USA* (169)

NICHOLAS A. PEPPAS, *Departments of Chemical and Biomedical Engineering, and Division of Pharmaceutics, CPE 3.466, The University of Texas at Austin, Austin, TX 78712-0231, USA* (75)

JENNIFER B. RECKNOR, *Department of Chemical Engineering, Iowa State University, Ames, IA 50011-2230, USA* (47)

MICHAEL V. SEFTON, *Institute of Biomaterials and Biomedical Engineering, Department of Chemical Engineering and Applied Chemistry, University of Toronto, Toronto, Ontario, M5S 3G9 Canada* (1)

PREFACE

Over the past forty years the field of Biomaterials Science and Engineering has grown from a small research area of no more than twenty researchers worldwide, to a robust discipline that has become a cornerstone of the field of Biomedical Engineering. During this time period, the field of biomaterials has found a welcome home in academic chemical engineering departments and in companies working with artificial organs, medical devices, and pharmaceutical formulations. The contributions of chemical engineers to the definition and the growth of the field have been important and at times seminal. It was therefore only natural for us to edit a volume that would highlight some of the major contributions of the chemical engineering world to biomaterials science and engineering.

In the mid 1960s biomaterials science was still at its infancy. The development of biomaterials was an evolving process. As Robert Langer of MIT and I indicated in a recent article (AIChE Journal, 49, 2990 (2003)), many biomaterials in clinical use were not originally designed as such but were off-the-shelf materials that clinicians found useful in solving a problem. Thus, dialysis tubing was originally made of cellulose acetate, a commodity plastic. The polymers initially used in vascular grafts, such as Dacron, were derived from textiles. The materials used for artificial hearts were originally based on commercial-grade polyurethanes. These materials allowed serious medical problems to be addressed. Yet, they also introduced complications. Dialysis tubing would activate platelets and the complement system. Dacron-based vascular grafts could only be used if their diameter exceeded about 6 mm. Otherwise occlusion could occur because of biological reactions at the blood–material and tissue–material interfaces. Blood–materials interactions could also lead to clot formation in an artificial heart, with the subsequent possibility of stroke and other complications.

In the last few years, novel synthetic techniques have been used to impart desirable chemical, physical, and biological properties to biomaterials. Materials have been synthesized either directly, so that desirable chain segments or functional groups are built into the material, or indirectly, by chemical modification of existing structures to add desirable segments or functional groups. It is possible to produce polymers containing specific hydrophilic or hydrophobic entities, biodegradable repeating units, or multifunctional structures that can become points for three-dimensional expansion of networks. Another synthetic approach involves genetic engineering for the preparation of artificial proteins of uniform structure. This enables the synthesis of periodic polypeptides that form well-defined lamellar crystals, polypeptides containing non-natural amino acids, and monodisperse helical rods. Important issues to be addressed include immunogenicity and purification from contaminants during large-scale production. If techniques were developed to produce polymers with the use of non-amide backbones, the versatility of this approach would be extended.

In this volume, we have collected a series of important critical articles on the present and future of biomaterials science as viewed by some of the leading chemical engineers of the field. It was not our intention to cover all aspects of biomaterials science but rather to unify certain synthetic, structural, and biological topics, and to point out the significant contributions of chemical engineers to the field. It is not a coincidence that this book is part of the well-known series of *Advances in Chemical Engineering*.

As I was commissioning the various chapters included in this volume, I wanted to highlight the main directions of this field: (i) novel methods of synthesis; (ii) advanced design; (iii) advanced characterization methods; (iv) better understanding of biomaterials/tissue interactions; and (v) a wealth of applications. Concerning this last point, it must be noted that just 25 years ago, the term biomaterials referred to materials in contact with the body but was restricted to materials for artificial organs and extracorporeal devices. The "explosion" of the fields of drug delivery and tissue engineering has led to new function and applications of biomaterials. The use of biomaterials in nanoscale technology requires added appreciation for the importance of chemical engineering principles in biomaterials science and engineering.

After a masterful introduction of the field and its new directions by Michael Sefton of the University of Toronto, Kristi Anseth of the University of Colorado offers a critical analysis of cell–materials interaction problems with emphasis on the nature of cell adhesions, adhesion ligands, and surface chemistry.

Surya Mallapragada of Iowa State University addresses questions related to the use of biomaterials in tissue engineering and nerve regeneration, while Anthony Lowman of Drexel University offers a detailed structural analysis of biological hydrogels used in biomaterials and drug delivery applications. Antonios Mikos of Rice University offers a critical review of biomaterials for gene therapy, whereas Balaji Narasimhan of Iowa State University pursues the question of biodegradability in materials, especially those used as drug delivery carriers.

As you read this book, I hope you will appreciate the infinite possibilities of biomaterials science in solving important medical problems.

If this book can influence young engineers and scientists to pursue a career in biomaterials science and engineering, it will have made a lasting impact. I want to thank Michael Sefton for coming to this project with an open mind and adding his advice as a co-editor and author of the first chapter. And I am indebted to the two early chemical engineering giants of the field, Edward Merrill of MIT and Alan Hoffman of the University of Washington, for having taken the first giant leaps in the tortuous road that is "biomaterials".

NICHOLAS A. PEPPAS
AUSTIN, TEXAS, USA
March 2004

THE NEW NEW BIOMATERIALS

Michael V. Sefton

Institute of Biomaterials and Biomedical Engineering, Department of Chemical Engineering and Applied Chemistry, University of Toronto, 4 Taddle Creek Rd, Suite 407, Toronto, Ontario, M5S 3G9 Canada
E-mail: sefton@chem-eng.utoronto.ca

I. What Happened to Inert Biomaterials?	1
II. Biocompatibility of Modern Biomaterials	2
References	5

I. What Happened to Inert Biomaterials?

In the beginning, there were metals and materials scientists. Plastics, polymers, and soft materials came later and then came the chemical engineers. The artificial heart program had a few (Artificial Heart Program Conference, 1969) but it was the artificial kidney program and the interest in new membranes that really started things off. Merrill at Massachusetts Institute of Technology (Merrill *et al.*, 1966) was a pioneer as was Leonard and Gregor (Friedman *et al.*, 1970) at Columbia and Hoffman at the University of Washington. Now almost every chemical engineering department has someone working on biomaterials or there is a bioengineering department nearby with chemical engineers on faculty. Several illustrations of this activity are apparent in this volume.

In the beginning the emphasis was on biocompatibility. Inertness was the key. We had our lists of no's (Table I) and the paradigm was focused on finding, synthesizing or surface modifying materials to make them fit these negative commandments. Interestingly, a large part of the early involvement of chemical engineers was to make materials that were not inert. Heparin immobilization was a hot topic in the late sixties and early seventies and the whole purpose was to make a surface that would actively interact with blood and prevent clotting. "Anti-thrombogenicity" was the keyword.

TABLE I

Commandments for inert biomaterials
No toxicity
No hemolysis
No pyrogens (endotoxin)
No protein or cell consumption
No thrombosis (and no emboli)
No inflammation
No infection
No immune response
No complement activation
No carcinogenicity and mutagenicity

Now with tissue engineering, regenerative medicine and combination products, active materials are the topic of interest of biomaterials specialists.

Some active materials are carriers for drugs (drug delivery systems), some have immobilized peptides to enable cell adhesion or migration, some are degradable by hydrolysis or by specific enzyme action. Some contain bioactive agents (e.g., heparin, thrombomodulin) to prevent coagulation or platelet activation while others incorporate bioactive groups to enhance osteo-conduction. Many include polyethylene oxide to retard protein adsorption and this is perhaps the closest we have come to a kind of inertness.

The advent of these materials has challenged the regulatory authorities since the materials are no longer being used simply for medical devices. Some include drugs and some include cells or biologicals. It was once sufficient to show that the material had no effect (i.e., it was inert) and then to get the blessing of the regulatory authorities. Now, it is the presence of an effect and a significant one at that, that needs to be regulated. The FDA has established an Office of Combination Products (http://www.fda.gov/oc/combination/) to deal with these products and every indication suggests that it is not long before these products are the norm. It is now not so simple to argue that the next generation of medical devices "does not achieve any of its primary intended purposes through chemical action within or on the body of man" as it is given in part of the FDA definition of a medical device.

II. Biocompatibility of Modern Biomaterials

When biomaterials were inert it was simple to think of biomaterials in terms of the absence of inflammation or the absence of thrombi. Now, with these newer combination materials we think of biocompatibility in more complex and subtle terms. The "appropriate host response" associated with the definition of biocompatibility has much more subtlety and complexity than we had hitherto considered. Blood compatibility may require some limited platelet adhesion and activation to passivate a material rather than the complete absence of adherent platelet deposits, especially if we want to limit embolization. What we now really mean by blood compatibility has been described in more detail elsewhere (Sefton et al., 2000).

We now recognize that blood compatibility is more complex than it was because we have to consider more than just platelets and coagulation factors and we have to consider the interactions among all the components of blood, including neutrophils, monocytes, and complement. This has led to the conclusion that thrombogenicity is really a special case of inflammation. That modern hematologists disregard Factor XII and the intrinsic coagulation system and focus on tissue factor (Jesty et al., 1995) and that tissue factor is expressed on activated monocytes (Gorbet et al., 2001) highlights further this linking of thrombogenicity and inflammation.

More fundamentally though the performance of these new biomaterials is challenging the entire concept of biocompatibility. A scaffold that promotes cell invasion may contain many of the attributes that in another context would lead to inflammation. Some constructs rely on a limited degree of inflammation to generate the enzymes that will cause the desired remodeling of the construct. Other uses of a biomaterial (e.g., as a vaccine adjuvant) is based on generating a local inflammatory response in order to boost the immune response, while immune responses to tissue constructs is an important, yet largely overlooked, element of the host response (Babensee et al., 1998). Some new angiogenic biomaterials (Gorbet et al., 2003) are designed to control the functional diversity of the monocyte (Riches, 1995), enabling a pro-angiogenic phenotype to emerge as the dominant functional form of these cells. The result is monocyte activation, but "good" activation: producing the blood vessels associated with granulation tissue but without the undesirable cytokines and other inflammatory mediators and proliferating fibroblasts. These new biomaterials are leading us to ask whether inflammation is bad or whether a little bit of inflammation can be a good thing?

Biomaterials are solid drugs. Rather than thinking of biomaterials as an inert contributor, my laboratory has taken to thinking about biomaterials as agonists of a biological response, much like drugs. However, biomaterials are solids and interact with cells and tissues through an interface, making the study of biomaterials more difficult than that of drugs, which are one-dimensional compared to the three-dimensional biomaterial. The biological responses we are interested in range from protein adsorption and platelet activation but extend to angiogenesis, matrix metalloproteinase secretion, immune recognition, and a wide variety of other biological phenomena. We can make use of the wealth of information, reagents, and assays that are available on these phenomena, but it is necessary to adapt them for the complexities of the interfaces and the differences between drugs and biologically active materials (Table II).

The differences in Table II are intended as broad generalities and readers can easily come up with exceptions or questions about what is meant by a biologically active material. For example, is the action of a drug delivery device always "local" or is a nanoparticle "large" and a DNA drug "small." Thus these characteristics must be interpreted and ringed with qualifiers to be strictly correct.

TABLE II

Biologically active materials	Drugs
Large, 3D objects	Small, 1D molecules
Immobile	Diffusible
Action is local	Action may be systemic, with side-effects a critical concern
Subject to foreign body reaction, coagulation, complement activation, etc.	Inflammation rarely a consideration
Interact across a cell membrane although endocytosis may occur	Act through a cell surface receptor or intracellularly
Limited surface area and ligand density	Even at nanomolar levels, there are many, many ligands (excess ligands?)
Action is often nonspecific	Specificity is key element
Protein adsorption influences cell response through altered ligand or receptor presentation or changes to microenvironment	No equivalent concept, although cell microenvironment affects drug action
Metabolism rarely relevant	Metabolized after an effect or to actually generate the effect
Effect is chronic	Effect is generally short-lived (half-life is a critical parameter)
Effect is generally permanent— pharmacokinetics and bioavailability are not normally considered	Effect is generally not permanent—pharmacokinetics and bioavailability are important
Can be engineered to be degradable and eliminated but many are not	Drug elimination is critical element of design

One of the more troubling characteristics is that of "specificity." Certainly a material that contains an immobilized growth factor or enzyme, contains much of the specificity of the immobilized agent. However, here I am thinking more about the biomaterial that has bioactivity (e.g., angiogenesis or osteoconduction), but without the obvious therapeutic agent within it. Here, the effect appears to be more nonspecific than that seen with drugs. This has been controversial, especially when presented in the form that many materials act the same (with occasional and important exceptions) resulting in questioning the importance of surface chemistry differences among materials (Sefton et al., 2001a). The implications of this with respect to hemocompatibility testing has also been discussed in reference Sefton et al., (2001b). The absence of substantive differences in platelet and leukocyte activation among many materials (Sefton et al., 2001a) suggests that the mechanism of these responses is fundamentally nonspecific in character.

The host response central to biocompatibility is to a 3D object, the chemistry of which does not appear to be terribly important. One way of thinking about this is that the biology does not really care if one changes the chemistry of a surface from one kind of nonspecific surface to another. Only when specificity is introduced through some sort of deliberate design can the biology "appreciate" what is happening. Hence it is little surprising that biomaterials specialists in 2003 speak of understanding the mechanism of biological response as much as they may tout a novel biomaterial. There is an extensive biological literature that we have only started to appreciate and exploit. The prospects for further basic research in biomaterials is correspondingly strong.

REFERENCES

Artificial Heart Program Conference; proceedings, Washington, D.C., June 9–13, 1969. Edited by Ruth Johnsson Hegyeli. National Institutes of Health.

Babensee, J. E., Anderson, J. M., McIntire, L. V., and Mikos, A. G., Host response to tissue engineered devices. *Adv. Drug Deliv. Rev.* **33**, 111–139 (1998).

Friedman, L. I., Liem, H., Grabowski, E. F., Leonard, E. F., and McCord, C. W., Inconsequentiality of surface properties for initial platelet adhesion. *Transactions—American Society for Artificial Internal Organs* **16**, 63–73 (1970).

Gorbet, M. B., and Sefton, M. V., Expression of procoagulant activities on leukocytes following contact with polystyrene and PEG grafted polystyrene beads. *J. Lab. Clin. Med.* **137**, 345–355 (2001).

Gorbet, M., Eckhaus*, A., Lawson-Smith, R., May, M., Sefton, M., and Skarja, G., Material-induced angiogenesis in impaired wound healing. Wound healing Society Abstract, May 2003.

Jesty, J., and Nemerson, Y., The pathways of blood coagulation, in "Williams Hematology" (E. Beutler, M. A. Lichtman, B. S. Coller, and T. J. Kipps Eds.), 5th Edition, pp. 1227–1238. McGraw-Hill, New York (1995).

Merrill, E. W., Salzman, E. W., Lipps, B. J., Jr., Gilliland, E. R., Austen, W. G., and Joison, J., Antithrombogenic cellulose membranes for blood dialysis. *Transactions—American Society for Artificial Internal Organs* **12**, 139–150 (1966).

Riches, D. W., Signalling heterogeneity as a contributing factor in macrophage functional diversity. *Semin. Cell Biol.* **6**(6), 377–384 (1995).

Sefton, M. V., Gemmell, Cynthia, H., and Gorbet, Maud B., What really is blood compatibility? *J. Biomater. Sci. Polymer Ed.* **11**, 1165–1182 (2000).

Sefton, M. V., Sawyer, A., Gorbet, M., Black, J. P., Cheng, E., Gemmell, C., and Pottinger-Cooper, E., "Does surface chemistry affect thrombogenicity of surface modified polymers?". *J. Biomed. Mater. Res.* **55**, 447–459 (2001a).

Sefton, M. V., Perspective on hemocompatibility testing. *J. Biomed. Mater. Res.* **55**, 445–446 (2001b).

CELL–MATERIAL INTERACTIONS

Kristyn S. Masters* and Kristi S. Anseth

Howard Hughes Medical Institute, Department of Chemical and Biological Engineering, University of Colorado, Boulder CO 80309, USA

I. Introduction	7
II. Cell Surface Receptors and their Ligands	8
A. Integrins	10
B. Proteoglycans and Selectins	13
C. Immunoglobulins	16
D. Anti-adhesive Matrix Molecules	17
III. Integrin–Ligand Binding and Signal Transduction	18
A. Focal Adhesions	19
B. Effect of Cell Adhesion and Shape on Cell Function	21
IV. Nonspecific Interactions of Cells with Materials	25
A. Dynamics of Protein Adsorption	26
B. Surface Chemistry	28
C. Surface Topography	31
V. Controlled Cell–Material Interactions	33
A. Ideal Surfaces	34
B. Adhesion Ligands	36
VI. Conclusion	41
References	42

I. Introduction

The nature of cell adhesion to substrate materials has a tremendous effect on cell function and tissue development. Signaling cascades initiated by cell adhesion have the ability to regulate a variety of events, including embryogenesis, tissue differentiation, and cell migration (Koenig and Grainger, 2002; Longhurst and Jennings, 1998). Signaling via receptor–ligand interactions provides the cell with vital information about its

---

*E-mail: kristi.anseth@colorado.edu

extracellular environment. Coordinated cellular responses to these signals enable cells to adapt their function to their specific environment.

Understanding how cells interact with a substrate is crucial in the development of functional biomaterials. The field of tissue engineering requires the creation of materials that are capable of directing tissue development, and one approach in achieving this control is through the manipulation of biological interactions between cell and material. A striking example of how cell–surface interactions influence cell function is the *in vitro* culture of mammary epithelial cells on tissue culture polystyrene (TCPS) vs laminin-coated surfaces. *In vivo*, epithelial cells are found as a monolayer on a basal lamina. When cultured on untreated TCPS *in vitro*, these cells lose their normal cuboidal morphology and ability to secrete milk proteins. However, upon addition of laminin to the surface, normal function and morphology are retained (Horwitz, 1997). Thus, in order to design and select appropriate polymeric scaffolds for tissue engineering, understanding the influence of the polymer surface chemistry on cell viability, growth, and function is critical.

Investigation of methods to control cell–material interactions is required in order to achieve the goal of developing ideal biomaterials and implants that can elicit specific, timely, and desirable responses from surrounding tissues. Study of cell–substrate interactions may also aid in analyzing differences between cell behavior *in vivo* vs *in vitro*. While *in vitro* experiments of cell–substrate interactions cannot reproduce the complex cascade of events and cellular responses that occur *in vivo*, they enable controlled, quantifiable experimental characterization that is difficult to obtain *in vivo*. Although this chapter discusses only the effects of receptor and ligand properties on cell–substrate interactions, these interactions may also be influenced by numerous co-factors such as cytokines and growth factors, thus greatly increasing their complexity. Because most cell–substrate interactions are mediated by biological molecules, a review of how cells adhere to their native extracellular matrix is first required.

II. Cell Surface Receptors and their Ligands

Whether on natural or synthetic materials, cell adhesion is mediated by protein interactions with cell surface receptors. There are several classes of cell surface receptors, and this chapter will discuss integrins, selectins, and immunoglobulins. These receptors bind their ligands with high affinity and specificity, and while each receptor family regulates separate cellular functions, there is some overlap between families. Each of these receptor families possesses a characteristic molecular structure, with every receptor normally consisting of an extracellular, transmembranous, and intracellular domain; this structure is illustrated in Fig. 1. The transmembrane region of receptors is generally hydrophobic and is roughly 6–8 nm in length, or approximately the thickness of the membrane (Hammer and Tirrell, 1996). The cell membrane itself is heterogeneous in composition and behaves like a fluid at physiological temperatures, where the viscosity of the membrane lipids can be 100–1000 times that of water, thus allowing receptor diffusion laterally within the membrane (Bussell et al., 1995a,b; Hammer and Tirrell, 1996). The membrane contains a two-dimensional suspension of proteins, where the area fraction of the membrane occupied by receptors may reach 0.4 (Hammer and Tirrell, 1996). Both proteins and lipids diffuse in the plane of the membrane, where the lipid diffusivity is approximately 10^{-8} cm^2/s, and receptor proteins exhibit a wide diffusivity range from 10^{-11} to 10^{-8} cm^2/s. The diffusion of receptors within a membrane is influenced by several factors, including hydrodynamic and

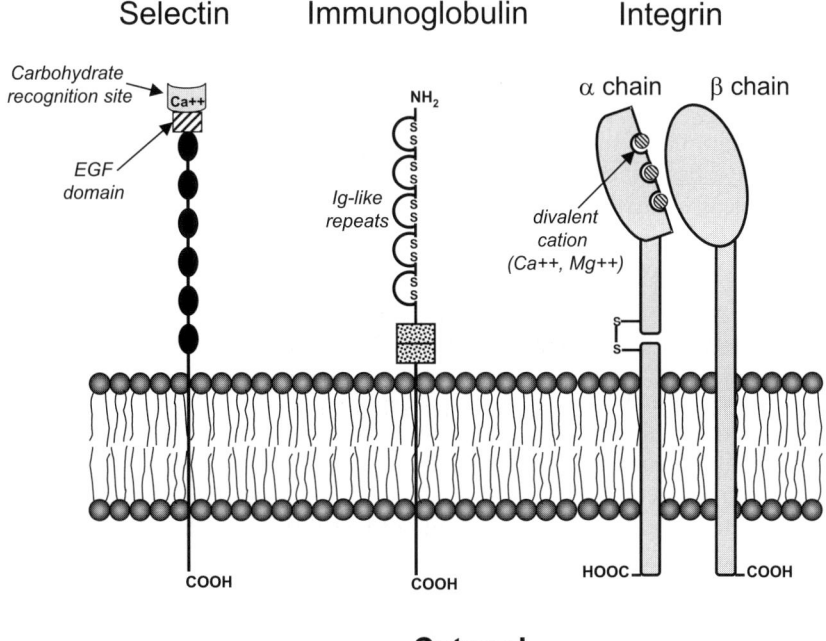

FIG. 1. Interaction of cells with the ECM is mediated by ligand binding to cell surface receptors, such as selectins, immunoglobulins, and integrins. Receptor–ligand binding allows cells to respond to changes in their extracellular environment. The general structure of these three types of receptors is illustrated here.

thermodynamic interactions between proteins, as well as obstruction or binding by cytoskeletal elements, all of which may reduce the receptor diffusivity (Bussell et al., 1995b).

This lateral mobility within the membrane is important because it participates in the regulation of receptor binding to ligands. Receptor diffusivity determines the rate at which receptors can find each other, thereby determining the transport-limited rate of binding. Under purely diffusive mechanisms, the rate of receptor collision, k_+ can be estimated according to the equation:

$$k_+ = 2\pi Ds \qquad (1)$$

where D is the sum of the lateral diffusivity of both interacting proteins and s is the radius of the encounter complex, or the distance at which the receptor and ligand are close enough to react (Bell, 1978). Because most proteins recognize and react with each other very rapidly, a diffusion-limited reaction rate is normal for many receptor interactions.

Most cellular interactions with the extracellular matrix (ECM) occur via integrins (Hynes, 2002). However, with the design of novel biomaterials in mind, the presence of other cell surface receptors such as proteoglycans and immunoglobulins may be exploited in order to create materials that elucidate a desired cellular response. Thus, while these receptor families are not typically highly involved in cell–substrate binding, their existence provides the bioengineer with more possibilities to achieve alteration of cell behavior via biomaterial modification.

A. Integrins

Integrins are the principal receptors on mammalian cells for binding most extracellular matrix proteins, including collagen, laminin, and fibronectin (Giancotti and Ruoslahti, 1999; Juliano, 2002). The integrin superfamily is comprised of homologous transmembrane linker proteins that mediate both cell–surface and cell–cell interactions. Each integrin receptor consists of a noncovalently assembled heterodimer of one α- and one β-subunit (Fig. 1; Longhurst and Jennings, 1998). In general, both subunits are N-glycosylated proteins with a large extracellular domain, a single hydrophobic transmembrane region, and a short cytoplasmic domain. There exist ~18 different α-subunits and 8 β-subunits, forming 24 different heterodimers (Hynes, 2002; van der Flier and Sonnenberg, 2001). Integrins differ from other cell surface receptors, such as those that bind to hormones and other soluble signaling molecules, in both their binding affinity and concentration. Integrins bind their ligand with a relatively low affinity ($K_a = 10^6 - 10^9$ liters/mole), and are present at 10- to 100-fold higher concentration on the cell surface (Alberts et al., 1994). This arrangement allows cells to weakly bind to a large number of matrix molecules, thus enabling it to explore its environment without losing attachment to it.

Integrins mediate cell adhesion through binding to a diverse array of ligands. These ligands include ECM proteins such as collagen, plasma proteins such as fibrinogen, and transmembrane immunoglobulins such as ICAM-1 (Longhurst and Jennings, 1998; Plow et al., 2000). The majority of ligands for integrin receptors are found as short peptide sequences within extracellular matrix proteins. The binding site in integrins for extracellular matrix ligands is composed of short regions in the N-termini of both subunits, with ligand specificity determined by the particular combination of α- and β-subunits (van der Flier and Sonnenberg, 2001). There are ~12 integrins that bind fibronectin and 7 that bind laminin (Plow et al., 2000; van der Flier and Sonnenberg, 2001). Many integrins can bind to more than one ligand, and several individual ligands can bind to more than one integrin. The most widely recognized and characterized ligand peptide motif is the RGD (Arginine–Glycine–Aspartic acid) sequence found in a variety of ECM proteins (Pierschbacher and Ruoslahti, 1984; Ruoslahti, 1996). Integrin recognition of this ligand occurs in almost all cell types and acts to promote their adhesion. However, some adhesive peptide sequences exhibit more cell selectivity, thereby encouraging the adhesion of only specific cell types. One example of this is REDV (Arginine–Glutamine–Aspartic acid–Valine), which is derived from the III-CS domain of human plasma fibronectin and has been shown to induce attachment and spreading of endothelial cells, but not fibroblasts, vascular smooth muscle cells, or platelets (Hubbell et al., 1991). Table I lists the major adhesive peptide sequences within several ECM proteins, as well as their receptors.

Integrin receptors are always present on the cell surface, although they often must be activated in order to bind a ligand (Hynes, 2002). Integrin expression does not necessarily increase with enhanced integrin-mediated adhesion, indicating the existence of other pathways by which the cell creates signals to change the affinity or avidity of the integrins. Activation of other surface receptors may induce an "inside-out" signaling cascade that results in conformational changes in integrins, altering their ability to bind ligands, a property known as receptor affinity (Bennett, 1998; van der Flier and Sonnenberg, 2001). Affinity is a measure of the binding strength between a single ligand and a single receptor; increases in integrin affinity mean that ligand binding can occur at lower ligand

TABLE I
Adhesive Peptide Sequences within ECM Proteins and their Receptors (For Review, See Yamada, 1991)

ECM protein	Adhesive peptide sequence	Major receptor(s)
Fibronectin	RGDS	$\alpha_v\beta_1$, $\alpha_v\beta_3$, $\alpha_v\beta_6$, $\alpha_{IIb}\beta_3$, $\alpha_3\beta_1$, $\alpha_5\beta_1$
	LDV	$\alpha_4\beta_1$, $\alpha_4\beta_7$
	REDV	$\alpha_4\beta_1$
	PHSRN	Synergistic for $\alpha_5\beta_1$ binding
Laminin	YIGSR	67-kDa binding protein
	PDGSR	Unknown
	LRGDN	$\alpha_v\beta_3$, $\alpha_5\beta_1$
	IKVAV	110-kDa binding protein
	LRE	Unknown
	IKLLI	$\alpha_3\beta_1$ and cell–surface heparan sulfate
Vitronectin	RGDV	$\alpha_v\beta_3$, $\alpha_v\beta_5$, $\alpha_{IIb}\beta_3$
Collagen I	RGDT	$\alpha_v\beta_3$
	DGEA	$\alpha_2\beta_1$
Fibrinogen	RGDS	$\alpha_v\beta_3$, $\alpha_{IIb}\beta_3$
	RGDF	$\alpha_{IIb}\beta_3$
	KQAGDV	$\alpha_{IIb}\beta_3$

Amino acid abbreviations: A = Arginine; D = Aspartic acid; E = Glutamate; F = Phenylalanine; G = Glycine; H = Histidine; I = Isoleucine; K = Lysine; L = Leucine; N = Asparagine; P = Proline; Q = glutamine; R = Arginine; S = Serine; T = Threonine; V = Valine; Y = Tyrosine.

concentrations. This occurrence may be due to changes in the rates of dissociation or association of the ligand as a result of agonist-induced conformational changes in the integrin itself. Modulation of integrin avidity can increase the number of integrin–ligand interactions, thereby strengthening cell adhesion. This behavior may occur via an agonist-induced rearrangement or clustering of integrins on the cell surface that is meant to increase the number of random encounters between integrin and ligand. As the cytoplasmic tail of the β-subunit is associated with the cell cytoskeleton, these changes in avidity likely occur due to a reorganization of cytoskeletal structures in response to other agonists or signals; it has been shown that Ca^{2+} induces the organization of the $\alpha_L\beta_2$ integrin into clusters that enhance the avidity of $\alpha_L\beta_2$-ligand binding interactions (Bennett, 1998; Binnerts et al., 1996). The concepts of integrin affinity and avidity and their effects on cell adhesion are illustrated in Fig. 2. Recent evidence also indicates that conformational activation and lateral clustering of integrins are closely and inextricably coupled (Li et al., 2003).

Just as the cytoplasmic domain of integrins is essential for transmitting intracellular signals that change integrin activity to achieve "inside-out"

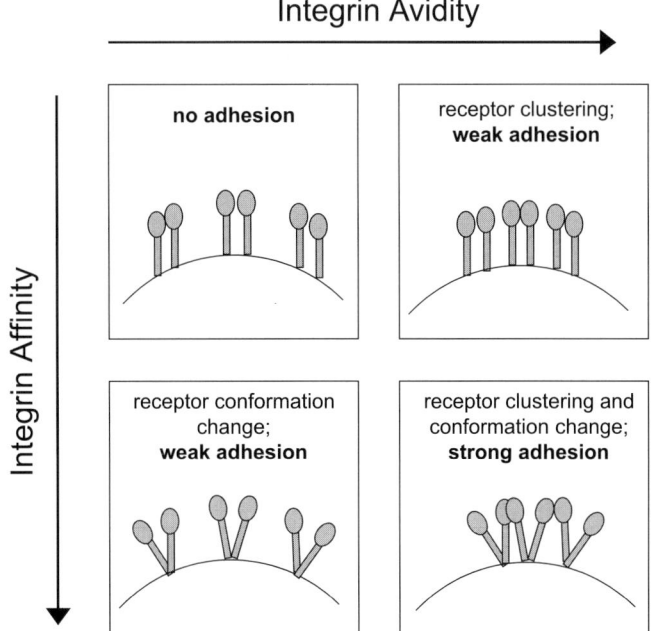

FIG. 2. Activation of cell surface receptors can initiate "inside-out" signaling, whereby the cell may alter its presentation of integrins. Integrin affinity and avidity may be modulated by a variety of agonists, resulting in alteration of ligand binding.

signaling, they are also required for communication in the opposite direction. This "outside-in" signaling allows cells to gain information about their extracellular environment through integrin–ligand binding and then transmit that information to the cytoplasm so that the cell function can appropriately respond to its surroundings. The implications of this signaling will be discussed later, in Section III.A; however, clearly, cell interactions with both synthetic and natural matrices are bi-directional and dynamic.

B. Proteoglycans and Selectins

All eucaryotic cells possess a carbohydrate-rich coating known as the glycocalyx, depicted in Fig. 3. Membrane proteins may be decorated or masked by these carbohydrates, which occur as oligosaccharide side chains covalently bound to membrane proteins or lipids, and as polysaccharide chains of integral membrane proteoglycans (Alberts et al., 1994).

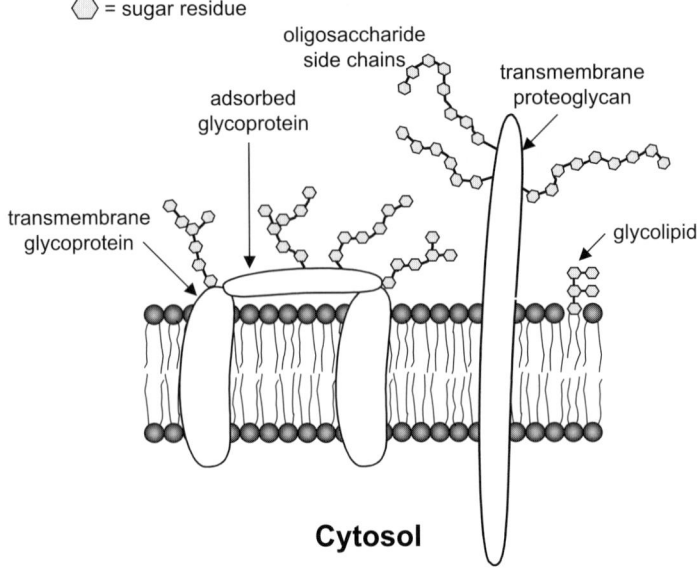

Fig. 3. Both adsorbed and transmembrane glycoproteins contribute to the formation of the cell glycocalyx. Once thought to function purely as a protective layer, cell surface oligosaccharides also participate in specific cell-recognition processes.

In addition to covalently bound saccharides, the glycocalyx also contains adsorbed glycoproteins and proteoglycans that have been secreted into the extracellular space.

It was originally believed that the sole function of the glycocalyx was to protect the cell against mechanical and chemical damage and to keep foreign objects and other cells at a distance. While this function of the glycocalyx is still valid, it has been discovered that these cell surface oligosaccharides also play a role in specific cell-recognition processes (Bertozzi and Kiessling, 2001; Sampson *et al.*, 2001). The oligosaccharides are composed of a diverse array of sugars, often branched, and covalently bound in a variety of linkages. This arrangement of diverse, exposed saccharides is well suited for mediating specific cell–cell adhesion processes, such as those occurring in sperm–egg interactions or inflammatory responses. The repulsive steric barrier created by the glycocalyx also functions to eliminate nonspecific adhesion while permitting specific interactions (Lauffenberger and Linderman, 1993). This means that the length of other cell surface adhesion molecules will play an important role, as the receptors must reach beyond the glycocalyx to bind to ligands.

The ligands for carbohydrate binding are known as lectins, which are often presented as components of the selectin family of cell–cell adhesion molecules. Selectins contain a carbohydrate-binding lectin domain connected to an epidermal growth factor-like motif, followed by a number of complement regulatory protein-like repeats, a transmembrane region, and a short cytoplasmic tail (Fig. 1; Furie and Furie, 1995). They bind to sialylated glycans, such as sialyl Lewis X, in a calcium-dependent manner (Juliano, 2002), and little is known about their association with the cell cytoskeleton. The selectin family consists of P–selectin, found in the α-granules of platelets and in the Weibel-Palade bodies of endothelial cells, E–selectin, which is expressed only by activated endothelial cells, and L–selectin, which is constitutively expressed on leukocytes (Mousa, 1998). The lectins have relatively low affinity for their carbohydrate ligands, and both the association and dissociation of the oligosaccharide with the lectin occurs very rapidly, resulting in only transient adhesion. Selectin binding is most prevalent in the bloodstream, where they are best known as the receptors that mediate the rolling on the blood vessel wall and subsequent extravasation of leukocytes and other inflammation-related molecules (McEver, 1995). The expression and function of selectins is tightly regulated such that they are only activated at specific times (Juliano, 2002). While primarily important in cell–cell interactions, this chemistry provides another opportunity to exploit and control cell surface interactions.

Membrane bound proteoglycans bind with low specificity relative to integrins. In addition to binding lectins, proteoglycans exhibit charge-mediated binding to ECM molecules. The glycosaminoglycann (GAG) blocks of proteoglycans are sulfated, resulting in a net negative charge that enables them to interact with clustered positive charges on proteins such as fibronectin. A higher degree of GAG sulfation causes tighter binding to these proteins. The positively charged protein regions may be described by the binding sequence, XBBXBX, where X is a hydrophobic amino acid and B is lysine or arginine (Cardin and Weintraub, 1989). Proteoglycan binding sequences of this nature have been identified in fibronectin, vitronectin, and laminin (West and Hubbell, 1997).

Lastly, monosaccharides may also participate in cell adhesion. Most commonly, galactose or lactose binds to the asialoglycoprotein receptor on hepatocytes (Geffen and Speiss, 1992). *In vivo*, this interaction serves to clear protein aggregates from the circulation. Regarding biomaterials synthesis, however, this mechanism has been exploited to create materials that induce hepatocyte-specific adhesion or enable liver-specific drug delivery (Cho *et al.*, 2001a; Gutsche *et al.*, 1994; Kobayashi *et al.*, 1994a).

C. IMMUNOGLOBULINS

The immunoglobulin (Ig) superfamily of receptors contains over 100 different molecules, and participates primarily in the mediation of cell–cell interactions (Buck, 1992). These receptors contain one or more Ig-like domains that are characteristic of antibody molecules (Fig. 1), and they function in a wide variety of cell types in which they are involved in many varied biological processes (Juliano, 2002). While Ig binding does initiate cytoplasmic signals, relatively little is known about the interactions of Ig receptors with cytoplasmic proteins. The most recognizable members of the Ig receptor family are ICAMs (intercellular adhesion molecules), VCAMs (vascular cell adhesion molecules), NCAM (neural cell adhesion molecule), and CD44s. This wide array of receptors is capable of binding in various manners; they commonly exhibit homophilic binding with identical Ig receptors, or they may bind to other different Ig receptors, nonIg family molecules such as integrins, and even some ECM components (Buck, 1992; Horton, 1996). NCAM is expressed on a variety of cell types, including most nerve cells, and binds cells together via a calcium-independent homophilic interaction. The binding interactions of NCAM are fairly versatile, however, as it may also bind to heparan sulfate and collagen (Brummendorf and Rathjen, 1996). Neural glial cell adhesion molecule (NgCAM) also exhibits a complex interaction pattern, binding to at least six different proteins including laminin and two integrin receptors responsible for fibronectin and vitronectin interactions (Brummendorf and Rathjen, 1996). Thus, even if an Ig receptor does not interact directly with the ECM, it can still regulate adhesion to the ECM substrate by signaling through the intermediate integrin receptor. These interactions of Ig receptors with ECM molecules and integrins have been shown to be important in events such as neurite outgrowth (Brummendorf and Rathjen, 1996).

Lastly, the CD44 receptors form a subgroup of the Ig family that is expressed on almost all cell types. CD44 is commonly overexpressed in cancer cells (Lesley et al., 1993) and assists in cell metastasis, indicating that the CD44–ligand interaction plays an important role in stimulating cell migration (Bartolazzi et al., 1994; Catterall et al., 1995). The principal ligand for CD44 is hyaluronic acid (HA), a glycosaminoglycan found in the ECM of many tissues, although CD44 may also bind to several other ECM proteins, including collagen, fibronectin, laminin, and osteopontin (Goodison et al., 1999). While all CD44 isoforms have the capability to bind HA, CD44 may be found in an active, an inducible, or an inactive state with respect to HA binding. CD44 appears to play a prominent role during embryogenesis, and it is involved primarily in the maintenance of

3D organ and tissue structure (Goodison et al., 1999). Binding of CD44 to hyaluronic acid mediates a multitude of cell functions, including cell aggregation, proliferation, migration, angiogenesis, and gene expression (Turley et al., 2002). Clearly, this degree of regulation makes hyaluronic acid-based chemistries attractive for many tissue engineering applications (Baier-Leach et al., 2003).

D. ANTI-ADHESIVE MATRIX MOLECULES

While a lack of cell adhesion will not promote cell survival or proliferation, there are several physiological processes that depend upon cell detachment from the ECM. Examples of this necessary de-adhesion can be found in normal development and tissue homeostasis, as anti-adhesive molecules cause different levels of de-adhesion ranging from complete cell detachment to the localized detachment required for cell migration. Investigation of these anti-adhesive molecules is important, as their use in biomaterials may provide a means to generate matrices that are conducive to cell migration by mimicking the adhesive/anti-adhesive nature of the native ECM.

In vivo, the ECM is composed of both adhesive and anti-adhesive components which interact both with cells and with each other in a complex manner. The principal molecules falling under the anti-adhesive classification are the tenascins, thrombospondins (TSPs), and secreted protein acidic and rich in cysteine (SPARC) (Sage and Bornstein, 1991; Sage, 2001). Several cell surface molecules, such as integrins, syndecans, and CD36, can serve as receptors of anti-adhesive ECM molecules (Orend and Chiquet-Ehrismann, 2000). Cells can exhibit varied adhesion responses to individual matrix components versus combinations of the same molecules. For instance, expression of metalloproteinases by synovial fibroblasts occurred when cultured on mixtures of tenascin-C and fibronectin, but not when either protein was presented alone (Tremble et al., 1994). Additionally, while these anti-adhesive proteins may antagonize the proadhesive activities of other matrix proteins, they have also been found to promote integrin-mediated cell adhesion under certain circumstances (Orend and Chiquet-Ehrismann, 2000).

Anti-adhesive molecules affect cell adhesion by changing the arrangement of cytoskeletal proteins and by altering signaling cascades. Specifically, tenascin-C, TSP-1, and SPARC all downregulate the actin stress fiber system and disrupt focal adhesions when added in solution to spread cells (Murphy-Ullrich, 2001; Orend and Chiquet-Ehrismann, 2000). Reorganization of the actin cytoskeleton is a major pathway by which anti-adhesive molecules modulate cell adhesion. Altering the state of actin polymerization has a great effect upon cell shape, and can also influence gene and protein expression profiles (Bissell *et al.*, 1999; Orend and Chiquet-Ehrismann, 2000). Several studies have explored the link between cell morphology and function, and this topic will be discussed later in the chapter (Section III.B).

III. Integrin–Ligand Binding and Signal Transduction

Integrin–ligand binding provides a critical pathway by which cells can explore and examine their extracellular environment. This interaction initiates signaling cascades that essentially control cell behavior, and these signals may change with cell substrate identity or conformation. Various ligand properties can affect cell signal transduction processes, including ligand surface concentration, strength of receptor–ligand adhesion, degree of receptor occupancy by ligand, and ligand affinity (Hammer and Tirrell, 1996). This relationship between substrate or ligand properties and cell function is illustrated in Fig. 4.

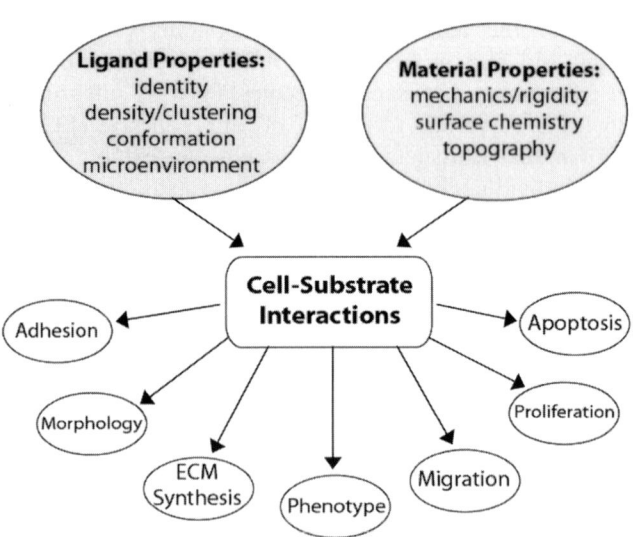

FIG. 4. Alterations in either ligand or material properties may alter the nature of cell–substrate interactions. These interactions, in turn, impact many aspects of cell function.

A. Focal Adhesions

The function of integrins is not solely to act as cell surface receptors for ECM ligands, but also to mediate interactions between the cell cytoskeleton and the ECM, thereby initiating signaling cascades in response to the extracellular environment. Thus, the integrins are transmembrane linkers, with the intracellular domain indirectly connected to bundles of actin filaments. In a 2D *in vitro* culture of fibroblasts, most of the cell is separated from the substrate by a > 50 nm gap. In some areas, however, clusters of adhesion sites form focal contacts, decreasing this gap to 10–15 nm and causing very strong cell attachment (Alberts *et al.*, 1994; Burridge *et al.*, 1988).

Focal adhesions are integrin-based structures that mediate strong cell–substrate adhesion and enable signal transduction between the ECM and cell cytoplasm (Boudreau and Jones, 1999; Wehrle-Haller and Imhof, 2002; Zamir and Geiger, 2001). The action of integrin–ligand binding initiates a sequence of events involving cytoplasmic attachment proteins that enables the integrin to link indirectly to actin filaments in the cell cortex. Following integrin–ligand binding, the cytoplasmic tail of the β-chain associates with cytoskeletal proteins, inducing the localized clustering of talin, vinculin, paxillin, and tensin, which participate in integrin linkage to actin filaments (Boudreau and Jones, 1999; Burridge *et al.*, 1988). This assembly and organization of actin filaments promotes more integrin clustering, which acts as a positive feedback system, as the ligand binding and cytoskeletal organization are further enhanced (Giancotti and Ruoslahti, 1999). The result of this sequence of events is the formation of aggregates of ECM proteins, integrins, and cytoskeletal proteins on either side of the cell membrane, and these components comprise the focal adhesion. This transmembrane attachment of ECM to the cytoskeleton via integrins is required for robust cell–substrate and cell–cell adhesions. In the absence of this anchorage, the attachment site may be ripped out of the cell (Alberts *et al.*, 1994). This cytoskeletal connection is also necessary for the formation of focal adhesions. Cells that have been modified to lack the cytoplasmic domain of the β-chain are still capable of binding ligands, but not able to cluster at focal contacts (Solowska *et al.*, 1989).

In addition to providing stable anchorage sites for cell–substrate interactions, focal adhesions can also serve as pathways for signal transduction. Integrin-mediated cell adhesion initiates a number of biochemical events, including cytoplasmic alkalinization due to activation of a Na^+–H^+ antiporter, increases in intracellular calcium, activation of tyrosine kinases, protein tyrosine phosphatases, and lipid kinases, and changes in gene expression (Bennett, 1998; Romer, 1995). Signaling molecules congregate at focal adhesions, suggesting that these contacts serve as foci for "outside-in" signaling cascades. For instance, several protein kinases are localized to focal adhesions, and there is evidence that their activity changes with substrate composition (Koenig and Grainger, 2002). Because protein kinases participate in phosphorylation of various intra- and extracellular proteins, they are thus capable of significantly affecting cell survival and function in response to the specific ECM environment.

It is well known that cell adhesion, and by consequence, cell signaling, depends upon the molecular identity of the ECM on which the cell is anchored. Different cell types exhibit preferential binding to some ECM components over others. However, the physical state of the ECM may also govern the formation of focal adhesions and modulation of cell function. Fibroblasts cultured on either covalently immobilized fibronectin (FN) or substrates coated with FN form different types of adhesion complexes (Katz et al., 2000). The FN did not vary in conformation or density; only its physical state was altered. Cells on nonimmobilized FN are capable of rearranging the ECM in fibrils, resulting in "fibrillar adhesions" which contain low levels of focal adhesion components such as paxillin, vinculin, and tyrosine-phosphorylated proteins, and bind primarily through the $\alpha_5\beta_1$ integrin. Yet, cells on immobilized FN displayed traditional focal contacts bound through the $\alpha_v\beta_3$ integrin and contained high amounts of cytoskeletal proteins normally associated with focal adhesion formation. These differences in the adhesion of a single cell type to a single ECM component illustrate the complexity of cell–substrate interactions, and imply that the deformability or rigidity of the ECM regulates local tension at adhesion sites, thus activating signaling such as local tyrosine phosphorylation.

However, it must be noted that our current understanding of focal adhesions is based primarily upon 2D *in vitro* studies, and we know very little about their 3D *in vivo* counterparts. Cell behavior exhibits differences even between 2D and 3D *in vitro* cultures. For example, fibroblasts cultured on flat surfaces exhibit an artificial polarity between the upper and lower surfaces of these normally nonpolar cells, yet when cultured in 3D collagen matrices, their morphology and migration patterns change significantly (Elsdale and Bard, 1972; Friedl and Brocker, 2000). Cell-derived 3D matrices have been used to examine how *in vivo* cell–substrate adhesion varies from the traditional planar environment normally used *in vitro*. Significant differences have been illustrated between 3D-matrix interactions relative to 2D substrates, thus challenging the use of traditional tissue culture conditions for understanding *in vivo* structure, function, and signaling of cell adhesions (Cukierman et al., 2001). *In vivo* 3D-matrix interactions not only display enhanced biological activity and narrowed integrin usage, but also differ in structure, localization, and function from 2D *in vitro* adhesions. Additionally, it was found that neither a 3D collagen gel fabricated *in vitro* nor a flattened, 2D cell-derived matrix could mimic the results obtained using the 3D cell-derived matrix (Cukierman *et al.*, 2001). This observation illustrates that both the biological composition and the 3D quality of these matrices are integral in creating the *in vivo* cell adhesions.

B. Effect of Cell Adhesion and Shape on Cell Function

Alterations in ECM–integrin interactions may cause changes in both cell shape and function (Boudreau and Jones, 1999; Folkman and Moscona, 1978). The intracellular signaling pathway activated by integrin binding has recently been implicated as playing a role in ECM-dependent changes in cell shape. Both the magnitude and duration of expression of signaling molecules, such as mitogen-activated protein kinases (MAPK), are affected by integrin binding (Boudreau and Jones, 1999), and alterations in MAPK expression often correlate with changes in cell morphology. The nature of these intracellular signals initiated by integrin–ligand binding ultimately controls cell function. As will be discussed in this section, cell–ECM interactions can determine cell fate, with respect to differentiation, apoptosis, and migration; these relationships are summarized in Fig. 4.

1. Differentiation

The mechanism by which cells switch between proliferative and differentiated phenotypes is important in creating systems that control tissue development. Numerous examples of how the ECM influences cell differentiation can be found *in vivo*; one such example was described in this chapter's introduction, where variations in substrate material were shown to have drastic effects on mammary epithelial cell function (Horwitz, 1997). Several studies have examined the relationship between cell shape and proliferation, where a proliferative phenotype is indicative of a dedifferentiated state. Increased spreading of both fibroblasts and endothelial cells proportionally stimulated DNA synthesis, and thus progression through the cell cycle (Folkman and Moscona, 1978). Substrate adhesivity and cell confluence were used to modulate cell shape, resulting in rounder cells synthesizing significantly less DNA than spread cells. Another study was performed in which cell spreading was increased without increasing the area of cell–substrate contacts (Chen et al., 1997), and this resulted in the same finding, where more highly spread cells displayed increased proliferation. Lastly, photolithographic methods were used to pattern adhesive islands of various sizes to further explore the relationship between hepatocyte spreading and function (Singhvi et al., 1994). When cells are restricted to a minimum spread area, they exhibit more differentiation markers than spread cells.

One cell-type that exhibits drastic switches between growth and differentiation is the hepatocyte. Numerous *in vitro* studies have been performed to investigate whether this alternation between differentiation and growth may be controlled via culture conditions or substrate materials. Some studies have concluded that differentiation can be controlled through the type of ECM presented (Caron, 1990; Sudhakaran et al., 1986; Tomomura et al., 1987), while others have implicated cell–cell interactions (Ben Ze'ev et al., 1988; Bissell et al., 1987), cell shape (Ben Ze'ev et al., 1988; Bissell et al., 1987), matrix rigidity (Opas, 1989), or presence of a 3D matrix environment (Dunn et al., 1989) as key in this modulation. To clarify these results, a study was performed in which cell spreading, ECM composition, and ECM geometry were controlled, enabling the analysis of how ECM molecules switch hepatocytes between growth and differentiation (Mooney et al., 1992). The degree of cell spreading on varying densities of several ECM coatings was identified as a critical determinant in cells switching to a differentiated state. Lower ECM coating densities induced a rounded cell morphology and inhibited proliferation while promoting expression of differentiation markers. Cells on higher density ECM coatings were significantly more spread and exhibited increased proliferation with decreased differentiation. These results also verified that neither cell–cell contact nor 3D culture was necessary to induce hepatocyte proliferation, as had been suggested by other studies.

The conformation of adsorbed proteins is also important in mediating cell differentiation, and implicates specific integrin receptors as playing crucial roles in this event (García et al., 1999). Fibronectin conformation was varied via adsorption to different substrate materials. Differences in FN conformation altered the presentation of the $\alpha_5\beta_1$ integrin binding site in FN, and presentation of this integrin controlled switching between proliferative and differentiated phenotypes in myoblasts. Differentiation of myoblasts occurred with the highest degree of $\alpha_5\beta_1$ binding and was completely inhibited by an antibody to α_5 (García et al., 1999). In a similar set of experiments, osteoblasts exhibited enhanced expression of several differentiation markers when cultured upon FN whose conformation allowed for the greatest presentation of the $\alpha_5\beta_1$ integrin binding site

(Stephansson et al., 2002). This modulation of differentiation is specific to the α_5 integrin, as antibodies to α_v did not inhibit differentiation (Stephansson et al., 2002).

The ability to understand the mechanism behind cellular differentiation is important not only to developmental biologists, but also to tissue engineers. Tissue engineering first requires the *in vitro* expansion of a cell population, followed by the seeding of these cells within a scaffold to form a functional tissue replacement. Thus, it is evident that knowledge of how to switch these cells from growth to differentiation is of paramount importance in this application. By employing our knowledge of how this phenotypic switch is modulated, we can tailor biomaterials design in order to promote cell growth or differentiation.

2. Apoptosis

Apoptosis, or programmed cell death, can occur following disruption of the ECM by pharmacologic or genetic mechanisms (Boudreau et al., 1995; Stupack and Cheresh, 2002). While apoptosis is necessary for proper tissue development, inappropriately triggered cell death can detrimentally affect tissue function. The survival of many cell types requires integrin-mediated adhesion to the ECM (Ruoslahti and Reed, 1994; Stupack and Cheresh, 2002), and when deprived of extracellular signals, nearly all cell types are susceptible to apoptosis (Meredith and Schwartz, 1997). It has even been suggested that apoptosis is a default pathway that cells enter in the absence of extracellular signals that instruct them otherwise (Raff, 1992). Cells exhibit varying sensitivities to apoptosis, such that no single treatment can effect apoptosis protection for all cell types. Death by apoptosis has been inhibited by exposing cells in suspension to immobilized integrin antibodies (Meredith et al., 1993). These results indicate a role for integrin signaling in the adhesion-dependent control of apoptosis. To further explore the relationship between cell adhesion and apoptosis, a nonadhesive substrate was patterned with small, closely spaced circular adhesive islands (3–5 μm island size), and the extent of cell spreading across these islands was controlled by changing the spacing between them (Chen et al., 1997). In this manner, the authors were able to keep the cell–substrate contact area constant while changing the area of the cell itself (i.e., the same number of adhesive islands per cell, but increased distance between these islands increases cell spreading). The results implicated cell shape as a critical determinant in apoptosis, as increased cell spreading caused decreased apoptosis, with cell–ECM contact area remaining constant. This relationship between cell shape and apoptosis was consistent, although cells cultured with ligands for the β_1 receptor were more sensitive to apoptosis than those cultured with the $\alpha_v\beta_3$ ligands, indicating the ability of different adhesion receptors to convey distinct death signals.

3. Migration

Cell migration across 2D surfaces occurs as a sequence of events. First, the leading edge of the cell protrudes, initiating interactions with the substrate. This step is followed by the contraction of the cell body and finally detachment of the trailing edge. Matrix proteins in the path of migration may force cells to adapt their morphology and/or enzymatically degrade the ECM components via contact-dependent proteolysis or protease secretion (Friedl and Brocker, 2000). The nature of cell–material interactions exhibits a profound effect on a cell's ability to migrate. Both theoretical and experimental evidence indicate that the average speed of cell locomotion exhibits a biphasic dependence on the strength of cell–substrate adhesion (DiMilla et al., 1993; Lauffenberger and Horwitz, 1996; Palecek et al., 1997; Palecek et al., 1999). Maximal cell migration is attained at intermediate cell adhesion strength. Either too weak or too strong adhesion forces induce reduced cell motility. In order to migrate, cells must generate traction forces through surface receptors bound to the ECM. These traction forces are generated by the cytoskeleton at sites of cell adhesion, specifically focal adhesion complexes. Thus, at low adhesiveness, cell–substrate bonds are disrupted by cytoskeletal forces, resulting in the cell's inability to generate the traction required for migration. At high adhesiveness, the cytoskeletal forces are not sufficient to disrupt the strong cell–substrate bonds, also leaving the cell unable to migrate. While integrin-mediated cell motility can be modulated by altering adhesion ligand surface density, cell integrin expression level, or integrin–ligand binding affinity, cell migration speed still ultimately depends upon the cell–substrate adhesion strength (Palecek et al., 1997).

Much investigation regarding the effects of cell–substrate interactions on cell migration has focused upon alterations in matrix rigidity. The strength of integrin–cytoskeleton linkages has been found to depend upon the substrate compliance, as cells sense the substrate elasticity and respond by strengthening these linkages proportionally with increases in matrix rigidity (Choquet et al., 1997). Cytoskeletal organization is affected by substrate rigidity, as fibroblast actin filaments on stiff substrates are well-defined and distributed throughout the cell, whereas cells on soft materials displayed are extremely fine and localized around the cell periphery (Wong et al., 2003). In general, cells cultured on flexible substrates exhibit increased migration rates, with irregular focal adhesions and reduced amounts of phosphotyrosine at adhesion sites (Choquet et al., 1997; Katz et al., 2000;

Pelham and Wang, 1997). Well-defined, stable focal adhesions are observed in cells cultured on stiff substrates, and this condition is accompanied by decreased cell motility (Pelham and Wang, 1997). The exact mechanism by which cells are able to sense and respond to the mechanics of their substrate has not been completely elucidated, although it is believed that the density and turnover of integrins in focal adhesions sense the elasticity and spacing of extracellular ligands (Wehrle-Haller and Imhof, 2002). The focal adhesion components act as mechanical transducing devices, relaying changes in intra- and extracellular tension into signaling pathways that modify the composition and behavior of focal adhesions, thereby regulating cell contractility and motility (Geiger and Bershadsky, 2001). This establishment of more stable focal adhesions may also lead to the preference of cells to grow on stiff substrates (Lo *et al.*, 2000). This concept of modulating cell adhesion and motility via changes in substrate rigidity has been exploited to synthesize gradient-compliant materials that enable directed cell migration (Wong *et al.*, 2003). Smooth muscle cells were found to migrate toward and accumulate on the stiff regions of the substrate, and the migration speed of cells on the soft regions was significantly higher than that of cells on more rigid areas (Wong *et al.*, 2003). This system illustrates the importance of understanding the mechanisms of focal adhesion regulation of cell function so that control over cell behavior can be achieved in order to synthesize novel materials for use in tissue engineering.

IV. Nonspecific Interactions of Cells with Materials

As discussed earlier in this chapter, cells express numerous types of receptors that mediate interactions with biological substrates. These interactions are specific, and the ligands for the cell receptors may exist as proteins, other receptors, or other biomolecules. Thus far, receptor–ligand interactions have been discussed in the context of cell interactions with components of the natural ECM. Synthetic materials are not intrinsically recognized by cell receptors; instead, their interactions are mediated by protein adsorption to the material, causing cells to interact with synthetic biomaterials via the same ligand–receptor interactions involved in normal binding to the ECM (Elbert and Hubbell, 1996). Even an entirely non biological material interacts with cells through biological pathways, as proteins adsorb to the material, essentially modifying its surface such that the cells recognize it as biological in nature (Castner and Ratner, 2002). In the case of interaction of cells with biomaterials, proteins or other biological signals may be either adsorbed or intentionally immobilized to the material surface. To control the extent of protein adsorption, material properties such as charge, roughness, and hydrophobicity may be modified. This type of cell–material interaction, which is regulated primarily by protein adsorption and not by the controlled presentation of biological signals, will be discussed as nonspecific cell–material interactions.

A. DYNAMICS OF PROTEIN ADSORPTION

Proteins play a critical role in regulating cell interactions with both biological and synthetic surfaces. The type and density of proteins presented on a surface are major determinants in cell function. Because proteins are present in all bodily fluids and most cell culture media, it is important to understand the dynamics of protein adsorption to biomaterials. Additionally, protein adsorption to materials impacts the overall performance of biomaterials in several manners, including regulation or inhibition of cell adhesion.

Proteins may adsorb to surfaces for both thermodynamic and electrostatic reasons. The kinetics and thermodynamics of protein adsorption have been reviewed in references Haynes and Norde, (1994); Horbett and Brash, (1995); Ramsden, (2003). The hydrophobic effect is the primary thermodynamic regulator in protein–material interactions, where changes occur in the interaction of water with both the hydrophobic material surface and with hydrophobic amino acid residues on the protein. Specifically, water is poorly bonded to hydrophobic surfaces and forms a more ordered surface layer as it more strongly hydrogen-bonds to itself. Thus, protein adsorption results in an entropic gain as water is released from the hydrophobic material surface and creates a polar surface capable of hydrogen bonding (Hubbell, 1995). Although virtually all surfaces are hydrophobic relative to water, the more hydrophobic materials tend to adsorb larger amounts of protein than hydrophilic ones. Proteins may also interact with surfaces by electrostatic mechanisms. Generally possessing a net negative charge, proteins have a greater tendency to adsorb to cationic surfaces (Horbett and Brash, 1995). However, because proteins contain both positively and negatively charged moieties, they interact to some extent with both cationic and anionic materials. Similarly charged proteins and surfaces may also interact via a soluble multivalent linker of opposite charge, such as Ca^{2+} (Elbert and Hubbell, 1996).

Proteins may adopt an altered conformation upon adsorption to a surface. In solution, hydrophobic sequences within proteins are folded such that contact with water is minimal. Adsorption on a hydrophobic surface, however, has the ability to cause unfolding of these regions, often resulting in irreversible adsorption of the protein (Kiaei et al., 1992, 1995). The conformation of the protein also affects cellular recognition and binding to the material. For example, the nature of a material's surface chemistry has the ability to modulate the conformation of adsorbed fibronectin (FN). Varying surface chemistries results in quantitative differences in the functional presentation of the major integrin-binding domain of FN (Keselowsky et al., 2003). Changes in FN conformation can significantly alter the bioavailability of the $\alpha_5\beta_1$ integrin binding site, thereby affecting cell adhesion, proliferation, differentiation, and the composition and localization of integrins in focal adhesion complexes (García et al., 1999; Keselowsky et al., 2003).

The irreversibility of adsorption of some proteins also emphasizes the importance of understanding the kinetics of the adsorption process. Given a situation where transport of the protein to the material surface is diffusion controlled, Eq. (2) can be used during initial stages of adsorption, where the amount of protein on the surface (Λ) is proportional to the product of the protein concentration in solution (C) and the square roots of protein diffusion coefficient (D) and time (t):

$$\Lambda \propto C(Dt)^{1/2} \qquad (2)$$

This relationship allows one to estimate the relative flux of proteins within a multicomponent solution to the material surface. In the case of irreversible protein adsorption, the first protein to arrive stays on the surface permanently, illustrating the importance of understanding the properties of the proteins in solution.

Protein diffusivity, however, is not always the main determinant in the composition of adsorbed protein layers. If this were the case, the composition of the adsorbed protein layer would be the same on different materials exposed to the same solution. This condition is not usually observed (Horbett, 1999), indicating that the affinity of each protein is influenced by the surface chemistry of the biomaterial (Horbett and Brash, 1995). Because proteins differ in affinity for various surface chemistries, the competitive protein adsorption process will also differ, leading to unique protein layer compositions upon different materials. Furthermore, the vast majority of protein adsorption studies have been carried out *in vitro*, assuming that this accurately mimics the *in vivo* environment. However, differences in implant site (i.e., blood-contacting devices vs solid tissue implants) will result in a different presentation of body proteins, presumably evoking differing cellular responses.

Protein–surface interactions are highly complex, complicating the ability to precisely control the concentration, conformation, and bioactivity of the adsorbed protein. Numerous materials have been modified in order to achieve better control over the adsorption process, thereby enabling better characterization of the material and greater control over cell function. A few of these modifications will be discussed in the following sections.

B. Surface Chemistry

1. Charge

Ionically charged surfaces have long been used to improve cell adhesion upon traditionally nonadhesive substrates. Adhesion and spreading of numerous cell types has been accomplished through the modification of materials to contain charged groups, and positive charges tend to elicit the best cellular response (Davies, 1998). As mentioned earlier, proteins generally possess a net negative charge, thereby leading to the tendency of proteins to adsorb to cationically charged surfaces, such as those created by amine modification.

A variety of methods have been employed to create charged surfaces for the purpose of increasing cell adhesion. These methods include photolithographic patterning (Ito, 1999) or adsorptive coating (Seyfert *et al.*, 1995) of charged chemicals, hydrolytic etching of a polymer surface (McAuslan and Johnson, 1987), or copolymerization with monomers containing ionizable functional groups (Bergethon *et al.*, 1989; van Wachem *et al.*, 1987). Glass slides treated with a variety of polycationic chemicals have been used to promote enhanced leukocyte adhesion (Seyfert *et al.*, 1995). Cell integrity was preserved on all surfaces, and the greatest increase in leukocyte adhesion was observed on materials with the most positive zeta potentials. Studies have examined not only differences in charge identity, but also the effects of charge density on cell behavior (Lee *et al.*, 1997). When both negatively or positively charged molecules were immobilized on surfaces to create a gradient of charge density, both the adhesion and proliferation of chinese hamster ovary (CHO) cells exhibited a biphasic response, with intermediate charge densities causing the greatest increase in both events. This result, however, may be due to changes in surface hydrophilicity with charge density, and not because of the effects of specific functional groups, as CHO cells have previously been shown to preferentially adhere on moderately hydrophilic surfaces (Lee and Lee, 1993).

Preferential attachment of cells has been demonstrated on multiple types of amine-modified surfaces patterned on hydrophobic substrates in the presence of serum. However, because charge and wettability are related properties, it is often difficult to separate the effects of material wettability from those of surface charge. Thus, it is questionable whether observations of cell behavior that involve varying charge density are actually attributable to the cellular response to changes in material hydrophilicity. In one study, use of either a positively charged quaternary amine or an unprotonated amine surface modification resulted in five-fold greater cell attachment over control or negatively charged surfaces (Webb et al., 1998). This suggests that the moderate wettability shared by the quaternary amine and amine surfaces is the major factor in determining cell attachment in the presence of serum proteins.

When cells are cultured in serum-free conditions, the cell response to charged surfaces can change dramatically. Cell attachment to quaternary amine surfaces was significantly higher than on all other materials, including the amine surface, which displayed four-fold less cell adhesion than the quaternary amine surface (Webb et al., 1998). This result suggests that positively charged functional groups possess an enhanced role in promoting cell adhesion in protein-free environments relative to when proteins are present. The accepted explanation for this phenomenon is that, in the absence of proteins, the negatively charged chondroitin sulfate within the cell glycocalyx exhibits electrostatic interactions with the positive charges upon the material surface. Chondroitinase ABC inhibits the adhesion of cells to normally adhesive amine surfaces, thus affirming the involvement of chondroitin sulfate in mediating the interactions between cells and cationic surfaces in a protein-free environment (Massia and Hubbell, 1992). Furthermore, negatively charged surfaces achieved the lowest levels of cell attachment in the absence of serum, indicating possible repulsion between the anionic cell surface chondroitin sulfate and the material surface. Single cationic amino acids such as arginine and lysine immobilized on polymer substrates were found to support cell adhesion and spreading via strong interactions with cell surface chondroitin sulfate, while interactions with heparan sulfate were weaker (Massia and Hubbell, 1992). There is potential for this interaction between cell-surface glycosaminoglycans and positively charged oligopeptides on adhesion proteins to be exploited for the design of biomaterials. For instance, using materials with specific cationic oligopeptides, it may be possible to achieve greater selectivity with respect to the type of cell-surface glycosaminoglycan or even the cell type.

2. Hydrophilicity/Hydrophobicity

As mentioned in the previous section, surface hydrophilicity can be closely linked to surface ionic charge. In general, either extreme in surface hydrophilicity results in decreased cell adhesion and spreading. Extremely hydrophilic surfaces inhibit protein adsorption, leading to inhibited cell adhesion to the substrate. On the other hand, very hydrophobic materials promote irreversible protein adsorption, with the proteins often so denatured such that they are not recognizable by cells (Williams et al., 1995). Several studies have concluded that optimal cell adhesion occurs on materials of moderate hydrophilicity, with water contact angle measurements averaging 40° (van Wachem et al., 1987; Webb et al., 1998). It has been shown that the conformation of adsorbed proteins can be directly controlled by surface wettability through defined alterations in material chemistry (Keselowsky et al., 2003). The central cell-binding domain of fibronectin was kept most intact when adsorbed on hydrophilic surfaces, and essentially destroyed on the most hydrophobic material, supporting previous studies that suggest protein denaturation occurs on highly hydrophobic surfaces. Thus, it is important to note that material hydrophilicity controls not only the amount or type of proteins adsorbed, but also determines the protein conformation. The more preserved protein conformation observed on hydrophilic materials results in enhanced functional presentation of ligands as well as improved cell adhesion (Keselowsky et al., 2003). This specific study demonstrated that well-characterized and controlled alterations in surface chemistry provide a method by which substrate-directed control of adsorbed protein activity may be achieved, with the goal of manipulating integrin binding to elicit a desired cellular response.

When materials are exposed to dilute serum conditions, hydrophilic surfaces promote greater cell attachment, spreading, and cytoskeletal organization relative to hydrophobic surfaces. Enhanced cell spreading has been observed on hydrophilic surfaces in multiple studies (Ruardy et al., 1995; Schakenraad et al., 1986; Webb et al., 1998). Cells on moderately hydrophilic surfaces have a greater cell area, highly organized actin stress fibers, and more focal adhesions than cells cultured on more hydrophobic materials (Webb et al., 1998). Within the various hydrophilic surfaces, alterations in charge and wettability changed cell attachment but neither spreading nor cytoskeletal arrangement. Cytoskeletal organization in particular appears to depend primarily upon general hydrophilicity or hydrophobicity, with little variation between materials within each category (Altankov et al., 1996; Webb et al., 1998).

C. Surface Topography

There are numerous factors involved in cellular responses to the extracellular environment, as many ECM properties are able to prompt cells to activate specific signaling cascades or function in a certain manner. The importance of protein composition and conformation has been discussed earlier in this chapter. Yet, cells also respond to the topography of their substrate material, as the nature of the topography may impart nonspecific biomechanical stimuli (Abrams et al., 2002). Study of native basement membranes from a variety of animal sources has demonstrated that these ECM layers possess a complex topography consisting of intertwining fibers mixed with elevations and pores of varying nanoscale dimensions (Abrams et al., 2002). The conserved nature of this topography implies that more than just the integrin–ligand interactions are responsible for directing cell behavior.

In the past, most studies have examined surfaces with topographical features on the microscale level, due to limitations in nanoscale fabrication. However, recent advances in creating surfaces with submicrometer surface features have allowed analysis of more biologically relevant features. Nanometer-size topographical features more closely mimic the natural ECM, thus enabling researchers to more accurately recreate a cell's *in vivo* environment.

Surfaces have been fabricated to contain a variety of types of topographical features, examples of which are listed in Table II [reviewed in Abrams et al. (2002) and Curtis and Wilkinson (1997)]. The features that have been most extensively investigated with respect to cell function are grooves. Culturing cells on grooved substrates generally results in significant alterations to cell morphology and cytoskeletal arrangement (Braber et al., 1998; Brunette, 1986b; Oakley and Brunette, 1993; Oakley and Brunette, 1995). Specifically, cells align along the long axis of the groove, with cytoskeletal elements such as actin and microtubules also organizing themselves parallel to grooves. This cell alignment is dependent upon not only groove width, but also groove depth. The degree of cell orientation increases with greater groove depth and decreases with increasing groove width (Braber et al., 1998; Brunette, 1986a; Clark et al., 1991). Grooves or ridges that are much wider than the cells tend to have little effect on cell orientation, although cells may align to one edge. When the width is in the order of the size of a cell, the effects on orientation become more pronounced. Multigrooved materials, which consist of a combination of macrogrooves and microgrooves, have been shown to not only control the alignment of cells, but also the orientation of the ECM (Yoshinari et al., 2003). Production and alignment of the ECM was

TABLE II
A Summary of Topographical Features and Cell Types that have been Investigated in the Literature

Topographical features	Cell type	Cell functions examined
Cliffs	Astrocytes	Adhesion strength
Cylinders	Cardiomyocytes	Bridging
Fibers	Chondrocytes	Cytoskeletal organization
General roughness	Dermal fibroblasts	Differentiation
Grooves	Dermal keratinocytes	ECM orientation
Nodes	Endothelial cells	ECM production/mineralization
Pits	Epithelial cells	Focal adhesion formation
Pores	Gingival fibroblasts	Migration
Ridges	Gingival keratinocytes	Morphology/elongation
Spheres	Heart fibroblasts	Orientation
Spikes	Leukocytes	Proliferation
Steps	Macrophages	
Waves	Monocytes	
Wells	Neurites	
	Neutrophils	
	Oligodendrocytes	
	Osteoblasts	
	Smooth muscle cells	

For reviews, see Abrams et al. (2002); Curtis et al. (1995); Flemming et al. (1999).

enhanced on multigrooved substrates when compared to microgrooves alone or smooth surfaces. Grooves are also capable of directing cell migration, with deeper grooves again showing greater efficacy. Extension of cells, specifically neurites, has also been stimulated by growth on grooved surfaces (Curtis et al., 1995).

Other features, such as pores or general roughness, have been shown to significantly alter cell behavior. Surfaces with greater texture can encourage cellular differentiation, causing increased mineralization and ECM synthesis by osteoblasts (Groessner-Screiber and Tuan, 1992) or formation of a stratified epidermis by keratinocytes (Pins et al., 2000). Surface roughness also tended to increase fibroblast alignment as well as the migration of vascular and corneal cells in comparison to smooth surfaces (Eisenbarth et al., 1996; Lampin et al., 1997).

Topographical features do not elicit the same response for all cell types tested. For instance, while all fibroblasts align in grooves, this alignment does not occur at all in either neutrophils or keratinocytes (Meyle et al., 1995). Furthermore, when a variety of materials, such as alumina, titania, and hydroxyapatite, were used to create nanophase (< 100 nm grain size) surface roughness, the effects on cell adhesion differed significantly with cell type. These results may be explained by the preferential adsorption of certain proteins on the nanophase ceramic surfaces; vitronectin preferentially adsorbed to these materials, thereby promoting the selective adhesion of osteoblasts over fibroblasts and endothelial cells (Webster *et al.*, 2000). However, laminin preferentially adsorbs to conventional ceramics, resulting in increased endothelial cell adhesion and decreased attachment of osteoblasts (Webster *et al.*, 2000). The presence of adsorbed proteins may also impact the alignment of cells on grooves. Cells cultured in the presence of serum exhibited greater alignment with topographical patterns than cells cultured in serum-free media (Abrams *et al.*, 2002). The possibility that proteins may preferentially adsorb to groove and ridge boundaries, thereby contributing to the induction of cell alignment, has been proposed (Braber *et al.*, 1998).

The variables in investigating cell interactions with topographical features include feature type, fabrication technique, material composition, feature dimensions, feature frequency, and cell type (Abrams *et al.*, 2002). A vast amount of literature is available on this topic, and a good review by Flemming *et al.*, (1999) discusses many more cell–substrate interactions that have not been described here. Combinations of these variables allow for thousands of possibilities, often making it difficult to analyze and compare multiple studies to achieve a general conclusion, as alterations in any of the available parameters may change cell behavior. For instance, while increased surface roughness appears to increase cell adhesion, migration and ECM production, this is not always the case (Anselme *et al.*, 2000), and these varying results may be due to fabrication technique, material composition, or cell type.

V. Controlled Cell–Material Interactions

In designing materials for biological applications, it is often desirable to create systems that enable precise control over cell adhesion and function. This goal is not easily accomplished by relying on adsorbed proteins to provide the appropriate biological cues. Composition and conformation of adsorbed protein layers are difficult to control, resulting in materials that do not exhibit specific regulation of cell behavior. These nonspecifically adsorbed protein layers have even been described as "the enemy" (Castner and Ratner, 2002) which must be defeated in order to develop surfaces that control the conformation and orientation of proteins so that the body will specifically recognize them. As displayed in Table I, several ECM proteins contain short peptide sequences that are sufficient for cell surface receptor recognition. Incorporation of well-characterized biological moieties, such as these peptide sequences, into biomaterials has enabled investigators to examine the effects of specific biological signals on cell function, and to tailor materials such that they contain a specified amount or spatial distribution of these signals. Materials containing specific biological sequences are able to interact directly with cell surface receptors, and do not require adsorbed proteins to mediate the cell–material interaction.

A. Ideal Surfaces

Controlled presentation of biological signals on a material begins with designing materials to which proteins do not readily adsorb. Given the mechanisms of protein adsorption discussed earlier, such a material would likely be very hydrophilic and uncharged. Various synthetic hydrogel materials meet this description, and it has been shown that protein adsorption on these materials is inhibited. Hydrogels consist of a crosslinked network of water-soluble polymers, where the structure of the water around the polymer hinders protein adsorption, as displacement of this water is energetically unfavorable. Several synthetic polymers have been used in the creation of hydrogels, including poly(ethylene glycol) (PEG), poly(vinyl alcohol) (PVA), polyacrylamide, and poly(hydroxyethyl methacrylate). These materials are all biocompatible, in addition to inhibiting protein adsorption.

The nonadsorptive nature of these materials allows for their modification in order to include specified biological signals. Cells will not adhere to hydrogels without chemical or biological modification of the material. While it may seem that lack of cell adhesion to materials intended for tissue engineering applications would not be a desirable property, this is not necessarily the case. This anti-adhesive property is beneficial, as it allows precise, defined modifications of the material to achieve a specific cellular response without interference by nonspecific cell or protein interactions.

Poly (ethylene glycol) (PEG) has been used to not only create scaffolds, but also to improve the material or molecule hydrophilicity and inhibit protein adsorption on a variety of materials (Elbert and Hubbell, 1996; Tirrell et al., 2002). Hydrogels consisting of PEG may be synthesized by modification of PEG to contain photopolymerizable acrylate groups, whose crosslinking to form a hydrogel is initiated by radical formation and propagation. In particular, photopolymerization has been exploited to make PEG gels under physiological conditions and in the presence of cells (Burdick and Anseth, 2002; Mann et al., 2001). A variety of chemistries are available in order to tailor the properties of PEG-containing hydrogels to suit the specific application. For instance, PEG may be combined with other photoactive polymers or monomers to form copolymer hydrogels. Block copolymers of PEG with other monomers may also be synthesized. Specifically, block copolymers of PEG with poly(lactic acid) (PLA) are commonly synthesized to design materials with a wide range of degradation times (Anseth et al., 2002; Sawhney et al., 1993). Biological molecules such as growth factors (Mann et al., 1999) and enzymatically degradable or adhesive peptide sequences (Burdick and Anseth, 2002; Hern and Hubbell, 1998; Mann et al., 2001) have also been attached to PEG and shown to retain their bioactivity.

Poly (ethylene glycol) (PEG) has been grafted to numerous materials, including polyurethane and poly(ethylene terephthalate), in order to reduce protein adsorption to the these materials, often for purpose of making them nonthrombogenic (Gombotz et al., 1991; Han et al., 1993). Longer PEG chains appear to be more effective at blocking protein adsorption, yet it becomes more difficult to achieve high graft densities with increasing PEG molecular weight. However, because PEG molecular weight is not expected to be a major determinant in protein adsorption, the observed molecular weight dependence may, in fact, be due to the inability to generate dense PEG packings with other immobilization schemes, and higher molecular weight PEGs somewhat compensate for this by occupying a larger surface area per attachment site (Elbert and Hubbell, 1996). Modification of surfaces via PEG adsorption has also been investigated. Treatment of surfaces with PEG surfactants has effectively reduced protein adsorption, inhibited platelet adhesion, and prevented white blood cell uptake (Elbert and Hubbell, 1996). Self-assembled monolayers have also been fabricated that contain PEG chains (Lopez et al., 1993). Alkane thiols terminated with oligo(ethylene glycols) were successful in virtually eliminating protein adsorption (Prime and Whitesides, 1993). In surfaces modified with PEG brushes, it was concluded that the graft density of the surface-bound polymer chains is the predominant factor in determining material nonadhesiveness (Tirrell et al., 2002).

The ability of hydrophilic polymers, specifically PEG, to provide a substrate material that is essentially a blank slate is extremely valuable in both investigations of the nature of cell–substrate interactions as well as in the creation of well-defined biomaterials and tissue engineering scaffolds. In this manner, PEG serves as an ideal material which can be modified to contain numerous biological signals.

B. ADHESION LIGANDS

1. Integrins

As discussed earlier, cells may interact with substrates via integrins specific for proteins adsorbed upon the material. However, a controlled adhesion environment is difficult to achieve when relying upon protein adsorption to encourage cell adhesion. Furthermore, protein adsorption may not be stable, as the proteins can desorb. To overcome these limitations, whole adhesive proteins and peptide segments of these proteins have been covalently immobilized upon and within biomaterials in order to promote and control cell adhesion (Mann *et al.*, 2001; Massia and Hubbell, 1990, 1991; Nuttelman *et al.*, 2001). When coupled to a normally nonadhesive material, such as PEG, these proteins can be used to control cell function, density, shape, and cell type adherent upon the material. Control of receptor-mediated cell behavior upon biomaterials requires controlling nonspecific interactions between cells and the material presenting the bioactive ligand; this allows the cell response to be attributed solely to the specific receptor–ligand interaction under study.

Extracellular matrix (ECM) proteins such as collagen and fibronectin have been covalently incorporated into poly(vinyl alcohol) polymer matrices (Kobayashi and Ikada, 1991; Nuttelman *et al.*, 2001) and polytetrafluoroethylene vascular grafts to render them cell adhesive (Seeger and Klingman, 1987). Using entire protein structures for covalent immobilization, however, can have several drawbacks. Proteins require relatively mild processing conditions, making it difficult to perform some organic synthesis methods which would be useful for their immobilization. Furthermore, proteins are subject to conformational changes, denaturation, or degradation following incorporation into a synthetic material. Yet, as displayed in Table I, matrix proteins contain short peptide sequences that are sufficient for cell adhesion. Covalent attachment of such sequences to substrates mimics attachment of the whole protein in the sense that it allows the conferral of biological properties to a synthetic polymer, yet it also overcomes several difficulties experienced by using the entire protein molecule. Oligopeptides are less susceptible to denaturation and proteolysis, and may be easier to use in organic syntheses.

Many materials have been modified to contain covalently immobilized adhesive peptide sequences, as summarized in Table III [reviewed in Harbers *et al.* (2002) and West and Hubbell (1997)]. Interaction of cells with peptide-modified surfaces can occur directly, without mediation by adsorbed proteins. Issues that affect selectivity in cellular attachment to peptide-modified surfaces include spacer length, peptide surface

TABLE III
EXAMPLES OF SEVERAL ADHESIVE PEPTIDES THAT HAVE BEEN
IMMOBILIZED TO A VARIETY OF SUBSTRATE MATERIALS

Peptide	Material
	Agarose
	Alginate
IKVAV	Collagen
KQAGDV	Glass
PHSRN	Poly(ethylene glycol)
REDV	Poly(ethylene terephthalate)
RGD	Polytetrafluoroethylene
VAPG	Poly(vinyl alcohol)
YIGSR	Polyacrylamide
	Polyurethane

concentration, and the particular peptide sequence that is immobilized. Since the identification of RGD as a ubiquitous peptide sequence that is capable of promoting cell adhesion, this short sequence has been the most widely investigated in terms of biomaterial modification. RGD interacts with a number of integrin receptors and can thus bind to most cell types (Humphries, 1990). Cell response to these peptides is extremely specific, as only a single amino acid change (i.e., RGE instead of RGD) can eliminate cell adhesion and reduce the peptide activity by 100-fold or more (Drumheller and Hubbell, 1994; Hautanen et al., 1989). RGD may also be combined with other fibronectin-derived sequences such as EILDV or PHSRN, the latter effecting a synergistic response (Aota et al., 1994; Komoriya et al., 1991). The extent of cell spreading on RGD-modified materials is determined in part by the RGD concentration, with increasing peptide density resulting in increased attachment and spreading (Burdick and Anseth, 2002; Massia and Hubbell, 1990; 1991; Rezania and Healy, 2000). Attachment of GRGDY to polymer-modified glass substrates demonstrated that a peptide concentration of 10 fmol/cm^2 was sufficient to support fibroblast adhesion and spreading, with clustering of integrins and organization of actin filaments (Massia and Hubbell, 1990; 1991). At a surface density of 1 fmol/cm^2, cells were spread, but did not form focal contacts and exhibited abnormal actin fiber organization.

Recent evidence, however, implies that ligand spacing, rather than concentration, is critical in determining the extent of cell adhesion (Griffith and Lopina, 1998). In a system where ligands were tethered to allow for independent variation of ligand concentration and spacing, cell spreading occurred as a function of both ligand concentration and tether length; spreading was enabled when it was possible for three adjacent ligands to assume positions corresponding to spacing in a high-affinity trivalent branched ligand (Griffith and Lopina, 1998). Many changes in the micro- or nano-environment of immobilized peptides have been shown to exhibit an effect on the nature of cell adhesion (Dori *et al.*, 2000; Houseman and Mrksich, 2001; Maheshwari *et al.*, 2000; Tirrell *et al.*, 2002). For example, peptides presented in clusters of 9 peptides/molecule or higher on materials such as albumin (Danilov and Juliano, 1989) or star-configured PEG (Maheshwari *et al.*, 2000) induce adhesion that is comparable to native matrix proteins and encourage formation of actin stress fibers, whereas presentation of single peptides results in poor cell spreading. Presentation of nonclustered RGD also significantly inhibits fibroblast migration, even when grafted at the same density as clustered ligands (Maheshwari *et al.*, 2000). By using the PEG star molecules, the number of peptides per star and the relative density of stars with and without peptides can be altered to control both the density and spatial arrangement of peptides on a 50 nm length scale (Maheshwari *et al.*, 2000). Other research has demonstrated the necessity of a ligand spacer arm in order to achieve ligand-specific cell adhesion (Hern and Hubbell, 1998). In this study, RGD immobilized with no spacer arm did not mediate ligand-specific cell adhesion and spreading compared to RGD immobilized with a spacer arm consisting of PEG, MW 3400. The reason given for this result was that RGD with no spacer is sterically unavailable; however, this occurrence could also be due to the ability of ligands on a flexible spacer arm to form clusters. Another variable in peptide immobilization is the amino acid conformation, which can be altered by immobilizing the peptide by either its carboxyl end, amino end, or as a looped sequence. Such changes in the nature of peptide immobilization can drastically alter the cellular response (Pakalns *et al.*, 1999). Peptide recognition by cellular integrins may also be controlled by altering the length of surrounding molecules, such as oligo(ethylene glycol) groups (Dori *et al.*, 2000; Houseman and Mrksich, 2001), thus selectively masking the peptides.

Utilization of cell-specific peptide sequences in biomaterials enables the selective adhesion of certain cell types, even in the presence of a mixture of many cell types. As mentioned earlier, REDV promotes the adhesion of endothelial cells, but not other vascular cell types (Hubbell *et al.*, 1991). This selectivity has great potential for endothelialization of vascular devices, where the growth of an endothelial cells, but not fibroblasts or smooth muscle cells, is desired. Another peptide sequence, KRSR, has been shown to selectively promote the adhesion of osteoblasts, which is useful in the rational design of better dental and orthopedic biomaterials (Dee *et al.*, 1998).

These immobilized peptide sequences are capable of controlling aspects of cell behavior that are influenced by cell adhesion and spreading, such as proliferation, differentiation, migration, and extracellular matrix production. As discussed earlier, cell migration can be altered by changing the ligand density, as a high ligand density may restrict cell motility. Matrix mineralization by osteoblasts was also enhanced by higher ligand densities compared to lower ligand concentrations (Rezania and Healy, 2000). However, enhanced cell adhesion and spreading may also be accompanied by decreased cell function. Extracellular matrix production by smooth muscle and endothelial cells was greatest on substrates that were the least cell adhesive, while cells on highly adhesive surfaces displayed significantly decreased ECM production (Mann et al., 1999). This result suggests a role of adhesion-mediated signaling events in the regulation of ECM synthesis. As matrix production is a critical part of creating engineered tissues, this study emphasizes the importance of tailoring materials to contain the optimal concentration of ligands such that the desired cellular response is effected.

2. Proteoglycans/Selectins

Relative to integrins, interactions of proteoglycans with their ligands have not been widely employed in the design of biomaterials that regulate cell adhesion or function. This lack of investigation is likely due to the fact that these interactions primarily participate in cell–cell contacts, thereby not playing a large role in *in vivo* cell adhesion. However, a few groups have demonstrated that proteoglycan or selectin interactions with ligands can be exploited to create unique biomaterials (Eniola and Hammer, 2003 Ozaki et al., 1993). Additionally, investigation of chemical approaches for the development of synthetic glycoconjugate mimics is an active field of study (Bertozzi and Kiessling, 2001; Marcaurelle and Bertozzi, 1999). The chemical synthesis of molecules such as glycopeptides is challenging, but the ability to generate defined glycoproteins on cell surfaces would have a tremendous impact on biological investigation of cells and their interactions with substrates. Research in this area also involves the design of materials that mimic the cell glycocalyx. Such substrates have been synthesized using oligosaccharide surfactant polymers in order to provide a biomimetic surface that suppresses protein adsorption (Holland et al., 1998).

Hepatocytes are a cell-type, of particular interest in tissue engineering due to the regenerative capacity of the liver and the quantity of waiting liver transplant recipients, for which there are too few available organ donors. While the asialoglycoprotein receptor on hepatocytes does not usually promote cell adhesion *in vivo*, monosaccharide asialoglycoprotein ligands have been employed as adhesive ligands in order to induce hepatocyte adhesion to polymer surfaces. Specifically, *N*-acetyllactosamine and *N*-acetylglucosamine have been immobilized on polymer surfaces and found to selectively encourage the adhesion of mammalian and aviane hepatocytes, respectively (Gutsche *et al.*, 1994; Kobayashi *et al.*, 1994a). When a galactose ligand was bound to particles, it was found that high saccharide surface densities led to internalization of the particles by hepatocytes, which occurs *in vivo* with biological molecules possessing the appropriate monosaccharide ligand (Adachi *et al.*, 1994). Lower ligand densities prevented particle internalization and encouraged cell attachment to the particle. Microparticles have also been modified with monosaccharides for the purpose of targeted drug delivery (Cho *et al.*, 2001a,b). These drug delivery carriers possess an immobilized saccharide such as galactose, which then localizes to hepatocytes through its unique interactions with asialoglycoprotein.

The use of lectins on biomaterial surfaces may also provide a means of achieving cell-selective adhesion. The lectin Ulex europaeus I (UEA I) has a high affinity for endothelial cell surface glycoproteins. Covalent immobilization of UEA I on poly(ethylene terephthalate) resulted in a 100-fold increase in endothelial cell attachment, while adhesion of monocytes, smooth muscle cells, and fibroblasts was decreased (Ozaki *et al.*, 1993). Endothelialization of vascular grafts and other blood-contacting devices is highly important in maintaining a nonthrombogenic implant, and these results indicate that UEA I may be a useful ligand in achieving this goal of selectively encouraging endothelialization *in vivo*. Furthermore, this study demonstrates the potential of lectin–carbohydrate interactions for biomaterial modifications.

Most material modifications with biological molecules involve alteration of a polymeric biomaterial such that it may be recognized by cells. A novel alternative to this scheme is the formation of biomimetic polymeric cells that recognize native tissues as their substrates. As discussed earlier, selectins mediate the rolling of inflammatory cells such as leukocytes on the vascular endothelium and their subsequent extravasation. Acute inflammatory indicators, such as histamine or thrombin, induce increased expression of P–selectin, thereby facilitating leukocyte binding. Chronic inflammation is accompanied by expression of E–selectin. The interaction of selectins with their carbohydrate ligands is transient, yet highly specific. Furthermore, selectin expression is carefully regulated and localized, making selectins excellent candidates for participation in targeted drug delivery (Juliano, 2002).

One group has modified the surfaces of degradable microspheres loaded with an anti-inflammatory drug to contain sialyl-Lewis^x (sLe^x), a sialylated fucosylated carbohydrate which mediates rolling on selectins (Eniola and Hammer, 2003). These sLe^x-modified microspheres specifically interacted with P-selectin-coated surfaces and exhibited similar interactions with the selectin surface as those observed *in vivo* between neutrophils and activated endothelial cells. The rolling velocity of the polymeric cells was controlled via changes in the sLe^x density or wall shear stress. Increasing sLe^x site density decreased rolling velocity, as an increase in ligand density results in the formation of more sLe^x–selectin bonds, thereby slowing down the rolling. Because this method delivers anti-inflammatory drugs via the same route used during *in vivo* recruitment of inflammatory molecules, it displays several advantages over conventional anti-inflammatory drug administration. This system enables localized, sustained delivery of a therapeutic molecule, thereby bypassing the transport limitations and gastrointestinal side effects associated with traditional drug therapy. Additionally, the chemistry used to attach the sLe^x ligands can be extended to develop several different artificial polymeric cell types, including lymphocytes, bone marrow cells, and macrophages.

VI. Conclusion

In order to synthesize rational biomaterials, it is necessary to understand the interactions between the cell and its external environment, specifically materials. Knowledge of how cells interact with native proteins and matrices contributes to the synthesis of biologically recognizable materials. These cell–matrix interactions may be regulated by protein adsorption to materials, as well as by various material physical properties such as surface charge, hydrophilicity, and topographical features. Additionally, materials may also be designed to display only specific biological molecules, such as certain cell adhesion peptides. These modifications create a controlled environment in which cell behavior can be regulated and examined to achieve the desired response. Aspects of cell function, such as differentiation, apoptosis, proliferation, and extracellular matrix production, may be regulated by the expression of specific adhesion molecules, as well as by their density and spatial organization, thus simulating the clustering that occurs upon attachment to native ECM proteins. Modification of materials with biological sequences also allows the creation of biomimetic materials that capture essential features of native matrices, but whose composition is well-defined and characterized.

Exploitation of our knowledge of cell–material interactions can allow the bioengineer to rationally design appropriate materials for applications such as tissue engineering.

REFERENCES

Abrams, G., Teixeira, A., Nealey, P., and Murphy, C., *in* "Biomimetic Materials and Design" (A. Dillow and A. Lowman Eds.), p. 91. Marcel Dekker, Inc., New York (2002).
Adachi, N., Maruyama, A., Ishihara, T., and Akaike, T. *J. Biomat. Sci. Polym. Ed.* **6,** 463 (1994).
Alberts, B., Bray, D., Lewis, J., Raff, M., Roberts, K., and Watson, J., "Molecular Biology of the Cell". Garland Publishing, Inc., New York (1994).
Altankov, G., Grinnell, F., and Groth, T. *J. Biomed. Mater. Res.* **30,** 385 (1996).
Anselme, K., Linez, P., Bigerelle, M., LeMaguer, D., LeMaguer, A., Hardouin, P., Hildebrand, H., Iost, A., and Leroy, J. *Biomaterials* **21,** 1567 (2000).
Anseth, K., Metters, A., Bryant, S., Martens, P., Elisseef, J., and Bowman, C. *J. Control. Rel.* **78,** 199 (2002).
Aota, S., Nomizu, M., and Yamada, K. *J. Biol. Chem.* **269,** 24756 (1994).
Baier-Leach, J., Bivens, K., Patrick, C., and Schmidt, C. *Biotechnol. Bioeng.* **82,** 578 (2000).
Bartolazzi, A., Peach, R., Aruffo, A., and Stamenkovic, I. *J. Exp. Med.* **180,** 53 (1994).
Bell, G. *Science* **200,** 618 (1978).
Ben Ze'ev, A., Robinson, S., Bucher, N., and Farmer, S. *Proc. Natl. Acad. Sci. USA* **85,** 1 (1988).
Bennett, J., *in* "Cell adhesion molecules and matrix proteins" (S. Mousa Ed.), p. 29. Springer-Verlag, Berlin (1998).
Bergethon, P., Trinkaus-Randall, V., and Franzblau, C. *J. Cell. Sci.* **92,** 111 (1989).
Bertozzi, C., and Kiessling, L. *Science* **291,** 2357 (2001).
Binnerts, M., Kooyk, Y. v., and Figdor, C., *in* "Molecular Biology of Cell Adhesion Molecules" (M. Horton Ed.), p. 17. John Wiley and Sons Ltd., West Sussex, England (1996).
Bissell, D., Arenson, D., Maher, J., and Roll, F. *Am. Soc. Clin. Invest.* **79,** 801 (1987).
Bissell, M., Weaver, V., Lelièvre, S., Wang, F., Petersen, O., and Schmeichel, K. *Cancer. Res.* **59,** 1757 (1999).
Boudreau, N., and Jones, P. *Biochem. J.* **339,** 481 (1999).
Boudreau, N., Sympson, C. J., Werb, Z., and Bissell, M. *J. Science* **267,** 891 (1995).
Braber, E. d., Ruitjer, J. d., Ginsel, L., Recum, A. v., and Jansen, J. *J. Biomed. Mater. Res.* **40,** 291 (1998).
Brummendorf, T., and Rathjen, F. *Curr. Opin. Neurobiol.* **6,** 584 (1996).
Brunette, D. *Exp. Cell Res.* **164,** 11 (1986a).
Brunette, D. *Exp. Cell Res.* **167,** 203 (1986b).
Buck, C. A. *Semin. Cell Biol.* **3,** 179 (1992).
Burdick, J., and Anseth, K. *Biomaterials* **23,** 4315 (2002).
Burridge, K., Fath, K., Kelly, T., Nuckolis, G., and Turner, C. *Annu. Rev. Cell. Biol.* **4,** 487 (1988).
Bussell, S., Koch, D., and Hammer, D. *Biophys. J.* **68,** 1828 (1995a).
Bussell, S., Koch, D., and Hammer, D. *Biophys. J.* **68,** 1836 (1995b).
Cardin, A., and Weintraub, H. *Arteriosclerosis* **9,** 21 (1989).

Caron, J. *Mol. Cell Biol.* **10,** 1239 (1990).
Castner, D., and Ratner, B. *Surf. Sci.* **500,** 28 (2002).
Catterall, J., Gardner, M., and Turner, G. *Cancer J.* **8,** 320 (1995).
Chen, C., Mrksich, M., Huang, S., Whitesides, G., and Ingber, D. *Science* **276,** 1425 (1997).
Cho, C. S., Cho, K. Y., Park, I. K., Kim, S. H., Sasagawa, T., Uchiyama, M., and Akaike, T. *J. Control. Rel.* **77,** 7 (2001a).
Cho, C. S., Kobayashi, A., Takei, R., Ishihara, T., Maruyama, A., and Akaike, T. *Biomaterials* **22,** 45 (2001b).
Choquet, D., Felsenfeld, D., and Sheetz, M. *Cell* **88,** 39 (1997).
Clark, P., Connolly, P., Curtis, A., Dow, J., and Wilkinson, C. *J. Cell Sci.* **99,** 73 (1991).
Cukierman, E., Pankov, R., Stevens, D., and Yamada, K. *Science* **294,** 1708 (2001).
Curtis, A., and Wilkinson, C. *Biomaterials* **18,** 1573 (1997).
Curtis, A., Wilkinson, C., and Wojciak-Stothard, B. *J. Cellular Eng.* **1,** 35 (1995).
Danilov, Y., and Juliano, R. *Exp. Cell. Res.* **182,** 186 (1989).
Davies, J., in "Surface Characterization of Biomaterials" (B. Ratner Ed.), p. 219. Elsevier, Amsterdam (1998).
Dee, K., Andersen, T., and Bizios, R. *J. Biomed. Mater. Res.* **40,** 371 (1998).
DiMilla, P., Stone, J., Quinn, J., Albelda, S., and Lauffenberger, D. *J. Cell Biol.* **122,** 729 (1993).
Dori, Y., Bianco-Peled, H., Satija, S., Fields, G., McCarthy, J., and Tirrell, M. *J. Biomed. Mater. Res.* **50,** 75 (2000).
Drumheller, P., and Hubbell, J. *Anal. Biochem.* **222,** 380 (1994).
Dunn, J., Yarmush, M., Koebe, H., and Tompkins, R. *FASEB J.* **3,** 174 (1989).
Eisenbarth, E., Meyle, J., Nachtigail, W., and Breme, J. *Biomaterials* **17,** 1399 (1996).
Elbert, D., and Hubbell, J. *Ann. Rev. Mater. Sci.* **26,** 365 (1996).
Elsdale, T., and Bard, J. *J. Cell Biol.* **54,** 626 (1972).
Eniola, A., and Hammer, D. *J. Control. Rel.* **87,** 15 (2003).
Flemming, R., Murphy, C., Abrams, G., Goodman, S., and Nealey, P. *Biomaterials* **20,** 573 (1999).
Folkman, J., and Moscona, A. *Nature* **273,** 345 (1978).
Friedl, P., and Brocker, E. B. *Cell Mol. Life Sci.* **57,** 41 (2000).
Furie, B., and Furie, B., in "Adhesion Molecules and Cell Signaling: Biology and Clinical Applications" (W. Siess, R. Lorenz, and P. Weber Eds.), p. 93. Raven Press, New York (1995).
García, A., Vega, M., and Boettiger, D. *Mol. Biol. Cell.* **10,** 785 (1999).
Geffen, I., and Speiss, M. *Int. Rev. Cytol.* **137B,** 181 (1992).
Geiger, B., and Bershadsky, A. *Curr. Opin. Cell Biol.* **13,** 584 (2001).
Giancotti, F., and Ruoslahti, E. *Science* **285,** 1028 (1999).
Gombotz, W., Wang, G., Horbett, T., and Hoffman, A. *J. Biomed. Mater. Res.* **25,** 1547 (1991).
Goodison, S., Urquidi, V., and Tarin, D. *J. Clin. Pathol: Mol. Pathol.* **52,** 189 (1999).
Griffith, L., and Lopina, S. *Biomaterials* **19,** 979 (1998).
Groessner-Screiber, B., and Tuan, R. *J. Cell Sci.* **101,** 209 (1992).
Gutsche, A., Parsons-Wigerter, P., Chand, D., Saltzman, W., and Leong, K. *Biotechnol. Bioeng.* **43,** 801 (1994).
Hammer, D., and Tirrell, M. *Annu. Rev. Mater. Sci.* **26,** 651 (1996).
Han, D., Ryu, G., Park, K., Jeong, S., Kim, Y., and Min, B. *J. Biomater. Sci. Polym. Ed.* **4,** 401 (1993).
Harbers, G., Barber, T., Stile, R., Sumner, D., and Healy, K., in "Biomimetic Materials and Design" (A. Dillow and A. Lowman Eds.), p. 55. Marcel Dekker, Inc., New York (2002).
Hautanen, A., Gailit, J., Mann, D., and Ruoslahti, E. *J. Biol. Chem.* **264,** 1437 (1989).

Haynes, C., and Norde, W. *Colloids Surf.* **2**, 517 (1994).
Hern, D., and Hubbell, J. *J. Biomed. Mater. Res.* **39**, 266 (1998).
Holland, N., Qiu, Y., Ruegsegger, M., and Marchant, R. *Nature* **392**, 799 (1998).
Horbett, T., and Brash, J., "Proteins at Interfaces II: Fundamentals and Applications". American Chemical Society, Washington, DC (1999).
Horbett, T. *BMES Bulletin* **23**, 5 (1999).
Horton, M., in "Molecular Biology of Cell Adhesion Molecules" (M. Horton Ed.), p. 221. John Wiley and Sons Ltd., West Sussex, England (1996).
Horwitz, A. *Sci. Am.* **276**, 68 (1997).
Houseman, B., and Mrksich, M. *Biomaterials* **22**, 943 (2001).
Hubbell, J., Massia, S., Desai, N., and Drumheller, P. *Biotechnol.* **9**, 568 (1991).
Hubbell, J. *Biotechnol.* **13**, 565 (1995).
Humphries, M. *J. Cell Sci.* **97**, 585 (1990).
Hynes, R. *Cell* **110**, 673 (2002).
Ito, Y. *Biomaterials* **20**, 2333 (1999).
Juliano, R. *Annu. Rev. Pharmacol. Toxicol.* **42**, 283 (2002).
Katz, B., Zamir, E., Bershadsky, A., Kam, Z., Yamada, K., and Geiger, B. *Mol. Biol. Cell* **11**, 1047 (2000).
Keselowsky, B., Collard, D., and García, A. *J. Biomed. Mater. Res.* **66A**, 247 (2003).
Kiaei, D., Hoffman, A., and Horbett, T. *J. Biomater. Sci. Polym. Ed.* **4**, 35 (1992).
Kiaei, D., Hoffman, A., Horbett, T., and Lew, K. *J. Biomed. Mater. Res.* **29**, 729 (1995).
Kobayashi, H., and Ikada, Y. *Biomaterials* **12**, 747 (1991).
Kobayashi, K., Kobayashi, A., and Akaike, T. *Meth. Enzymol.* **247**, 409 (1994a).
Koenig, A., and Grainger, D., in "Biomimetic Materials and Design" (A. Dillow and A. Lowman Eds.), p. 187. Marcel Dekker, Inc., New York (2002).
Komoriya, A., Green, L., Mervic, M., Yamada, S., Yamada, K., and Humphries, M. *J. Biol. Chem.* **266**, 15075 (1991).
Lampin, M., Warocquier-Clerout, R., Legris, C., Degrange, M., and Sigot-Luizard, M. *J. Biomed. Mater. Res.* **36**, 99 (1997).
Lauffenburger, D., and Horwitz, A. *Cell* **84**, 359 (1996).
Lauffenburger, D., and Linderman, J., "Receptors: Models for Binding, Trafficking, and Signaling". Oxford Press, New York (1993).
Lee, J., and Lee, H. *J. Biomater. Sci. Polym. Ed.* **4**, 467 (1993).
Lee, J., Lee, J., Khang, G., and Lee, H. *Biomaterials* **18**, 351 (1997).
Lesley, J., Hyman, R., and Kincade, P. W. *Adv. Immunol.* **54**, 271 (1993).
Li, R., Mitra, N., Gratkowski, H., Vilaire, G., Litvinov, R., Nagasami, C., Weisel, J., Lear, J., DeGrado, W., and Bennett, J. *Science* **300**, 795 (2003).
Lo, C., Wang, H., Dembo, M., and Wang, Y. *Biophys. J.* **79**, 144 (2000).
Longhurst, C., and Jennings, L. *Cell Mol. Life Sci.* **54**, 514 (1998).
Lopez, G., Albers, M., Schreiber, S., Carroll, R., Peralta, E., and Whitesides, G. *J. Amer. Chem. Soc.* **115**, 5877 (1993).
Maheshwari, G., Brown, G., Lauffenburger, D., Wells, A., and Griffith, L. *J. Cell. Sci.* **113**, 1677 (2000).
Mann, B., Tsai, A., Scott-Burden, T., and West, J. *Biomaterials* **20**, 2281 (1999).
Mann, B., Gobin, A., Tsai, A., Schmedlen, R., and West, J. *Biomaterials* **22**, 3045 (2001).
Marcaurelle, L., and Bertozzi, C. *Chem. Eur. J.* **5**, 1384 (1999).
Massia, S., and Hubbell, J. *J. Biol. Chem.* **267**, 10133 (1992).
Massia, S., and Hubbell, J. *J. Cell Biol.* **114**, 1089 (1991).
Massia, S., and Hubbell, J. *Anal. Biochem.* **187**, 292 (1990).
McAuslan, B., and Johnson, G. *J. Biomed. Mater. Res.* **21**, 921 (1987).

McEver, R., *in* "Adhesion Molecules and Cell Signaling: Biology and Clinical Applications" (W. Siess, R. Lorenz, and P. Weber Eds.), p. 85. Raven Press, New York (1995).
Meredith, J., and Schwartz, M. *Trends Cell Biol.* **7,** 146 (1997).
Meredith, J., Fazeli, B., and Schwartz, M. *Mol. Biol. Cell.* **4,** 953 (1993).
Meyle, J., Gutlig, K., and Nisch, W. *J. Biomed. Mater. Res.* **29,** 81 (1995).
Mooney, D., Hansen, L., Vacanti, J., Langer, R., Farmer, S., and Ingber, D. *J. Cell. Physiol.* **151,** 497 (1992).
Mousa, S., *in* "Cell Adhesion Molecules and Matrix Proteins" (S. Mousa Ed.), p. 1. Springer-Verlag, Berlin (1998).
Murphy-Ullrich, J. *J. Clin. Invest.* **107,** 785 (2001).
Nuttelman, C., Mortisen, D., Henry, S., and Anseth, K. *J. Biomed. Mater. Res.* **57,** 217 (2001).
Oakley, C., and Brunette, D. *J. Cell. Sci.* **106,** 343 (1993).
Oakley, C., and Brunette, D. *Biochem. Cell Biol.* **73,** 473 (1995).
Opas, M. *Dev. Biol.* **131,** (1989).
Orend, G., and Chiquet-Ehrismann, R. *Exp. Cell. Res.* **261,** 104 (2000).
Ozaki, C., Phaneuf, M., Hong, S., Quist, W., and LoGerfo, F. *J. Vasc. Surg.* **18,** 486 (1993).
Pakalns, T., Haverstick, K., Fields, G., McCarthy, J., Mooradian, D., and Tirrell, M. *Biomaterials* **20,** 2265 (1999).
Palecek, S., Loftus, J., Ginsberg, M., Lauffenberger, D., and Horwitz, A. *Nature* **385,** 537 (1997).
Palecek, S., Horwitz, A., and Lauffenberger, D. *Ann. Biomed. Eng.* **27,** 219 (1999).
Pelham, R., and Wang, Y. *Proc. Natl. Acad. Sci. USA* **94,** 13,661 (1997).
Pierschbacher, M., and Ruoslahti, E. *Nature* **309,** 30 (1984).
Pins, G., Toner, M., and Morgan, J. *FASEB J.* **14,** 593 (2000).
Plow, E., Haas, T., Zhang, L., Loftus, J., and Smith, J. *J. Biol. Chem.* **275,** 21,785 (2000).
Prime, K., and Whitesides, G. *J. Amer. Chem. Soc.* **115,** 10,714 (1993).
Raff, M. *Nature* **356,** 397 (1992).
Ramsden, J. *Surfactant Sci Ser.* **110,** 199 (2003).
Rezania, A., and Healy, K. *J. Biomed. Mater. Res.* **39,** 63 (2000).
Romer, L., *in* "Adhesion Molecules and Cell Signaling: Biology and Clinical Applications" (W. Siess, R. Lorenz, and P. Weber Eds.), p. 37. Raven Press, New York (1995).
Ruardy, T., Schakenraad, J., Mei, H. v. d., and Busscher, H. *J. Biomed. Mater. Res.* **29,** 1415 (1995).
Ruoslahti, E., and Reed, J. *Cell* **77,** 477 (1994).
Ruoslahti, E. *Annu. Rev. Cell Dev. Biol.* **12,** 697 (1996).
Sage, E., and Bornstein, P. *J. Biol. Chem.* **266,** 14,831 (1991).
Sage, E. *J. Clin. Invest.* **107,** 781 (2001).
Sampson, N., Mrksich, M., and Bertozzi, C. *Proc. Natl. Acad. Sci. USA* **98,** 12,870 (2001).
Sawhney, A., Pathak, C., and Hubbell, J. *Macromolecules* **26,** 581 (1993).
Schakenraad, J., Busscher, H., Wildevuurr, C., and Arends, J. *J. Biomed. Mater. Res.* **20,** 773 (1986).
Seeger, J., and Klingman, N. *J. Vasc. Surg.* **8,** 476 (1987).
Seyfert, S., Voigt, A., and Kabbeck-Kupijai, D. *Biomaterials* **16,** 201 (1995).
Singhvi, R., Kumar, A., Lopez, G. P., Stephanopoulos, G. N., Wang, D. I. C., Whitesides, G. M., and Ingber, D. E. *Science* **264,** 696 (1994).
Solowska, J., Guan, J., Marcantonio, E., Trevithick, J., Buck, C., and Hynes, R. *J. Cell Biol* **109,** 853 (1989).
Stephansson, S. N., Byers, B. A., and García, A. J. *Biomaterials* **23,** 2527 (2002).
Stupack, D., and Cheresh, D. *J. Cell. Sci.* **115,** 3729 (2002).
Sudhakaran, P., Stamataglou, S., and Hughes, R. *Exp. Cell. Res.* **167,** 505 (1986).

Tirrell, M., Kokkoli, E., and Biesalski, M. *Surf. Sci.* **500,** 61 (2002).
Tomomura, A., Sawada, N., Sattler, G., Kleinman, H., and Pitot, H. *J. Cell. Physiol.* **130,** 221 (1987).
Tremble, P., Chiquet-Ehrismann, R., and Werb, Z. *Mol. Biol. Cell* **5,** 439 (1994).
Turley, E., Noble, P., and Bourguignon, L. *J. Biol. Chem.* **277,** 4589 (2002).
van der Flier, A., and Sonnenberg, A. *Cell Tissue Res.* **305,** 285 (2001).
van Wachem, P., Hogt, A., Beugeling, T., Feijen, J., Bantjes, A., Detmers, J., and van Aken, W. *Biomaterials* **8,** 323 (1987).
Webb, K., Hlady, V., and Tresco, P. *J. Biomed. Mater. Res.* **41,** 422 (1998).
Webster, T. J., Ergun, C., Doremus, R. H., Siegel, R. W., and Bizios, R. *J. Biomed. Mater. Res.* **51,** 475 (2000).
Wehrle-Haller, B., and Imhof, B. *Trends Cell Biol.* **12,** 382 (2002).
West, J., and Hubbell, J., *in* "Synthetic Biodegradable Polymer Scaffolds" (A. Atala and D. Mooney Eds.), p. 81. Birkhäuser, Boston (1997).
Williams, R., Hunt, J., and Tengvall, P. *J. Biomed. Mater. Res.* **29,** 1545 (1995).
Wong, J., Velasco, A., Rajagopalan, P., and Pham, Q. *Langmuir* **19,** 1908 (2003).
Yamada, K. *J. Biol. Chem.* **256,** 12,809 (1991).
Yoshinari, M., Matsuzaka, K., Inoue, T., Oda, Y., and Shimono, M. *J. Biomed. Mater. Res.* **65A,** 359 (2003).
Zamir, E., and Geiger, B. *J. Cell. Sci.* **114,** 3583 (2001).

POLYMERIC BIOMATERIALS FOR NERVE REGENERATION

Surya K. Mallapragada* and Jennifer B. Recknor

Department of Chemical Engineering, Iowa State University, Ames, IA 50011-2230, USA

I. Introduction	47
II. Polymers for Regeneration in the Peripheral Nervous System	48
A. Nondegradable Polymers for Entubulization	50
B. Degradable Polymers for Entubulization	52
C. Comparative Studies	57
III. Polymers for Regeneration in the Central Nervous Systems	60
IV. Polymers for Controlled Release	64
V. Cell Encapsulation	66
VI. Conclusions	68
Acknowledgments	68
References	68

I. Introduction

Each year, over 10,000 Americans sustain spinal cord injuries (Teng et al., 2002). In addition, numerous surgeries are performed every year to try to repair peripheral nerve damage (Miller et al., 2001a). Central nervous system repair is impeded partly by myelin-associated inhibitors and if the axons can traverse the injury site, there is a possibility of regrowth in the unscarred areas and of functional recovery (Teng et al., 2002). Grafting is a common approach to facilitate peripheral nerve regeneration to provide guidance to the regenerating axons. Grafting methods include autografts and allografts (Ide et al., 1983; Keeley et al., 1993; Wang et al., 1992). However, a major drawback of autografts is that they partially deinnervate the donor site to repair the injury site. Problems with allografts include tissue rejection and lack of donor tissue. These problems could eventually

*Tel.: +1-515-294-7407; Fax: +1-515-294-2689; E-mail: suryakm@iastate.edu

be minimized by tissue engineered nerve grafts based on polymers for transplantation and alternative methods to engineer an artificial environment to mimic the physical and chemical stimulus that promotes nerve regeneration.

Polymers are being extensively investigated to help facilitate nerve regeneration (Bellamkonda and Aebischer, 1994). Entubulization methods involving polymers where a conduit is used to connect the nerve endings has great potential as a repair method for peripheral nerve regeneration. The conduit allows for neurotropic and neurotrophic communication between the nerve stumps and also provides physical guidance for the regenerating axons similar to the grafts (Fig. 1) (Heath and Rutkowski, 1998). The closely fitting tubes facilitate axonal regeneration by inducing rapid development of a highly organized capsule that isolates the repair site and guides and aligns endoneurial components (Stensaas et al., 1989). Entubulization minimizes unregulated axonal growth at the site of injury by providing a distinct environment, and allows for trophic factors emitted from the distal stump to reach the proximal segment, which enhances physiological conditions for nerve regeneration. The spatial cues also induce a change in tissue architecture, with the cabling of cells within the microconduit (Pearson et al., 2003). The conduits can also be environmentally enhanced with chemical stimulants like laminin and nerve growth factor (NGF), biological cues such as from Schwann cells and astrocytes, the satellite cells of the peripheral and central nervous systems, and lastly, physical guidance cues.

Another area where polymers are making a significant difference in nerve regeneration is the use of polymers to encapsulate and release trophic factors, or encapsulate cells that release nerve growth factor or other agents that enhance the regeneration process. This chapter details the advances in the use of polymeric biomaterials that have been explored for nerve regeneration in the peripheral and central nervous systems.

II. Polymers for Regeneration in the Peripheral Nervous System

Current polymeric entubulization repair methods for peripheral nerve regeneration use various nondegradable and biodegradable materials. The most common nondegradable material investigated has been silicone rubber. Medical grade silicone rubber, polydimethylsiloxane, maintains its shape and can be filled with neurotrophic factors or extracellular

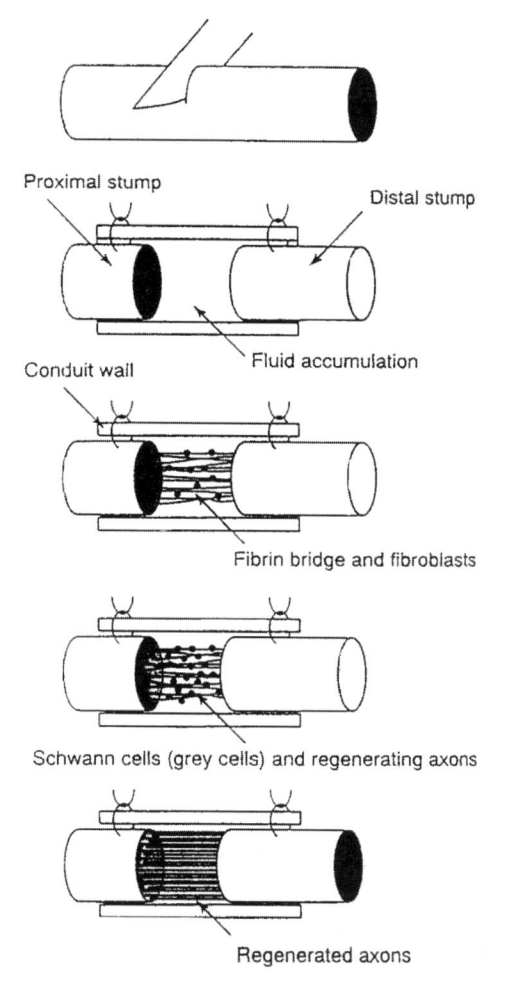

FIG. 1. Silicone-chamber model showing the progression of events during peripheral-nerve regeneration. After bridging the proximal and distal nerve stumps, the silicone tube becomes filled with serum and other extracellular fluids. A fibrin bridge containing a variety of cell types connects the two stumps. Schwann cells and axons processes migrate from the proximal end to the distal stump along the bridge. The axons continue to regenerate through the distal stump to their final contacts. [Reproduced with permission from Heath and Rutkowski (1998).]

matrix (ECM) components. The silicone tubes provide an impermeable conduit for endoneurial fluid that creates an environment favoring the regeneration of axons and Schwann cells. Unfortunately, the nerve guide remains in the body and can cause a chronic immune response.

A second surgery is required after regeneration to prevent secondary nerve injury due to compression (den Dunnen et al., 1996a).

Biodegradable materials such as collagen, poly(glycolic acid) and poly(lactic acid) have been used to make conduits for entubulization repairs. These polymers completely degrade in the body eliminating the need for a second surgery. One problem with some biodegradable polymers is that they tend to swell and can deform causing compression to the regenerating nerve (den Dunnen et al., 1996b; Henry et al., 1985).

A. Nondegradable Polymers for Entubulization

Silicone has been one of the most commonly investigated nondegradable polymer for nerve entubulization, especially for peripheral nerve regeneration in animal models (Wang-Bennett and Coker, 1990). Some of the earliest studies have shown that silicone tubes sutured to the proximal and distal ends of a severed nerve can promote directed growth (Seckel et al., 1986) and regeneration to bridge a 6–10 mm gap in the nerve (Luo and Lu, 1996). However, in human studies with a small 3–4 mm gap between nerve endings, the silicone tubes did not exhibit a significant improvement in regeneration compared to conventional microsurgical repair of the nerve trunk (Lundborg et al., 1997).

1. Chemical Cues

The fluid filling these cylindrical chambers was found to contain trophic factors (Lundborg et al., 1982a,b,c), but local application of the accumulated fluid to silicone chambers at the time of implantation did not have any significant effect on nerve elongation rates (Sebille and Becker, 1988). One of the components of the fluid, fibrin, was injected into silicone chambers prior to implantation and was found to enhance regeneration in the short-term, but no difference was observed after five weeks (Chen, 1992). However, filling the silicone chambers with a resorbable fibrin sponge matrix was found to enable axons to bridge a 10-mm gap in a sciatic nerve transection within 14 days under appropriate substrate conditions (Dubovy and Bednarova, 1996). Similarly, filling the silicone compartment with a collagen gel prior to implantation led to more rapid and directed outgrowth of sprouting axons towards the distal side, but led to fewer fibroblasts and Schwann cells (Satou et al., 1986). An extracellular gel containing collagen, laminin, and fibronectin was filled into silicone, tubes to enhance regeneration and both qualitative and quantitative histology of the regenerated nerves revealed a more mature ultrastructural organization with larger cross-sectional area and higher number of myelinated axons in the combination gel group than the controls (Chen et al., 2000). Similar results were observed with polyethylene tubes filled with pure collagen or collagen–NGF mixtures (Da-Silva and Langone, 1989). Relative adhesiveness of various chemically modified substrates was however not a good predictor of the rate of axon growth or the degree of axon fasciculation (Lemmon et al., 1992). However, a conduit made of a perm-selective material such as an acrylic copolymer that allows solute transport was found to promote much better peripheral nerve regeneration compared to an impermeable silicone conduit (Aebischer et al., 1988). Gore-Tex has also been explored as a conduit material with limited success (Young et al., 1984).

Various chemical cues have been used in conjunction with the silicone chambers to accelerate regeneration (Liu, 1996). Using a nitrocellulose strip soaked in fibroblast growth factor (FGF) to partition the silicone chamber into two compartments was found to lead to faster migration of all cellular elements including perineurial-like cells, vasculature, and Schwann cells and revealed that two separate nerve structures had formed, one on either side of the partition (Danielsen et al., 1988a,b). Nerve growth factor added to silicone chambers has also been shown to promote regeneration in the short-term of facial and sciatic nerves (Chen et al., 1989; Rich et al., 1989). However, over 10 weeks, ultrastructural analysis demonstrated no difference in the distribution of axonal diameters or myelin thickness between the regenerated groups, and there was essentially complete regeneration of both the NGF and control regenerative groups demonstrating that NGF provides an early but limited neurotrophic effect on nerve regeneration (Hollowell et al., 1990; Spector et al., 1993). This could be due to the short half-life of NGF *in vivo*. Use of silicone chambers filled with thyroid hormones have also been found to significantly increase the number, the mean diameter of myelinated axons, and the thickness of myelin sheaths compared to control samples, even after eight weeks of peripheral nerve regeneration (Voinesco et al., 1998).

2. Electrical Cues

Electrical stimuli have also been investigated to promote neurite outgrowth. Neurons cultured on electrically charged piezoelectric polymers such as poly(vinylidene fluoride) exhibited significantly greater levels of process outgrowth and neurite lengths than the control samples (Valentini et al., 1992). An electrically conductive polymer, oxidized polypyrrole, was found to significantly enhance neurite outgrowth of PC12 cells when they were subjected to an electrical stimulus (Schmidt et al., 1997; Shastri et al., 1997).

3. Directed Growth

Several methods have been developed to control neuronal outgrowth on substrates (Buettner, 1996; Clark, 1996; Tessier-Lavigne, 1994). Oriented growth of the axons was promoted by filling silicone tubes with longitudinal fibers made of nonabsorbable polyamide or absorbable materials such as polyglactin and catgut. No axons were found growing in direct contact with the filaments and the filaments did not seem to disturb axonal growth across the tube (Terada *et al.*, 1997). Silicone tubes prefilled with oriented collagen and laminin gels produced by gravitational or magnetic forces were found to increase the success and the quality of regeneration in long nerve gaps. The laminin gel was found to perform better than the collagen gel in promoting sciatic nerve regeneration (Verdu *et al.*, 2002). Silicone tubes were also filled with collagen or poly(lactide) fibers to enhance regeneration (Itoh *et al.*, 2001). To avoid problems associated with removing a nondegradable material after nerve regeneration, silicone tubes were used to create pseudo nerves, which contain longitudinal Schwann cell columns without axons and surrounded by perineurium-like tissue (Zhao *et al.*, 1992). These pseudo-nerves were applied as a graft to repair nerve defects in rats and were found to induce nerve repair to a similar extent as a real graft (Zhao *et al.*, 1997). Alternative approaches involve the use of degradable materials as conduits for nerve regeneration, as discussed in the following section.

B. Degradable Polymers for Entubulization

In order to avoid common problems associated with nondegradable polymeric conduits such as chronic immune response and a second surgery to prevent nerve injury due to compression, degradable polymers have been investigated extensively for entubulization applications. The degradable polymers can be either synthetic or biological. The most commonly used synthetic degradable polymers for entubulization have been poly(L-lactide), poly(glycolide), and their copolymers (Schugens *et al.*, 1996; Widmer *et al.*, 1998) and the most commonly used biological polymer has been collagen (Tong *et al.*, 1994). The biological polymers such as collagen have also been used extensively in conjunction with the synthetic biodegradable as well as nondegradable polymers.

When using synthetic polymers, the use of copolymers enables tailoring of the degradation rates to periods varying from a few days to a few months. The degradation of the polymers eliminates the need for a second surgery after the regeneration is complete. The degradation products are usually biocompatible and have been found to cause no adverse reactions: however, in some cases where synthetic polymers are used, there is a local drop in pH inside the conduit due to acidic degradation products. But studies with poly(lactic acid) devices affixed to divided nerves have shown that even though there are significant amounts of degradation products formed, there was no adverse reaction to the biodegradable substance or its metabolites (de Medinaceli et al., 1995). The natural polymers suffer from disadvantages associated with increase immunogenicities compared to synthetic polymers (Navarro et al., 1996), and variability based on source.

Polyglactin mesh tubes were used to bridge defects 7–9 mm in length and were found to reduce formation of neuromas and growth of scar tissue from surrounding structures (Molander et al., 1982). Copolymers of lactic and glycolic acid were used to bridge peripheral nerve transections (Nyilas et al., 1983) and the local environment was manipulated further by the addition of the proteins collagen, fibrinogen, and anti-Thy-1 antibody to the nerve guide lumens at the time of operation (Madison et al., 1984). The results for poly(L-lactide) (PLLA) were significantly improved over those for 75:25 poly(DL-lactic-co-glycolic acid) (PLGA) and suggest that PLLA porous conduits may serve as a better scaffold for peripheral nerve regeneration (Evans et al., 1999). However, longer evaluation of polymer degradation is warranted (Evans et al., 2000). Laminin-containing gels filled in the bioresorbable conduits enabled improved initial regeneration compared to empty conduits (Madison et al., 1985) at two weeks, but was found to be inhibitory at six weeks (Madison et al., 1987). For PLGA nerve guides, studies revealed a reduction in the total axon count and the number of myelinated axons in the presence of exogenously added Schwann cells compared to saline controls. In contrast, the addition of glial growth factor (GGF) alone enhanced the total number of axons and significantly increased the number of blood vessels. Although combining GGF with Schwann cells negated this effect, this combination resulted in the highest myelination index and the fastest conduction velocities recorded, demonstrating a potential role for GGF in nerve regeneration (Bryan et al., 2000). These results can be explained by a simple reaction–diffusion model that was developed to describe the mass transport of nutrients and nerve growth factor within a bioartificial nerve graft (Rutkowski and Heath, 2002b). The results suggest that at higher porosities, more growth factors diffuse out of the conduit, while at low porosities there is competition for nutrients. Increasing the Schwann cell seeding density enhances growth but also leads to an increase in the number of axons along the length of the conduit. This is indicative of branching of the axons, which requires additional resources to maintain and can lead to painful neuroma formation (Rutkowski and Heath, 2002a).

Biodegradable conduits made of poly(L-lactide-*co*-epsilon-caprolactone) (PLC) polymers have been evaluated long-term and found to enable sciatic nerve regeneration with very mild foreign body reaction for two years (den Dunnen *et al.*, 1993; Nicoli Aldini *et al.*, 1996; Perego *et al.*, 1994). The diameter of the nerve guide was seen to have a significant role as nerve guides with smaller lumens showed nerve compression due to a pronounced swelling of the degrading tube and increased foreign body reaction (den Dunnen *et al.*, 1995; Meek *et al.*, 1997, 1999). To minimize diffusion limitations, a nerve guide comprised of an inner microporous layer of PLC (pore size 0.5–1 μm) and an outer microporous layer (pore size 30–70 μm) of polyurethane/poly(L-lactide) mixture was investigated (Hoppen *et al.*, 1990). These conduits were filled with denatured muscle tissue in order to enable slightly faster regeneration than the empty conduits, and also enable regeneration across longer nerve gaps of 15-mm (Meek *et al.*, 1996, 2001). Syngeneic, isogeneic, and autologous Schwann cells were suspended in Matrigel and seeded in permeable PLC guides. Transplants of autologous Schwann cells resulted in slightly lower levels of reinnervation than autografts, but higher recovery and number of regenerated fibers reaching the distal nerve than transplants of isologous and syngeneic Schwann cells, although most of the differences were not statistically significant (Rodriguez *et al.*, 2000). The main problem with PLC nerve conduits is their propensity to swell, especially in the first three months, and that can have a negative influence on the regenerating nerve. Therefore, PLC nerve guides are most suited for clinical situations involving short nerve gaps in small nerves (den Dunnen *et al.*, 2000).

Poly-3-hydroxybutyrate (PHB), a polymer obtained from bacterial sources, has also shown promise in peripheral nerve regeneration as a conduit material and demonstrated good regeneration in comparison with nerve grafts (Hazari *et al.*, 1999b; Young *et al.*, 2002). Transected radial nerves were also wrapped in PHB sheets to promote regeneration (Hazari *et al.*, 1999a). Polymers made of noncrystallizable blocks of poly(glycolide-*co*-(epsilon-caprolactone))-diol and crystallizable blocks of poly((R)-3-hydroxybutyric acid-*co*-(R)-3-hydroxyvaleric acid)-diol were used to fabricate nerve conduits since they have elastomeric properties and their degradation rates can be modulated. These conduits were seen to promote sciatic nerve regeneration in the majority of the cases (Borkenhagen *et al.*, 1998). Polyphosphazenes have also demonstrated success similar to those seen with PLLA and PLC conduits in peripheral nerve regeneration (Aldini *et al.*, 1999; Nicoli Aldini *et al.*, 2000). Poly(phospho esters) have been found to promote peripheral nerve regeneration and have advantages over some other biodegradable polymers due to their lack of swelling and no crystallization after implantation.

However, the mechanical strength of the polymers tested was lacking since tube fragmentation and even breakage was observed less than five days after implantation (Wang et al., 2001).

Enhancement of regeneration was observed following subcutaneous priming of bioresorbable PLGA guides in vivo. Four weeks after nerve reconstruction, regeneration of the peripheral nerve through the cell-infiltrated guides displayed a significant increase in the total axon number and myelination status recorded in primed over unprimed guides, demonstrating the importance of cell-mediated events in the regeneration process. Factors capable of eliciting Schwann-cell migration were identified, providing a rationale for selection and use of exogenous factors for the enhancement of peripheral-nerve regeneration (Bryan et al., 2003).

The ECM protein laminin was covalently coupled to agarose hydrogels and was found to significantly enhance neurite extension from three-dimensionally cultured embryonic chick dorsal root ganglia and PC12 cells (Yu et al., 1999). However, fibronectin was shown to induce greater Schwann cell proliferation than laminin, making it a potentially important component of nerve guidance channels (Chafik et al., 2003). Sciatic nerve regeneration was facilitated by laminin–fibronectin double coated biodegradable collagen grafts in rats (Tong et al., 1994).

1. Localized and Directed Cell Placement and Growth

Several methods have been developed to control positioning and directed growth of cells on biodegradable polymeric substrates. Axonal guidance has also been achieved using diffusible repellants and attractants (Cao and Shoichet, 2001; Tessier-Lavigne, 1994). In order to provide better control of interactions between scaffolds and cells, poly(lactic acid-co-amino acid) graft copolymers with poly(lysine), poly(aspartic acid), and poly(alanine) side chains of varying lengths were synthesized (Harkach et al., 1996). A tubular nerve guidance conduit possessing the macroarchitecture of a polyfascicular peripheral nerve was created. Methods of generating micron-scale patterns of any biotinylated ligand on the surface of a biodegradable polylactide-poly(ethylene glycol) block copolymers were developed. These were used to obtain spatial control over nerve cells (Patel et al., 1998; Shakesheff et al., 1999).

Control of axonal growth was also achieved by forming two-dimensional adherent patterns of collagen. The axons grew along the collagen-adsorbed pathways and completed the honeycomb-like patterning, as designed (Matsuda et al., 1992). Following implantation of any absorbable device there occurs a proliferation of fibrous tissue, which along with material from the degrading implant forms a composite membranous structure called a neomembrane. Neomembranes have been proposed as potential candidates that can be used for guiding tissue regeneration, including nerve regeneration (Ashammakhi, 1996). Tubular nerve guidance conduits possessing the macroarchitecture of a polyfascicular peripheral nerve were created using a dip coating method and preseeded with Schwann cells to enable more robust and more precisely directed nerve regeneration (Hadlock et al., 1998). A biohybrid nerve guide containing fibers or microfilaments of poly(lactic acid) (Ngo et al., 2003) coated with Schwann cells (Steuer et al., 1999) or laminin (Rangappa et al., 2000) were fabricated and shown to greatly improve nerve regeneration.

A magnetically aligned collagen gel filling a collagen nerve guide was found to enhance peripheral-nerve regeneration (Ceballos et al., 1999; Dubey et al., 1996). Collagen conduits, filled with collagen fibers or sheets to provide guided nerve regeneration, were effective in providing a scaffold for regenerating nerve tissue (Itoh et al., 2001). Two types of pore structures in PLLA foams—oriented or interconnected pores, were produced depending on the mechanism of phase separation. Microscopic observations of the cells seeded onto the polymer foams showed that the interconnected pore networks were more favorable to cell attachment than the anisotropic ones. In the oriented pores, abundant cell migration was observed at the outer surface of the polymer implant, but not within the macrotubes (Maquet et al., 2000).

To address this issue of directional growth, micropatterned biodegradable polymer films were fabricated and inserted on the inside of poly(D,L-lactide) (PDLA) conduits. The micropatterned surfaces were preseeded with Schwann cells in order to provide guidance to axons at the cellular level. Over 95% alignment of the axons and Schwann cells was observed on the micropatterned surfaces with laminin selectively attached to the microgrooves (Miller et al., 2002). Acceleration of neurite extension from rat dorsal root ganglia was also observed within micron-scale tubes in the range of 200 to 635 microns. Within these hydrogel-filled conduits, neurites were observed to extend more rapidly than when cultured within the hydrogel alone and a change in tissue architecture was observed with the cabling of cells within the microconduit (Pearson et al., 2003). Various fabrication techniques have been used for these biodegradable polymer conduits as described in the following section.

2. Fabrication Methods

A common method of fabricating porous conduits is to use a combined solvent casting (Luciano et al., 2000; Widmer et al., 1998) and extrusion technique involving salt mixed in with the polymer. The salt is then leached out leaving a conduit with an open ended pore structure. Using this method, PLGA and PLLA conduits were fabricated and the modulus and failure strength of PLLA conduits were approximately 10 times higher than those of PLGA conduits (Widmer et al., 1998).

Tubes of poly-L-lactic acid or polylactic-co-glycolic acid copolymer were formed using a dip-molding technique and were created containing 1, 2, 4, or 5 sublumina, or "fascicular analogs" (Hadlock et al., 1998). Liquid–liquid phase separation of solutions of amorphous PDLA and semicrystalline PLLA in solvent mixtures was used to produce a porous scaffold for cell transplantation. Freeze–drying of phase-separated polylactide solutions was found to produce flexible and tough foams with an isotropic morphology. Interconnected pores of 1–10 microns in diameter resulted from the spinodal decomposition of the polylactide solutions with formation of co-continuous phases (Schugens et al., 1996). A thermally induced polymer–solvent phase separation was used to create PLLA foams with two types of pore structures—oriented or interconnected pores, depending on the mechanism of phase separation, which in turn depends on the thermodynamics of the polymer–solvent pair (Maquet et al., 2000).

Poly(phosphoester) conduits were fabricated by immersing mandrels coated with a solution of the polymer in chloroform into nonsolvent immersion baths, followed by freeze or vacuum–drying (Wan et al., 2001) (Fig. 2). To control micropositioning of neural cells and guidance of extending axons in a given region, a novel surface photoprocessing method was developed. Ultraviolet irradiation with the use of a photomask placed on a substrate hydrophilically modified the irradiated regions. Collagen was adsorbed only on the nonirradiated hydrophobic portions to guide axonal growth (Matsuda et al., 1992). Microcontact printing techniques have also been developed to attach protein selectively to certain regions of the substrate (James and Davis, 2000). A novel transfer patterning method was developed to fabricate biodegradable films with microgrooves with laminin selectively adsorbed to the grooves. A combination of photolithography, reactive ion etching, solvent casting, and surface-tension-based techniques were used to fabricate these films to provide guidance to axons at the cellular level (Miller et al., 2001a,b, 2002) (Fig. 3).

C. COMPARATIVE STUDIES

In order to compare the relative performance of various types of conduit materials, several studies have been conducted as described in this section.

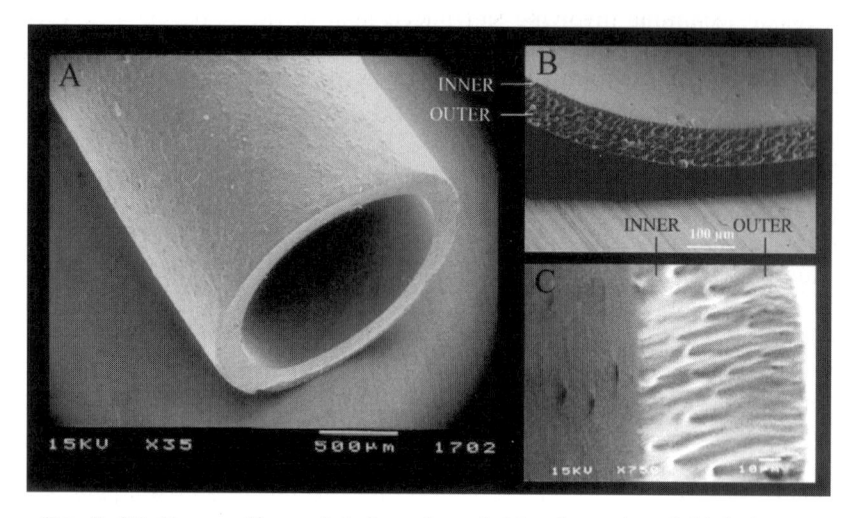

FIG. 2. (A) Nerve guide conduit from the poly(phosphoester), poly(bis(hydroxyethyl) terepthalate-ethyl ortho-phosphate/terephthaloyl chloride) (M_w: 14,900, solution concentration: 34% (w/w), immersion bath: water, drying method: freeze–drying); (B) cross-section of conduit showing distinct coating layers; (C) cross-section of conduit with finger-like cavities. [Reproduced with permission from Wan *et al.* (2001).]

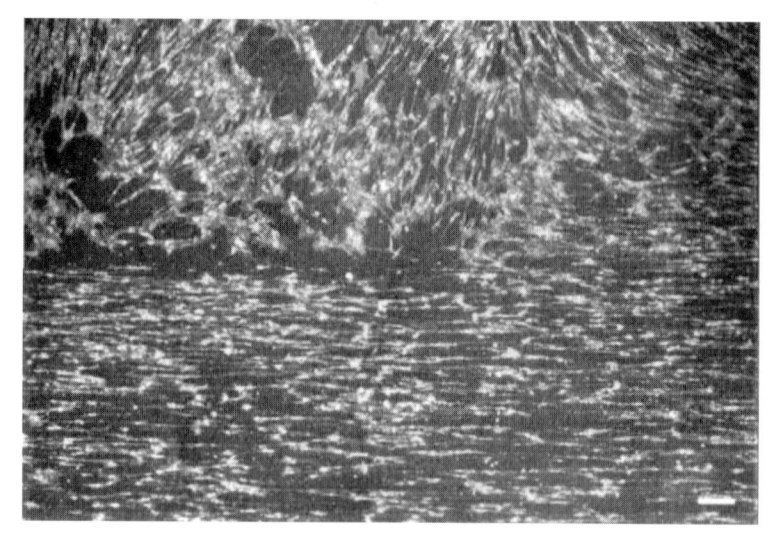

FIG. 3. Half smooth (top) and half 10/20/3 μm patterned laminin coated (200 μg/mL) PDLA solvent-cast substrate with DiI-labeled neurons and Schwann cells showing nonaligned and aligned cells, respectively. Bar = 50 μm. [Reproduced with permission from Miller *et al.* (2001a).]

Silicone tubes prefilled with NGF were compared to autologous nerve grafts in their ability to bridge an 8-mm nerve gap in rabbit facial nerves. The number of regenerating myelinated axons in the autologous nerve grafts at five weeks was significantly greater than the number of myelinated axons in the silicone tubes. But in the nerve grafts, majority of the axons were found in the extrafascicular connective tissue and did not find their way into the distal nerve stump. Thus, functional recovery of autologous nerve graft repairs may not be superior to that of entubulization repairs (Spector *et al.*, 1995).

Comparative studies of biodegradable conduits and silicone conduits have been conducted with various polymers. Peripheral nerve repair using degradable poly(organo)phosphazene tubular conduits was found to be enhanced compared to the regenerated nerve fiber bundle obtained with the silicone conduits (Langone *et al.*, 1995). Recordings of compound muscle action potential (CMAP) after sciatic nerve regeneration was found to be similar with autografts and with PLC tubes but lower with silicone tubes. The number of neurons with multiple projections was also lower in autografts and PLC tubes compared to silicone tubes, thereby indicating that the PLC tubes and superior to silicone tubes for peripheral nerve regeneration (Navarro *et al.*, 1996; Valero-Cabre *et al.*, 2001). However, a study designed to compare regeneration of rat peroneal nerve across a 0.5-cm gap repaired with a sutured autograft versus an artificial nerve graft of PGA filled with collagen showed using electrophysiological analyses that the axonal regeneration was statistically inferior to that in the autograft (Rosen *et al.*, 1989).

Schwann cells incorporated in a collagen matrix and injected into PLLA conduits were found to demonstrate comparable SFI values compared to isograft controls, but showed a statistically lower number of axons for both the high and low density Schwann cells groups and the collagen samples compared to the isograft controls (Evans *et al.*, 2002). These results can be explained by a simple reaction diffusion model (Rutkowski and Heath, 2002b) described earlier.

A comparative study conducted with two different types of conduits, one biological, obtained with homologous glutaraldehyde preserved vein segments and the other synthetic bioabsorbable, made with PLC, were evaluated as guides for nerve repair. Nerve regeneration was effective with both conduits, but the count of myelinated axons showed a significant difference between the synthetic and biological tubes. Synthetic conduits were found to be better than those obtained with preserved vein segments for peripheral nerve reconstruction (Giardino *et al.*, 1995).

Poly(L-lactide-*co*-epsilon-caprolactone) (PLC) nerve guides were found to yield faster and higher levels of nerve innervation compared to conduits made of collagen, silicone, or teflon. Resorbable tubes promoted regeneration in a higher proportion of mice than durable tubes. There was only minimal inflammatory reaction within the remnants of collagen tubes, but not in the other materials (Navarro et al., 1996). PLC nerve guides were found to be superior to autologous nerve grafts in enabling faster as well as qualitatively better nerve regeneration to bridge a 1-cm gap (den Dunnen et al., 1996a,b). In another study, the highest number of regenerated myelinated fibers at mid tube and distal nerve were found in highly permeable PLC guides. Impermeable PLC guides allowed slightly worse levels of regeneration, while low-permeable PLC guides promoted neuroma and limited distal regeneration. The lowest number of regenerated fibers were found in permanent polysulfone tubes (Rodriguez et al., 1999). Therefore, resorbable permeable polymeric nerve guides with chemical cues seem to show the best potential for peripheral nerve regeneration.

III. Polymers for Regeneration in the Central Nervous Systems

In addition to the use of polymeric conduits for peripheral nerve regeneration, polymers, specifically hydrogels, have been used extensively to help rectify central nervous system disorders and promote regeneration. Oriented growth has been achieved not just in the peripheral nervous system, but also in the central nervous system using silicone tubes. Electrically mediated guidance of axonal growth has also been achieved using silicone tubes containing a cathodal electrode (Fig. 4). A robust regeneration of spinal cord axons into the tube was observed in more than half the cases with the imposed electric field, while there were rarely any axons found in the control guidance channels (Borgens, 1999).

Nitrocellulose implants treated with biological materials were introduced into neonatal rat spinal cords before the arrival of corticospinal tract (CST) axons. Implants with living cells from spinal cord primary cultures and acellular implants coated with laminin supported the adhesion and growth of CST axons. This suggests that laminin or some other adhesive factor produced by immature neuroglial cells may be normally involved in CST axon growth and guidance (Schreyer and Jones, 1987). Nerve growth factor (NGF)-treated nitrocellulose implants were used to promote growth across a complete transection lesion of a rat spinal cord and were found to be significantly better than the nontreated implants at promoting regrowth (Houle and Ziegler, 1994).

Solid fetal spinal cord tissue seeded into semipermeable mini guidance channels and implanted into a lesion site in the rat adult spinal cord

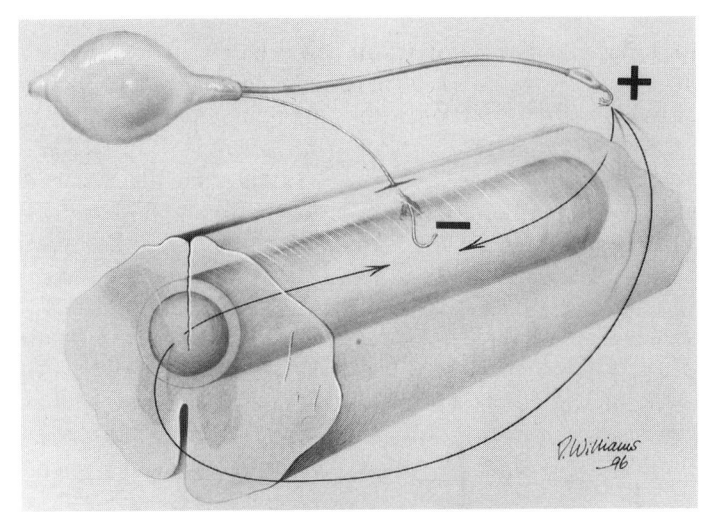

FIG. 4. Artist's drawing of the stimulator, silicone rubber tube or guidance channel, and the electrical circuit within the spinal cord. The tube was implanted into the dorsal spinal cord. The uninsulated tip of the cathodal electrode (negative) was sealed within the center of the tube, while the anodal electrode (positive) remained outside the vertebral column, sutured to paravertebral musculature. The body of the stimulator was surgically placed within the fat pad at the base of the guinea-pig's neck. To complete a circuit, current must flow initially into each end of the hollow tube as diagrammed. For diagrammatic purposes, the drawing is not made to scale. [Reproduced with permission from Borgens (1999).]

was found to serve as a permissive bridge for longitudinally directed axonal growth (Bamber *et al.*, 1999). Instead of autografts, a dual scaffold structure made of biodegradable polymers and seeded with neural stem cells was developed to address the issues of spinal cord injury. Unique biodegradable polymer scaffolds were fabricated where the general design of the scaffold was derived from the structure of the spinal cord with an outer section that mimics the white matter with long axial pores to provide axonal guidance and an inner section seeded with neural stem cells for cell replacement and mimic the general character of the gray matter (Lavik *et al.*, 2001). The seeded scaffold led to improved functional recovery as compared with the lesion control or cells alone following spinal cord injury. Implantation of the scaffold-neural stem cells unit into an adult rat hemisection model of spinal cord injury promoted long-term improvement in function (persistent for one year in some animals) relative to a lesion-control group (Teng *et al.*, 2002) (Fig. 5).

Poly(alpha-hydroxy acids) with seeded Schwann cells or Schwann cell grafts were also found to be effective candidates for spinal cord

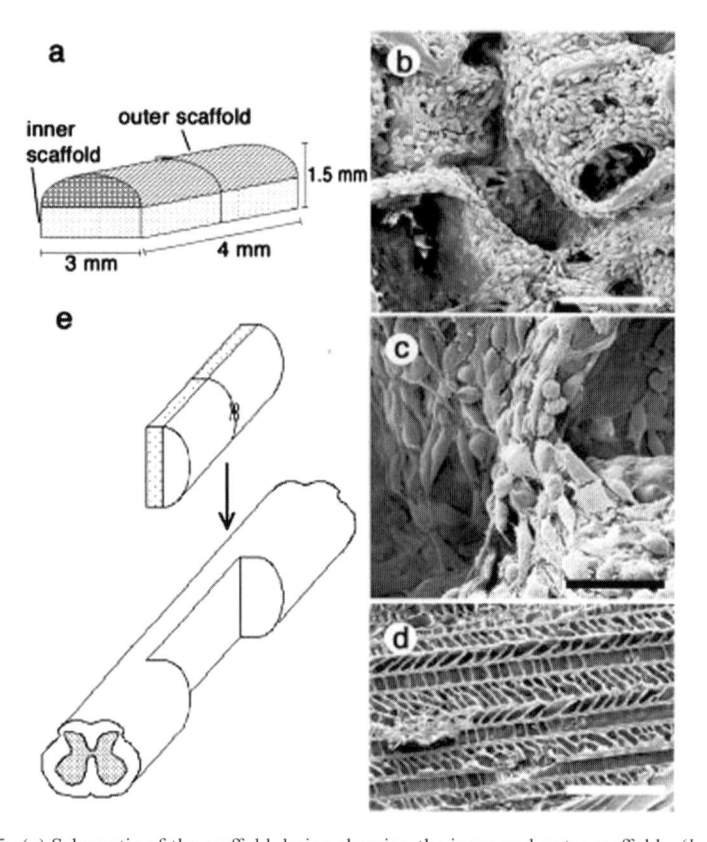

Fig. 5. (*a*) Schematic of the scaffold design showing the inner and outer scaffolds. (*b* and *c*) Inner scaffolds seeded with NSCs. (Scale bars: 200 µm and 50 µm, respectively.) The outer section of the scaffold was created by means of a solid–liquid phase separation technique that produced long, axially oriented pores for axonal guidance as well as radial pores to allow fluid transport and inhibit the ingrowth of scar tissue (*d*; scale bar, 100 µm). (*e*) Schematic of surgical insertion of the implant into the spinal cord. [Reproduced with permission from Teng *et al.* (2002).]

regeneration (Gautier *et al.*, 1998; Oudega *et al.*, 2001). PDLLA mixed with poly(ethylene oxide)-block-poly(D,L-lactide) (PELA) copolymers were made into foams by freeze drying and the ability of these foams to be integrated and to promote tissue repair and axonal regeneration in transected rat spinal cords was investigated. The polymer construct was able to bridge the cord stumps by forming a permissive support for cellular migration, angiogenesis, and axonal regrowth (Maquet *et al.*, 2001). Unsintered hydroxyapatite/poly-L-lactide (u-HA/PLLA) composite films were found to have good biocompatibility, osteoconductivity, and a fast primary degradation rate, with potential application to spinal surgery (Matsumoto et al., 2002).

Synthetic hydrogels have been used to serve as artificial matrices for neural tissue reconstruction, for the delivery of cells and for the promotion of axonal regeneration required for successful neurotransplantation. Cultured neurons were found to attach to hydrogel substrates prepared from poly(2-hydroxyethylmethacrylate) (PHEMA) but grow few nerve fibers unless fibronectin, collagen, or nerve growth factor was incorporated into the hydrogel. This provides a mechanism to provide controlled growth on hydrogel surfaces (Carbonetto et al., 1982). Ionic poly(glyceryl methacrylate) p(GMA)–collagen hydrogels containing polar chemical groups, either basic amino groups or acidic carboxyl groups, were evaluated after long-term implantation in the cerebral cortex. This approach was found to be a new avenue to modulate the brain scar formation (Woerly et al., 1992). Hydrogels have been created with bioactive characteristics for neural cell adhesion and growth (Woerly, 1993). Arg–Gly–Asp peptides (RGD) were synthesized and chemically coupled to the bulk of poly(N-(2-hydroxypropyl) methacrylamide) (PHPMA) based polymer hydrogels. These RGD-grafted polymers implanted into the striata of rat brains promoted and supported the growth and spread of glial tissue onto and into the hydrogels (Woerly et al., 1995). Cultured Schwann cells, neonatal astrocytes or cells dissociated from embryonic cerebral hemispheres were also dispersed within PHPMA hydrogel matrices and found to promote cellular ingrowth *in vivo* (Woerly et al., 1996). These polymer hydrogel matrices were found to have neuroinductive and neuroconductive properties and the potential to repair tissue defects in the central nervous system by promoting the formation of a tissue matrix and axonal growth by replacing the lost of tissue (Woerly et al., 1998, 1999, 2001a,b). Biocompatible porous PHMPA hydrogels (NeuroGels) were used to provide a permissive environment across a 3-mm gap in cat spinal cord to promote regeneration. Results indicated that functional deficit, as assessed by treadmill training, and morphological changes following double transection of the spinal cord can be modified by the implantation of NeuroGel. Most of the regenerating axons were found to be myelinated and were found to have grown at least 12-mm into the dorsal cord tissue 15 months after surgery (Woerly et al., 2001a,c).

The mechanical properties of the substrate were found to have a significant influence on neurite behavior. Neurons grown on softer substrates formed more than three times as many branches as those grown on stiffer gels (Flanagan et al., 2002). PHEMA hydrogels, coated with collagen and infiltrated *in vitro* with cultured Schwann cells, were implanted into lesioned optic tracts to act as prosthetic bridges to promote axonal regeneration (Lesny et al., 2002; Plant et al., 1995, 1998). Collagen impregnated PHEMA sponges were found to provide a safe supportive material for regenerating spinal cord axons (Giannetti et al., 2001). Hydrogel tubes of poly(2-hydroxyethyl methacrylate-*co*-methyl methacrylate) (p(HEMA-*co*-MMA)) were investigated as potential nerve guidance channels in the central nervous system since their mechanical properties were similar to those of the spinal cord, where they were implanted (Dalton et al., 2002). Hydrogel tubes of (p(HEMA-*co*-MMA)) were made by liquid–liquid centrifugal casting to yield tubes that were soft and flexible, consisting of a gel-like outer layer, and an interconnected macroporous, inner layer, and with mechanical properties similar to that of spinal cord (Dalton et al., 2002). Photochemical methods were developed to bind NGF to microporous PHEMA hydrogels to build stable concentration gradients and control cell growth (Kapur and Shoichet, 2003).

Poly-3-hydroxybutyrate (PHB) fibers coated with alginate gels and fibronectin were implanted into lesion cavities after cervical spinal cord injury in rats. Implantation of the PHB graft reduced cell loss by 50%, a rescuing effect similar to that obtained after treatment with brain-derived neurotrophic factor or neurotrophin-3 (NT-3). In the absence of PHB support, implants of only alginate hydrogel or fibronectin, or their combination had no effect on neuronal survival. After addition of neonatal Schwann cells to the PHB graft, regenerating axons were seen to enter the graft from both ends and to extend along its entire length (Mosahebi et al., 2003; Novikov et al., 2002).

Even though early success has been demonstrated with the use of polymers for peripheral and central nerve regeneration, it can be enhanced further by providing site-specific release of growth factors and other chemical cues to the regenerating axons, as described in the next section.

IV. Polymers for Controlled Release

Growth factor administration may also be a useful treatment for neurodegenerative diseases, such as Alzheimer's disease or Parkinson's disease, which are characterized by the degeneration of neuronal cell populations. It was found that the NGF promoted nerve regeneration within conduits at an early stage, but the effect did not last after one month. This was attributed to the rapid decline in NGF concentrations in the conduit due to degradation in aqueous media and leakage from the conduit (Hollowell et al., 1990). This limitation can be overcome by providing controlled release of NGF. Controlled-release polymer delivery systems may be an important technology in enabling the prevention of neuronal degeneration, or even the stimulation of neuronal regeneration, by providing a sustained release of growth factors to promote the long-term survival of endogenous or transplanted cells (Haller and Saltzman, 1998).

Basic fibroblast growth factor (b-FGF), for instance, has been shown to enhance the *in vitro* survival and neurite extension of various types of neurons including dorsal root ganglia. One of the earliest studies involved controlled release of b-FGF and Alpha 1-glycoprotein (alpha 1-GP) from synthetic nerve guidance channels. After an initial burst, linear release was obtained from the conduits for a period of at least two weeks and four weeks postimplantation. The dip molding technique was used to fabricate tubes containing b-FGF, bovine serum albumin (BSA), alpha 1-GP, etc., for controlled release. Only the tubes releasing b-FGF or b-FGF and alpha 1-GP displayed regenerated cables bridging both nerve stumps, which contained nerve fascicles with myelinated and unmyelinated axons (Aebischer et al., 1989).

Polymeric implants providing controlled release of nerve growth factor (NGF) for one month were developed and found to improve neurite extension in cultured PC12 cells (Powell et al., 1990). Neurotrophic factors such as glial cell line-derived neurotrophic factor (GDNF) and neurotrophin-3 (NT-3) were released from synthetic guidance channels for facial nerve regeneration. Nerve cables regenerated in the presence of GDNF showed a large number of myelinated axons while no regenerated axons were observed in the absence of growth factors, demonstrating that GDNF, as previously described for the sciatic nerve, a mixed sensory and motor nerve, is also very efficient in promoting regeneration of the facial nerve, an essentially pure motor nerve (Barras et al., 2002). Inosine, a purine analog that promotes axonal extension, was loaded into PLGA conduits for controlled release during sciatic nerve regeneration. Inosine loaded PLGA foams were fashioned into cylindrical nerve guidance channels using a novel low pressure injection molding technique. After 10 weeks, a higher percentage cross sectional area composed of neural tissue was found in the inosine-loaded conduits compared with controls (Hadlock et al., 1999). Biodegradable polymer foams for controlled release and to provide a permissive environment for spinal cord regeneration were formed by freeze–drying (Maquet et al., 2001).

To provide for prolonged, site-specific delivery of NGF to the tissue in a convenient manner without affecting the properties of the conduit, biodegradable polymer microspheres of poly(L-lactide)*co*-glycolide containing NGF were fabricated. Biologically active NGF was released from the microspheres, as assayed by neurite outgrowth in a dorsal root ganglion tissue culture system (Camarata et al., 1992; Pean et al., 1998, 1999) NGF co-encapsulated in PLGA microspheres along with ovalbumin was found to be bioactive for over 90 days (Cao and Schoichet, 1999). NGF release from biodegradable poly(phosphoester) microspheres produced using a double emulsion technique exhibited a lower burst effect but similar protein entrapment levels and efficiencies when compared with those made of PLGA (Xu et al., 2002). These NGF-loaded poly(phosphoester) microspheres were successfully implanted to bridge a 10-mm gap in a rat sciatic nerve model (Xu et al., 2003).

Biodegradable polymeric microspheres for controlled delivery of growth factors are commonly produced using the water-in-oil-in-water emulsion method. The use of sodium chloride in the dispersing phase of the double emulsion markedly reduced the burst effect from PLGA microspheres loaded with NGF by making the microparticle morphology more compact. Unfortunately, it was found to induce pronounced NGF denaturation (Pean et al., 1998). Co-encapsulation of PEG 400 improved the stability of NGF and allowed a continuous release from PLGA microspheres produced using a double emulsion method because the PEG reduced contact of NGF with the organic phase (Pean et al., 1999).

A pharmacotectonics concept was illustrated by researchers, in which drug-delivery systems were arranged spatially in tissues to shape concentration fields for potent agents. NGF-releasing implants placed within 1–2 mm of the treatment site enhanced the biological function of cellular targets, whereas identical implants placed ~3 mm from the target site of treatment produced no beneficial effect (Mahoney and Saltzman, 1999). Because of some limitations with controlled delivery systems, alternatives such as encapsulation of cells that secrete these factors are discussed in the next section.

V. Cell Encapsulation

A significant use of polymers has been to encapsulate cells that secrete growth and neurotrophic factors and implant them as a treatment for neurodegenerative disorders and to promote nerve regeneration. For instance, neural transplantation as an experimental therapy for Parkinsonian patients has been shown to be effective in several clinical trials. However, grafting combined with a treatment of neurotrophic factors improves the survival and growth of grafted embryonic dopaminergic neurons.

Continuous trophic support may be needed requiring long-term delivery of neurotrophic factors to the brain (Sautter *et al.*, 1998). A number of proteins have specific neuroprotective activities *in vitro*; however, the local delivery of these factors into the central nervous system over the long term at therapeutic levels has been difficult to achieve. Direct administration at the target site is a logical alternative, particularly in the central nervous system, but the limits of direct administration have not been defined clearly. For instance NGF must be delivered within several millimeters of the target to be effective in treating Alzheimer's disease (Mahoney and Saltzman, 1999). Cells engineered to express the neuroprotective proteins, encapsulated in immunoisolation polymeric devices and implanted at the site of lesions have the potential to alter the progression of neurodegenerative disorders. The polymers used for encapsulation should allow transport of nutrients and oxygen to the cells, but also afford immunoprotection. Long-term cell viability *in vivo* in these constructs due to diffusional limitations has been the major drawback of this approach.

An expression vector containing the human nerve growth factor gene (hNGF) was transfected into a baby hamster fibroblast cell line (BHK). Using an immunoisolatory polymeric device, encapsulated BHK-control cells and those secreting hNGF (BHK–hNGF) were transplanted unilaterally into rat lateral ventricles. Human nerve growth factor gene (hNGF) was found to be released by the encapsulated BHK-hNGF cells for over a year (Winn *et al.*, 1996) suggesting that implantation of polymer-encapsulated hNGF-releasing cells can be used to protect neurons from excitotoxin damage (Emerich *et al.*, 1994a,b). In the lesioned rat brain, chronic delivery of human nerve growth factor by the encapsulated BHK cells provided nearly complete protection of axotomized medial septal cholinergic neurons for up to six months *in vivo* and long-term encapsulated cell survival was confirmed by histologic analysis (Winn *et al.*, 1994). Encapsulated hNGF-secreting BHK cells were also found to promote the functional recovery of hemi-Parkinsonian rats (Date *et al.*, 1996a,b). Instead of fibroblasts, a Schwannoma cell line derived from a transgenic mouse, was transfected with a human NGF cDNA and encapsulated in a polymer capsule. The hNGF transgene was expressed for at least three weeks after implantation and the cells did not overgrow the capsule (Schinstine *et al.*, 1995). Transplantation of polymer-encapsulated cells genetically engineered to release nerve growth factor was found to allow a normal functional development of the visual cortex in dark-reared rats (Pizzorusso *et al.*, 1997).

Ciliary neurotrophic factor (CNTF) decreases naturally occurring and axotomy-induced cell death and has been evaluated as a treatment for neurodegenerative disorders such as amyotrophic lateral sclerosis (ALS) and Huntington's disease (Emerich et al., 1997). Effective administration of this protein to motoneurons has been hampered by the exceedingly short half-life of CNTF, and the inability to deliver effective concentration into the central nervous system after systemic administration in vivo. BHK cells stably transfected with a plasmid construct containing the gene for human or mouse CNTF were encapsulated in polymer fibers and found to continuously release CNTF and slow down motoneuron degeneration following axotomy (Tan et al., 1996). Implantation of polymer-encapsulated cells genetically engineered to continuously secrete glial cell line-derived neurotrophic factor to the adult rat striatum was found to improve dopaminergic graft survival and function (Sautter et al., 1998). Therefore cell encapsulation is a potentially important method in nerve regeneration, and can be used alone or in conjunction with other methods such as entubulization.

VI. Conclusions

Polymeric materials have great potential in facilitating nerve regeneration. The use of polymeric conduits in facilitating peripheral nerve regeneration has been demonstrated successfully and polymers have shown great promise in addressing spinal cord injuries as well. This regeneration process with various polymers, both degradable as well as nondegradable, has been enhanced further by promoting directed growth and by the addition of chemical cues such as laminin, nerve growth factors and other agents incorporated in the conduits to be released in a controlled fashion. Polymers also play an important role in encapsulating cells that release factors to promote nerve regeneration.

ACKNOWLEDGMENTS

The authors would like to acknowledge funding from the National Science Foundation (BES 9983735).

REFERENCES

Aebischer, P., Guenard, V., Winn, S. R., Valentini, R. F., and Galletti, P. M. *Brain Res.* **454**, 179 (1988).
Aebischer, P., Salessiotis, A. N., and Winn, S. R. *J. Neurosci. Res.* **23**, 282 (1989).

Aldini, N. N., Fini, M., Rocca, M., Giavaresi, G., Guzzardella, G. A., Di Denia, P., Caligiuri, G., and Giardino, R. *Acta Biomed. Ateneo. Parmense.* **70,** 49 (1999).
Ashammakhi, N. A. *J. Biomed. Mater. Res.* **33,** 297 (1996).
Bamber, N. I., Li, H., Aebischer, P., and Xu, X. M. *Neural. Plast.* **6,** 103 (1999).
Barras, F. M., Pasche, P., Bouche, N., Aebischer, P., and Zurn, A. D. *J. Neurosci. Res.* **70,** 746 (2002).
Bellamkonda, R., and Aebischer, P. *Biotechnol. Bioeng.* **43,** 543 (1994).
Borgens, R. B. *Neuroscience* **91,** 251 (1999).
Borkenhagen, M., Stoll, R. C., Neuenschwander, P., Suter, U. W., and Aebischer, P. *Biomaterials* **19,** 2155 (1998).
Bryan, D. J., Holway, A. H., Wang, K. K., Silva, A. E., Trantolo, D. J., Wise, D., and Summerhayes, I. C. *Tissue Eng.* **6,** 129 (2000).
Bryan, D. J., Tang, J. B., Holway, A. H., Rieger-Christ, K. M., Trantolo, D. J., Wise, D. L., and Summerhayes, I. C. *J. Reconstr. Microsurg.* **19,** 125 (2003).
Buettner, H. M., in "Nanofabrication and Biosystems: Integrating Materials Science, Engineering and Biology" (H. C. Hoch, L. W. Jelinski, and H. G. Craighead, Eds.), p. 300. Cambridge University Press, Cambridge, UK (1996).
Camarata, P. J., Suryanarayanan, R., Turner, D. A., Parker, R. G., and Ebner, T. J. *Neurosurgery* **30,** 313 (1992).
Cao, X., and Shoichet, M. S. *Biomaterials* **20,** 329 (1999).
Cao, X., and Shoichet, M. S. *Neuroscience* **103,** 831 (2001).
Carbonetto, S. T., Gruver, M. M., and Turner, D. C. *Science* **216,** 897 (1982).
Ceballos, D., Navarro, X., Dubey, N., Wendelschafercrabb, G., Kennedy, W. R., and Tranquillo, R. T. *Exp. Neurol.* **158,** 290 (1999).
Chafik, D., Bear, D., Bui, P., Patel, A., Jones, N. F., Kim, B. T., Hung, C. T., and Gupta, R. *Tissue Eng.* **9,** 233 (2003).
Chen, Y. S. *J. Formos. Med. Assoc.* **91** Suppl 3, S246 (1992).
Chen, Y. S., Hsieh, C. L., Tsai, C. C., Chen, T. H., Cheng, W. C., Hu, C. L., and Yao, C. H. *Biomaterials* **21,** 1541 (2000).
Chen, Y. S., Wang-Bennett, L. T., and Coker, N. J. *Exp. Neurol.* **103,** 52 (1989).
Clark, P., in "Nanofabrication and Biosystems: Integrating Materials Science, Engineering and Biology" (H. C. Hoch, L. W. Jelinski, and H. G. Craighead, Eds.), p. 357. Cambridge University Press, Cambridge, UK (1996).
Dalton, P. D., Flynn, L., and Shoichet, M. S. *Biomaterials* **23,** 3843 (2002).
Danielsen, N., Pettmann, B., Vahlsing, H. L., Manthorpe, M., and Varon, S. *J. Neurosci. Res.* **20,** 320 (1988a).
Danielsen, N., Vahlsing, H. L., Manthorpe, M., and Varon, S. *Exp Neurol.* **99,** 622 (1988b).
Da-Silva, C. F., and Langone, F. *Braz. J. Med. Biol. Res.* **22,** 691 (1989).
Date, I., Ohmoto, T., Imaoka, T., Ono, T., Hammang, J. P., Francis, J., Greco, C., and Emerich, D. F. *J. Neurosurg.* **84,** 1006 (1996a).
Date, I., Ohmoto, T., Imaoka, T., Shingo, T., and Emerich, D. F. *Neuroreport* **7,** 1813 (1996b).
de Medinaceli, L., al Khoury, R., and Merle, M. *J. Reconstr. Microsurg.* **11,** 43 (1995).
den Dunnen, W. F., van der Lei, B., Schakenraad, J. M., Blaauw, E. H., Stokroos, I., Pennings, A. J., and Robinson, P. H. *Microsurgery* **14,** 508 (1993).
den Dunnen, W. F., van der Lei, B., Robinson, P. H., Holwerda, A., Pennings, A. J., and Schakenraad, J. M. *J. Biomed. Mater. Res.* **29,** 757 (1995).
den Dunnen, W. F., van der Lei, B., Schakenraad, J. M., Stokroos, I., Blaauw, E., Bartels, H., Pennings, A. J., and Robinson, P. H. *Microsurgery* **17,** 348 (1996a).
den Dunnen, W. F., Stokroos, I., Blaauw, E. H., Holwerda, A., Pennings, A. J., Robinson, P. H., and Schakenraad, J. M. *J. Biomed. Mater. Res.* **31,** 105 (1996b).

den Dunnen, W. F., Meek, M. F., Grijpma, D. W., Robinson, P. H., and Schakenraad, J. M. *J. Biomed. Mater. Res.* **51,** 575 (2000).
Dubey, N., Letourneau, P., and Tranquillo, R. *FASEB J.* **10,** 2233 (1996).
Dubovy, P., and Bednarova, J. *Acta Histochem.* **98,** 123 (1996).
Emerich, D. F., Hammang, J. P., Baetge, E. E., and Winn, S. R. *Exp. Neurol.* **130,** 141 (1994a).
Emerich, D. F., Winn, S. R., Harper, J., Hammang, J. P., Baetge, E. E., and Kordower, J. H. *J. Comp. Neurol.* **349,** 148 (1994b).
Emerich, D. F., Winn, S. R., Hantraye, P. M., Peschanski, M., Chen, E. Y., Chu, Y., McDermott, P., Baetge, E. E., and Kordower, J. H. *Nature* **386,** 395 (1997).
Evans, G. R., Brandt, K., Katz, S., Chauvin, P., Otto, L., Bogle, M., Wang, B., Meszlenyi, R. K., Lu, L., Mikos, A. G., and Patrick, C. W., Jr. *Biomaterials* **23,** 841 (2002).
Evans, G. R., Brandt, K., Niederbichler, A. D., Chauvin, P., Herrman, S., Bogle, M., Otta, L., Wang, B., and Patrick, C. W., Jr. *J. Biomater. Sci. Polym. Ed.* **11,** 869 (2000).
Evans, G. R., Brandt, K., Widmer, M. S., Lu, L., Meszlenyi, R. K., Gupta, P. K., Mikos, A. G., Hodges, J., Williams, J., Gurlek, A., Nabawi, A., Lohman, R., and Patrick, C. W., Jr. *Biomaterials* **20,** 1109 (1999).
Flanagan, L. A., Ju, Y. E., Marg, B., Osterfield, M., and Janmey, P. A. *Neuroreport* **13,** 2411 (2002).
Gautier, S. E., Oudega, M., Fragoso, M., Chapon, P., Plant, G. W., Bunge, M. B., and Parel, J. M. *J. Biomed. Mater. Res.* **42,** 642 (1998).
Giannetti, S., Lauretti, L., Fernandez, E., Salvinelli, F., Tamburrini, G., and Pallini, R. *Neurol. Res.* **23,** 405 (2001).
Giardino, R., Nicoli Aldini, N., Perego, G., Cella, G., Maltarello, M. C., Fini, M., Rocca, M., and Giavaresi, G. *Int. J. Artif. Organs* **18,** 225 (1995).
Hadlock, T., Elisseeff, J., Langer, R., Vacanti, J., and Cheney, M. *Arch. Otolaryngol. Head Neck Surg.* **124,** 1081 (1998).
Hadlock, T., Sundback, C., Koka, R., Hunter, D., Cheney, M., and Vacanti, J. *Laryngoscope* **109,** 1412 (1999).
Haller, M. F., and Saltzman, W. M. *J. Control Rel.* **53,** 1 (1998).
Harkach, J. S., Schmidt, C., and Langer, R., *Book of Abstracts, 211th ACS National Meeting, New Orleans, LA, March 24–28.* BIOT (1996).
Hazari, A., Johansson-Ruden, G., Junemo-Bostrom, K., Ljungberg, C., Terenghi, G., Green, C., and Wiberg, M. *J. Hand. Surg. [Br]* **24,** 291 (1999a).
Hazari, A., Wiberg, M., Johansson-Ruden, G., Green, C., and Terenghi, G. *Br. J. Plast. Surg.* **52,** 653 (1999b).
Heath, C. A., and Rutkowski, G. E. *Trends in Biotechnology* **16**(4), 163–168 (1998).
Henry, E. W., Chiu, T. H., Nyilas, E., Brushart, T. M., Dikkes, P., and Sidman, R. L. *Exp. Neurol.* **90,** 652 (1985).
Hollowell, J. P., Villadiego, A., and Rich, K. M. *Exp. Neurol.* **110,** 45 (1990).
Hoppen, H. J., Leenslag, J. W., Pennings, A. J., van der Lei, B., and Robinson, P. H. *Biomaterials* **11,** 286 (1990).
Houle, J. D., and Ziegler, M. K. *J. Neural. Transplant. Plast.* **5,** 115 (1994).
Ide, C., Tohyama, K., Yokota, R., Nitatori, T., and Onodera, S. *Brain Res.* **288,** 61 (1983).
Itoh, S., Takakuda, K., Ichinose, S., Kikuchi, M., and Schinomiya, K. *J. Reconstr. Microsurg.* **17,** 115 (2001).
James, C. D., and Davis, R. *IEEE Trans. Biomed. Eng.* **47,** 17 (2000).
Kapur, T. A., and Shoichet, M. S. *J. Biomater. Sci. Polym. Ed.* **14,** 383 (2003).
Keeley, R. T., Atagi, T., Sabelman, E., Padilla, J., Kadlcik, S., Keeley, A., Nguyen, K., and Rosen, J. *J. Reconstruc. Microsurg.* **9,** 349 (1993).

Langone, F., Lora, S., Veronese, F. M., Caliceti, P., Parnigotto, P. P., Valenti, F., and Palma, G. *Biomaterials* **16**, 347 (1995).
Lavik, E., Teng, Y. D., Zurakowski, D., Qu, X., Snyder, E., and Langer, R. *Materials Research Society Symposium Proceedings* **662**, OO1.2/1 (2001).
Lemmon, V., et al. *J. Neurosci.* **12**, 818–826 (1992).
Lesny, P., De Croos, J., Pradny, M., Vacik, J., Michalek, J., Woerly, S., and Sykova, E. *J. Chem. Neuroanat.* **23**, 243 (2002).
Liu, H. M. *J. Peripher. Nerv. Syst.* **1**, 97 (1996).
Luciano, R. M., de Carvalho Zavaglia, C. A., and de Rezende Duek, E. A. *Artif. Organs* **24**, 206 (2000).
Lundborg, G., Dahlin, L. B., Danielsen, N., Gelberman, R. H., Longo, F. M., Powell, H. C., and Varon, S. *Exp. Neurol.* **76**, 361 (1982a).
Lundborg, G., Gelberman, R. H., Longo, F. M., Powell, H. C., and Varon, S. *J. Neuropathol. Exp. Neurol.* **41**, 412 (1982b).
Lundborg, G., Longo, F. M., and Varon, S. *Brain Res.* **232**, 157 (1982c).
Lundborg, G., Rosen, B., Dahlin, L., Danielsen, N., and Holmberg, J. *J. Hand. Surg. [Am]* **22**, 99 (1997).
Luo, Z. J., and Lu, S. B. *J. Hand. Surg. [Br]* **21**, 660 (1996).
Madison, R., Sidman, R. L., Nyilas, E., Chiu, T. H., and Greatorex, D. *Exp. Neurol.* **86**, 448 (1984).
Madison, R. D., da Silva, C. F., Dikkes, P., Chiu, T. H., and Sidman, R. L. *Exp. Neurol.* **88**, 767 (1985).
Madison, R. D., da Silva, C., Dikkes, P., Sidman, R. L., and Chiu, T. H. *Exp. Neurol.* **95**, 378 (1987).
Mahoney, M. J., and Saltzman, W. M. *Proc. Natl. Acad. Sci. USA* **96**, 4536 (1999).
Maquet, V., Martin, D., Malgrange, B., Franzen, R., Schoenen, J., Moonen, G., and Jerome, R. *J. Biomed. Mater. Res.* **52**, 639 (2000).
Maquet, V., Martin, D., Scholtes, F., Franzen, R., Schoenen, J., Moonen, G., and Jerome, R. *Biomaterials* **22**, 1137 (2001).
Matsuda, T., Sugawara, T., and Inoue, K. *Asaio J.* **38**, M243 (1992).
Matsumoto, M., Chosa, E., Nabeshima, K., Shikinami, Y., and Tajima, N. *J. Biomed. Mater. Res.* **60**, 101 (2002).
Meek, M. F., den Dunnen, W. F., Schakenraad, J. M., and Robinson, P. H. *Microsurgery* **17**, 555 (1996).
Meek, M. F., den Dunnen, W. F., Robinson, P. H., Pennings, A. J., and Schakenraad, J. M. *Int. J. Artif. Organs* **20**, 463 (1997).
Meek, M. F., den Dunnen, W. F., Schakenraad, J. M., and Robinson, P. H. *Microsurgery* **19**, 247 (1999).
Meek, M. F., Robinson, P. H., Stokroos, I., Blaauw, E. H., Kors, G., and den Dunnen, W. F. *Biomaterials* **22**, 1177 (2001).
Miller, C. A., Jeftinija, S., and Mallapragada, S. K. *Tissue Eng.* **7**, 705 (2001a).
Miller, C. A., Rutkowski, G., Shanks, H., Witt, A., and Mallapragada, S. K. *Biomaterials* **22**, 1263 (2001b).
Miller, C., Jeftinija, S. K., and Mallapragada, S. K. *Tissue Eng.* **8**, 367 (2002).
Molander, H., Olsson, Y., Engkvist, O., Bowald, S., and Eriksson, I. *Muscle Nerve* **5**, 54 (1982).
Mosahebi, A., Wiberg, M., and Terenghi, G. *Tissue Eng.* **9**, 209 (2003).
Navarro, X., Rodriguez, F. J., Labrador, R. O., Buti, M., Ceballos, D., Gomez, N., Cuadras, J., and Perego, G. *J. Peripher. Nerv. Syst.* **1**, 53 (1996).
Ngo, T. T., Waggoner, P. J., Romero, A. A., Nelson, K. D., Eberhart, R. C., and Smith, G. M. *J. Neurosci. Res.* **72**, 227 (2003).

Nicoli Aldini, N., Perego, G., Cella, G. D., Maltarello, M. C., Fini, M., Rocca, M., and Giardino, R. *Biomaterials* **17,** 959 (1996).
Nicoli Aldini, N., Fini, M., Rocca, M., Giavaresi, G., and Giardino, R. *Int. Orthop.* **24,** 121 (2000).
Novikov, L. N., Novikova, L. N., Mosahebi, A., Wiberg, M., Terenghi, G., and Kellerth, J. O. *Biomaterials* **23,** 3369 (2002).
Nyilas, E., Chiu, T. H., Sidman, R. L., Henry, E. W., Brushart, T. M., Dikkes, P., and Madison, R. *Trans. Am. Soc. Artif. Intern. Organs* **29,** 307 (1983).
Oudega, M., Gautier, S. E., Chapon, P., Fragoso, M., Bates, M. L., Parel, J. M., and Bunge, M. B. *Biomaterials* **22,** 1125 (2001).
Patel, N., Padera, R., Sanders, G. H. W., Cannizzaro, S. M., Davies, M. C., Langer, R., Roberts, C. J., Tendler, S. J. B., Williams, P. M., and Shakesheff, K. M. *FASEB J.* **12,** 1447 (1998).
Pean, J. M., Boury, F., Venier-Julienne, M. C., Menei, P., Proust, J. E., and Benoit, J. P. *Pharm Res.* **16,** 1294 (1999).
Pean, J. M., Venier-Julienne, M. C., Boury, F., Menei, P., Denizot, B., and Benoit, J. P. *J. Control. Rel.* **56,** 175 (1998).
Pearson, R. G., Molino, Y., Williams, P. M., Tendler, S. J., Davies, M. C., Roberts, C. J., and Shakesheff, K. M. *Tissue Eng.* **9,** 201 (2003).
Perego, G., Cella, G. D., Aldini, N. N., Fini, M., and Giardino, R. *Biomaterials* **15,** 189 (1994).
Pizzorusso, T., Porciatti, V., Tseng, J. L., Aebischer, P., and Maffei, L. *Neuroscience* **80,** 307 (1997).
Plant, G. W., Chirila, T. V., and Harvey, A. R. *Cell Transplant.* **7,** 381 (1998).
Plant, G. W., Harvey, A. R., and Chirila, T. V. *Brain Res.* **671,** 119 (1995).
Powell, E. M., Sobarzo, M. R., and Saltzman, W. M. *Brain Res.* **515,** 309 (1990).
Rangappa, N., Romero, A., Nelson, K. D., Eberhart, R. C., and Smith, G. M. *J. Biomed. Mater. Res.* **51,** 625 (2000).
Rich, K. M., Alexander, T. D., Pryor, J. C., and Hollowell, J. P. *Exp. Neurol.* **105,** 162 (1989).
Rodriguez, F. J., Gomez, N., Perego, G., and Navarro, X. *Biomaterials* **20,** 1489 (1999).
Rodriguez, F. J., Verdu, E., Ceballos, D., and Navarro, X. *Exp. Neurol.* **161,** 571 (2000).
Rosen, J. M., Pham, H. N., Abraham, G., Harold, L., and Hentz, V. R. *J. Rehabil. Res. Dev.* **26,** 1 (1989).
Rutkowski, G. E., and Heath, C. A. *Biotechnol. Prog.* **18,** 362 (2002a).
Rutkowski, G. E., and Heath, C. A. *Biotechnol. Prog.* **18,** 373 (2002b).
Satou, T., Nishida, S., Hiruma, S., Tanji, K., Takahashi, M., Fujita, S., Mizuhara, Y., Akai, F., and Hashimoto, S. *Acta. Pathol. Jpn.* **36,** 199 (1986).
Sautter, J., Tseng, J. L., Braguglia, D., Aebischer, P., Spenger, C., Seiler, R. W., Widmer, H. R., and Zurn, A. D. *Exp. Neurol.* **149,** 230 (1998).
Schinstine, M., Fiore, D. M., Winn, S. R., and Emerich, D. F. *Cell Transplant* **4,** 93 (1995).
Schmidt, C. E., Shastri, V. R., Vacanti, J. P., and Langer, R. *Proc. Natl. Acad. Sci. USA* **94,** 8948 (1997).
Schreyer, D. J., and Jones, E. G. *Brain Res.* **432,** 291 (1987).
Schugens, C., Maquet, V., Grandfils, C., Jerome, R., and Teyssie, P. *J. Biomed. Mater. Res.* **30,** 449 (1996).
Sebille, A., and Becker, C. *Exp. Neurol.* **99,** 765 (1988).
Seckel, B. R., Ryan, S. E., Gagne, R. G., Chiu, T. H., and Watkins, E., Jr. *Plast. Reconstr. Surg.* **78,** 793 (1986).
Shakesheff, K., Patel, N., Cannizzaro, S. M., and Langer, R. S., PCT Int. Appl. 9936107 (1999).
Shastri, V. R., Schmidt, C. E., Langer, R. S., and Vacanti, J. P., PCT. Int. Appln., 9716545 (1997).

Spector, J. G., Lee, P., Derby, A., Frierdich, G. E., Neises, G., and Roufa, D. G. *Laryngoscope* **103**, 548 (1993).
Spector, J. G., Lee, P., Derby, A., and Roufa, D. G. *Ann. Otol. Rhinol. Laryngol.* **104**, 875 (1995).
Stensaas, L., Bloch, L. M., Garcia, R., and Sotelo, J., Jr. *Exp. Neurol.* **103**, 135 (1989).
Steuer, H., Fadale, R., Muller, E., Muller, H. W., Planck, H., and Schlosshauer, B. *Neurosci. Lett.* **277**, 165 (1999).
Tan, S. A., Deglon, N., Zurn, A. D., Baetge, E. E., Bamber, B., Kato, A. C., and Aebischer, P. *Cell Transplant.* **5**, 577 (1996).
Teng, Y. D., Lavik, E. B., Qu, X., Park, K. I., Ourednik, J., Zurakowski, D., Langer, R., and Snyder, E. Y. *PNAS* **99**, 3024 (2002).
Terada, N., Bjursten, L. M., Dohi, D., and Lundborg, G. *Scand. J. Plast. Reconstr. Surg. Hand Surg.* **31**, 1 (1997).
Tessier-Lavigne, M. *Curr. Opin. Gene Dev.* **4**, 596 (1994).
Tong, X. J., Hirai, I., Shimada, H., Mizutani, Y., Izumi, T., Toda, N., and Yu, P. *Brain Res.* **663**, 155 (1994).
Valentini, R. F., Vargo, T. G., Gardella, J. A., Jr., and Aebischer, P. *Biomaterials* **13**, 183 (1992).
Valero-Cabre, A., Tsironis, K., Skouras, E., Perego, G., Navarro, X., and Neiss, W. F. *J. Neurosci. Res.* **63**, 214 (2001).
Verdu, E., Labrador, R. O., Rodriguez, F. J., Ceballos, D., Fores, J., and Navarro, X. *Restor. Neurol. Neurosci.* **20**, 169 (2002).
Voinesco, F., Glauser, L., Kraftsik, R., and Barakat-Walter, I. *Exp. Neurol.* **150**, 69 (1998).
Wan, A. C., Mao, H. Q., Wang, S., Leong, K. W., Ong, L. K., and Yu, H. *Biomaterials* **22**, 1147 (2001).
Wang, G., Hirai, K., and Shimada, H. *Brain Res.* **570**, 116 (1992).
Wang, S., Wan, A. C., Xu, X., Gao, S., Mao, H. Q., Leong, K. W., and Yu, H. *Biomaterials* **22**, 1157 (2001).
Wang-Bennett, L. T., and Coker, N. J. *Exp. Neurol.* **107**, 222 (1990).
Widmer, M. S., Gupta, P. K., Lu, L., Meszlenyi, R. K., Evans, G. R., Brandt, K., Savel, T., Gurlek, A., Patrick, C. W., Jr., and Mikos, A. G. *Biomaterials* **19**, 1945 (1998).
Winn, S. R., Hammang, J. P., Emerich, D. F., Lee, A., Palmiter, R. D., and Baetge, E. E. *Proc. Natl. Acad. Sci. USA* **91**, 2324 (1994).
Winn, S. R., Lindner, M. D., Lee, A., Haggett, G., Francis, J. M., and Emerich, D. F. *Exp. Neurol.* **140**, 126 (1996).
Woerly, S. *Biomaterials* **14**, 1056 (1993).
Woerly, S., Doan, V. D., Evans-Martin, F., Paramore, C. G., and Peduzzi, J. D. *J. Neurosci. Res.* **66**, 1187 (2001a).
Woerly, S., Doan, V. D., Sosa, N., de Vellis, J., and Espinosa, A. *Int. J. Dev. Neurosci.* **19**, 63 (2001b).
Woerly, S., Laroche, G., Marchand, R., Pato, J., Subr, V., and Ulbrich, K. *J. Neural. Transplant. Plast.* **5**, 245 (1995).
Woerly, S., Lavallee, C., and Marchand, R. *J. Neural. Transplant. Plast.* **3**, 21 (1992).
Woerly, S., Petrov, P., Sykova, E., Roitbak, T., Simonova, Z., and Harvey, A. R. *Tissue Eng.* **5**, 467 (1999).
Woerly, S., Pinet, E., De Robertis, L., Bousmina, M., Laroche, G., Roitback, T., Vargova, L., and Sykova, E. *J. Biomater. Sci. Polym. Ed.* **9**, 681 (1998).
Woerly, S., Pinet, E., de Robertis, L., Van Diep, D., and Bousmina, M. *Biomaterials* **22**, 1095 (2001c).
Woerly, S., Plant, G. W., and Harvey, A. R. *Neurosci Lett.* **205**, 197 (1996).

Xu, X., Yee, W. C., Hwang, P. Y., Yu, H., Wan, A. C., Gao, S., Boon, K. L., Mao, H. Q., Leong, K. W., and Wang, S. *Biomaterials* **24,** 2405 (2003).
Xu, X., Yu, H., Gao, S., Ma, H. Q., Leong, K. W., and Wang, S. *Biomaterials* **23,** 3765 (2002).
Young, B. L., Begovac, P., Stuart, D. G., and Goslow, G. E., Jr. *J. Neurosci. Methods* **10,** 51 (1984).
Young, R. C., Wiberg, M., and Terenghi, G. *Br. J. Plast. Surg.* **55,** 235 (2002).
Yu, X., Dillon, G. P., and Bellamkonda, R. B. *Tissue Eng.* **5,** 291 (1999).
Zhao, Q., Dahlin, L. B., Kanje, M., and Lundborg, G. *Brain Res.* **592,** 106 (1992).
Zhao, Q., Lundborg, G., Danielsen, N., Bjursten, L. M., and Dahlin, L. B. *Brain Res.* **769,** 125 (1997).

STRUCTURAL AND DYNAMIC RESPONSE OF NEUTRAL AND INTELLIGENT NETWORKS IN BIOMEDICAL ENVIRONMENTS

Anthony M. Lowman[1], Thomas D. Dziubla[2], Petr Bures[3], and Nicholas A. Peppas[3]

[1]Department of Chemical Engineering, Drexel University,
Philadelphia, PA 19104, USA
[2]Institute for Environmental Medicine, University of Pennsylvania School of Medicine,
Philadelphia, PA 19104, USA
[3]Departments of Chemical and Biomedical Engineering, and Division of Pharmaceutics, CPE 3.466, The University of Texas at Austin,
Austin, TX 78712-0231, USA

I. Introduction	75
II. Structure of Three-dimensional Polymeric Networks as Biomaterials	76
A. Hydrogel Classification	77
B. Network Structure of Hydrogels	77
C. Solute Transport in Hydrogels	83
D. Environmentally Responsive Hydrogels	88
E. Complexation in Polymers	92
F. Tissue Engineering Aspects of Neutral Networks	98
III. Applications of Hydrogels	105
A. Neutral Hydrogels	105
B. Responsive Networks	110
C. Oral Insulin Delivery Systems	119
D. Protein Based Hydrogels	120
E. Other Promosing Applications	121
References	122

I. Introduction

As biomedical materials are becoming more advanced and sophisticated, advanced techniques of combinatorial chemistry and molecular design are becoming of utmost importance in order to achieve better design and desirable response to the biological environment. In particular, hydrophilic polymer networks have attained new importance in this field as they are particularly prone to molecular or structural changes. Indeed, their structure can be modified by copolymerization to achieve hydrophilicity or hydrophobicity. In addition, the presence of selected functional groups can make these networks responsive to environmental changes. In this chapter, a detailed analysis of the structural and biological properties of polymer networks, both neutral and responsive, is given with an emphasis placed upon the significance of these properties in biomedical applications. As such, an overview of currently pursued hydrogels technologies is also provided at the end of the chapter.

II. Structure of Three-dimensional Polymeric Networks as Biomaterials

Hydrogels are three-dimensional, hydrophilic, polymeric networks capable of imbibing large amounts of water or biological fluids (Brannon-Peppas and Harland, 1990; Peppas and Mikos, 1986). The networks are composed of hydrophilic homopolymers or copolymers, which are rendered insoluble by the presence of chemical crosslinks (tie-points, junctions) or physical crosslinks such as entanglements or crystallites (Hickey and Peppas, 1995; Peppas, 1986a; Peppas and Merrill, 1976a,b; Peppas and Mongia, 1997; Stauffer and Peppas, 1992). These crosslinks define the network structure and the physical integrity of the hydrogel. Due to the hydrophilic nature of the polymer chains, hydrogels exhibit a thermodynamic compatibility with water which allows them to swell in aqueous media (Brannon-Peppas and Harland, 1990; Flory, 1953; Flory and Rehner 1943a,b; Peppas and Mikos, 1986).

There are numerous applications of these hydrogels, in particular in the medical and pharmaceutical sectors (Peppas, 1986b; Peppas and Langer, 1994; Ratner and Hoffman, 1976). Since they possess high water content and a soft, elastic consistency, hydrogels more closely resemble natural living tissue than any other class of synthetic biomaterial (Ratner and Hoffman, 1976). As a result of their high water content, hydrogels are typically very biocompatible. Thus, hydrogels can be used as contact lenses, membranes for biosensors, linings for artificial hearts, materials for artificial skin, and drug delivery devices (Park, 1997; Peppas, 1986b, 1997; Peppas and Langer, 1994; Ratner and Hoffman, 1976).

A. Hydrogel Classification

Hydrogels (Brannon-Peppas and Harland, 1990; Peppas and Mikos, 1986) can be neutral or ionic based on the nature of the side groups. They can also be classified based on the network morphology as amorphous, semicrystalline, hydrogen-bonded structures, supermolecular structures, and hydrocolloidal aggregates. Additionally, in terms of their network structures, hydrogels can be classified as macroporous, microporous, or nonporous (Brannon-Peppas and Harland, 1990; Peppas and Merrill, 1976a; Peppas and Mikos, 1986). A convenient way to classify hydrogels is based on the nature of the pendent groups, which can be either neutral or ionic. The chemical nature and number of these pendent groups can be precisely controlled by the choice of the monomers used in the polymer synthesis. Depending on the type and organization of the monomers in the polymer network, they can be further classified as neutral, biodegradable, complexing, and/or responsive hydrogels.

The literature on synthesis of new polymer materials has exploded since the discovery of poly(hydroxyethyl methacrylate) (PHEMA) by Wichterle and Lim (1960). Instead of utilizing "off-the-shelf" polymeric materials designed for use in consumer applications and adapting them for medical purposes, researchers are attempting to molecularly control material properties in order to elicit desired cellular and biological interactions. An extension of such molecular design is in the field of molecular imprinting, where specific substrate recognition sites are incorporated into a network by polymerization in the presence of the desired solute. An illustration of this process is shown in Fig. 1.

B. Network Structure of Hydrogels

One of the primary features of a hydrogel is its solute permeability properties, which is of key importance in drug delivery, controlled release, and tissue engineering. The performance of a hydrogel in any of these applications depends largely on its bulk structure. A number of excellent reviews discuss this topic in great detail. The most important parameters used to characterize the network structure of hydrogels are the polymer volume fraction in the swollen state, $v_{2,s}$, molecular weight of the polymer chain between two neighboring crosslinking points, $\overline{M}_c$ and the corresponding mesh size, ξ (Peppas and Barr-Howell, 1986).

The polymer volume in the swollen state, $v_{2,s}$, is a measure of the amount of fluid imbibed and retained by the hydrogel. The molecular weight between two consecutive crosslinks, which can be either of chemical

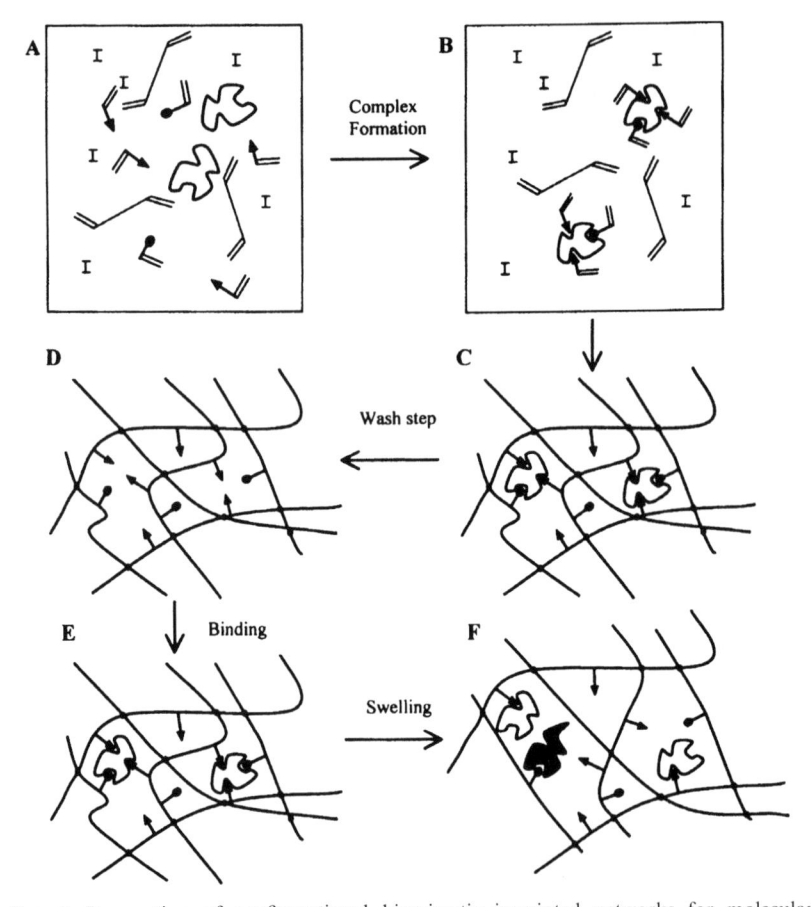

FIG. 1. Preparation of configurational biomimetic imprinted networks for molecular recognition of biological substrates. **A**: Solution mixture of template, functional monomer(s) (triangles and circles), crosslinking monomer, solvent, and initiator (I). **B**: The prepolymerization complex is formed via covalent or noncovalent chemistry. **C**: The formation of the network. **D**: Wash step where original template is removed. **E**: Rebinding of template. **F**: In less crosslinked systems, movement of the macromolecular chains will produce areas of differing affinity and specificity (filled molecule is isomer of template).

or physical nature, is a measure of the degree of crosslinking of the polymer. It is important to note that due to the random nature of the polymerization process itself only average values of $\overline{M}_c$ can be calculated. The correlation distance between two adjacent crosslinks, ξ, provides measure of the space available between the macromolecular chains available for the drug diffusion; again, it can be reported only as an average value. These parameters, which are related to one another, can be determined theoretically or through the use of variety of experimental techniques. The two most prominently used methods among the growing number of techniques utilized to elucidate the structure of hydrogels are the equilibrium swelling theory and the rubber elasticity theory.

1. Equilibrium Swelling Theory

The structure of hydrogels that do not contain ionic moieties can be analyzed by the Flory–Rehner theory (Flory and Rehner 1943a). This combination of thermodynamic and elasticity theories states that a crosslinked polymer gel which is immersed in a fluid and allowed to reach equilibrium with its surroundings is subject only to two opposing forces, the thermodynamic force of mixing and the retractive force of the polymer chains. At equilibrium, these two forces are equal. Equation (1) describes the physical situation in terms of the Gibbs free energy.

$$\Delta G_{total} = \Delta G_{elastic} + \Delta G_{mixing} \tag{1}$$

Here, $\Delta G_{elastic}$ is the contribution due to the elastic retractive forces developed inside the gel and ΔG_{mixing} is the result of the spontaneous mixing of the fluid molecules with the polymer chains. The term ΔG_{mixing} is a measure of the compatibility of the polymer with the molecules of the surrounding fluid. This compatibility is usually expressed by the polymer–solvent interaction parameter, χ_1 (Flory, 1953).

Differentiation of Eq. (1) with respect to the number of solvent molecules while keeping temperature and pressure constant, results in Eq. (2):

$$\mu_1 - \mu_{1,o} = \Delta\mu_{elastic} + \Delta\mu_{mixing} \tag{2}$$

In Eq. (2), μ_1 is the chemical potential of the solvent in the polymer gel and $\mu_{1,o}$ is the chemical potential of the pure solvent. At equilibrium, the difference between the chemical potentials of the solvent outside and inside the gel must be zero. Therefore, changes of the chemical potential due to mixing and elastic forces must balance each other. The change of chemical potential due to mixing can be expressed using heat and entropy of mixing.

The change of chemical potential due to the elastic retractive forces of the polymer chains can be determined from the theory of rubber elasticity (Flory, 1953; Treloar, 1958). Upon equaling these two contributions an expression for determining the molecular weight between two adjacent crosslinks of a neutral hydrogel prepared in the absence of a solvent can be written:

$$\frac{1}{\overline{M}_c} = \frac{2}{\overline{M}_n} \frac{(\bar{v}/V_1)\left[\ln(1-v_{2,s}) + v_{2,s} + \chi_1 v_{2,s}^2\right]}{\left(v_{2,s}^{1/3} - \frac{v_{2,s}}{2}\right)} \quad (3)$$

Here, $\overline{M}_n$, is the molecular weight of the polymer chains prepared under identical conditions but in the absence of the crosslinking agent, $\bar{v}$ is the specific volume of the polymer and V_1 is the molar volume of water.

Peppas and Merrill (1977) modified the original Flory–Rehner theory for hydrogels prepared in the presence of water. The presence of water effectively modifies the change of chemical potential due to the elastic forces. This term must now account for the volume fraction density of the chains during crosslinking. Equation (4) predicts the molecular weight between crosslinks in a neutral hydrogel prepared in the presence of water.

$$\frac{1}{\overline{M}_c} = \frac{2}{\overline{M}_n} \frac{(\bar{v}/V_1)\left[\ln(1-v_{2,s}) + v_{2,s} + \chi_1 v_{2,s}^2\right]}{v_{2,r}\left[\left(\frac{v_{2,s}}{v_{2,r}}\right) - \left(\frac{v_{2,s}}{2v_{2,r}}\right)\right]} \quad (4)$$

Here, $v_{2,r}$ is the polymer volume fraction in the relaxed state, which is defined as the state of the polymer immediately after crosslinking but before swelling.

The presence of ionic moieties in hydrogels makes the theoretical treatment of swelling much more complex. In addition to the ΔG_{mixing} and $\Delta G_{elastic}$ in Eq. (1), there is an additional contribution to the total change in Gibbs free energy due to the ionic nature of the polymer network, ΔG_{ionic}.

$$\Delta G_{total} = \Delta G_{elastic} + \Delta G_{mixing} + \Delta G_{ionic} \quad (5)$$

Upon differentiating Eq. (5) with respect to the number of moles of solvent keeping T and P constant, expression similar to Eq. (2) for the chemical potential can be derived.

$$\mu_1 - \mu_{1,o} = \Delta\mu_{elastic} + \Delta\mu_{mixing} + \Delta\mu_{ionic} \quad (6)$$

Here, the $\Delta\mu_{ionic}$ is the change of chemical potential due to the ionic character of the hydrogel. Expressions for the ionic contribution to the chemical potential have been also developed (Brannon-Peppas and Peppas,

1991a; Katchalsky and Michaeli, 1955; Ricka and Tanaka, 1984). They exhibit strong dependencies on the ionic strength of the surrounding media and on the nature of the ions present in the solvent. Equations (7) and (8) are expressions that have been derived for swelling of anionic and cationic hydrogels, respectively, prepared in the presence of a solvent.

$$\frac{V_1}{4IM_r}\left(\frac{v_{2,s}^2}{v}\right)\left(\frac{K_a}{10^{-pH}-K_a}\right)^2$$
$$=\left[\ln(1-v_{2,s})+v_{2,s}+\chi_1 v_{2,s}^2\right]+\left(\frac{V_1}{v\overline{M}_c}\right)\left(1-\frac{2\overline{M}_c}{\overline{M}_n}\right)v_{2,r}\left[\left(\frac{v_{2,s}}{v_{2,r}}\right)^{1/3}-\left(\frac{v_{2,s}}{2v_{2,r}}\right)\right] \tag{7}$$

$$\frac{V_1}{4IM_r}\left(\frac{v_{2,s}^2}{v}\right)\left(\frac{K_b}{10^{pH-14}-K_a}\right)^2$$
$$=\left[\ln(1-v_{2,s})+v_{2,s}+\chi_1 v_{2,s}^2\right]+\left(\frac{V_1}{v\overline{M}_c}\right)\left(1-\frac{2\overline{M}_c}{\overline{M}_n}\right)v_{2,r}\left[\left(\frac{v_{2,s}}{v_{2,r}}\right)^{1/3}-\left(\frac{v_{2,s}}{2v_{2,r}}\right)\right] \tag{8}$$

In these expressions, I is the ionic strength, K_a and K_b are the dissociation constants for the acid and base, respectively, M_r is the molecular weight of the repeating unit.

2. Rubber Elasticity Theory

Hydrogels resemble natural rubbers in their remarkable property to elastically respond to applied stresses. A hydrogel subjected to a relatively small deformation, less than 20%, will fully recover to its original dimension in a rapid fashion. This elastic behavior of hydrogels can be used to elucidate their structure by utilizing the rubber elasticity theory originally developed by Treloar (1958) and Flory (Peppas and Moynihan 1985; Peppas and Reinhart 1983) for vulcanized rubbers and modified to polymers by Flory (1953). However, the original theory or rubber elasticity does not apply to hydrogels prepared in the presence of a solvent. Such expressions were developed by Silliman (1972) and later modified by Peppas and Merrill (1977).

Here, only the form of rubber elasticity theory used to analyze the structure of hydrogels prepared in the presence of a solvent is presented and it is left up to the reader to consult the original reference for detailed derivations.

$$\tau = \frac{\rho RT}{\overline{M}_c}\left(1 - \frac{2\overline{M}_c}{\overline{M}_n}\right)\left(\alpha - \frac{1}{\alpha^2}\right)\left(\frac{v_{2,s}}{v_{2,r}}\right)^{1/3} \qquad (9)$$

Here, τ is the stress applied to the polymer sample, ρ is the density of the polymer, R is the universal gas constant, T is the absolute experimental temperature, and $\overline{M}_c$ is the desired molecular weight between crosslinks.

In order to perform analysis of the structure of hydrogels using the rubber elasticity theory, experiments need to be performed using a tensile testing system. Interestingly, the rubber elasticity theory has not been used to analyze only chemically but also physically crosslinked hydrogels (Anseth et al., 1996; Mark, 1982; Patterson et al., 1982), as well as hydrogels exhibiting temporary crosslinks due to hydrogen bonding (Lowman and Peppas, 1997).

3. Analysis of Structural Characteristics of Networks

The primary mechanism of release of many drugs from hydrogels is diffusion occurring through the space available between macromolecular chains. This space is often regarded as the "pore." Depending upon the size of these pores, hydrogels can be conveniently classified as (i) macroporous; (ii) microporous; and (iii) nonporous. A structural parameter that is often used in describing the size of the pores is the correlation length, ξ, which is defined as the linear distance between two adjacent crosslinks and can be calculated using the following equation:

$$\xi = \alpha\left(\overline{r}_o^2\right)^{1/2} \qquad (10)$$

Here, α is the elongation ratio of the polymer chains in any direction and $\left(\overline{r}_o^2\right)^{1/2}$ is the root-mean-square, unperturbed, end-to-end distance of the polymer chains between two neighboring crosslinks (Canal and Peppas, 1989). For isotropically swollen hydrogel, the elongation ratio, α, can be related to the swollen polymer volume fraction, $v_{2,s}$, using Eq. (11).

$$\alpha = v_{2,s}^{-1/3} \qquad (11)$$

The unperturbed end-to-end distance of the polymer chain between two adjacent crosslinks can be calculated using Eq. (12) where C_n is the Flory characteristic ratio, l is the length of the bond along the polymer backbone (for vinyl polymers 1.54 Å) and N is the number of links per chain that can be calculated by Eq. (13).

$$(\bar{r}_o^2)^{1/2} = l(C_n N)^{1/2} \tag{12}$$

$$N = \frac{2\overline{M}_c}{M_r} \tag{13}$$

In Eq. (13) M_r is the molecular weight of the repeating units from which the polymer chain is composed. Finally, when one combines Eqs. (10) through (13), the correlation distance between two adjacent crosslinks in a swollen hydrogel can be obtained:

$$\xi = v_{2,s}^{-1/3} \left(\frac{2C_n \overline{M}_c}{M_r} \right)^{1/2} l \tag{14}$$

A detailed theoretical characterization of the network structure of the polymer carrier in terms of the correlation length, ξ, in combination with diffusion studies of model drugs and proteins provide an invaluable insight into the very complex structure of polymer networks and aid in the design of drug delivery carriers (Narasimhan and Peppas, 1997a).

C. Solute Transport in Hydrogels

One of the most important and challenging areas of use of such biomaterials is as carriers in drug delivery. In this field it is important to predict the release of the active agent as a function of time using physical and mathematical models. The importance of such models lies in their utility during both the design stage of a pharmaceutical formulation and the experimental verification of a release mechanism (Narasimhan and Peppas, 1997b).

In order to design a particular release mechanism, experimental data of statistical significance are compared to a solution of the theoretical model. It is therefore clear that only a combination of accurate and precise data with models accurately depicting the physical situation will provide an insight into the actual mechanism of release.

The vast majority of theoretical models are based on diffusion equations. The phenomenon of diffusion is intimately connected to the structure of the material through which the diffusion takes place thus the morphology of the polymeric materials should be accounted for in a successful model. There have been a limited number of reviews that have addressed these aspects of controlled release formulations (Langer and Peppas, 1983; Narasimhan and Peppas, 1997b; Narasimhan et al., 1999). The mechanisms of drug release offer a convenient way to categorize controlled release systems into (i) diffusion-controlled; (ii) chemically-controlled; and (iii) swelling-controlled (Hennink et al., 1997). Due to the fact that ordinary diffusion takes place in each one of these mechanisms to a certain degree and since most of the models used are based on diffusion equations, the next two sections are devoted to the fundamentals of diffusion in matrix systems and how they pertain to solute transport.

1. Fundamentals of Ordinary Diffusion

The release of an active agent from a polymeric carrier consists of the movement of the drug through the bulk of the polymer. This phenomenon known as diffusion is to a large degree controlled by the mass transfer limitations at the boundary between the polymer carrier and its surroundings. On a macroscopic level the diffusion of drug molecules through the polymer carrier can be described by Fick's law of diffusion, which is mathematically stated by Eqs. (15) and (16) for transport in one dimension (Crank and Park, 1968):

$$j_i = -D_{ip}\frac{dc_i}{dx} \qquad (15)$$

$$\frac{\partial c_i}{\partial t} = D_{ip}\frac{\partial^2 c_i}{\partial x^2} \qquad (16)$$

Here, the concentration and mass flux of species i are designated c_i, and j_i, respectively; D_{ip} is the diffusion coefficient of species i in the polymer matrix, and x and t stand for the independent variables of position and time, respectively.

Several important assumptions have been implicitly incorporated in Eqs. (15) and (16). First, these equations describe the release of a drug from a carrier of a thin planar geometry, equivalent equations for release from thick slabs, cylinders, and spheres have been derived (Crank and Park, 1968). It should also be emphasized that in the above written form of Fick's law, the diffusion coefficient is assumed to be independent of concentration. This assumption, while not conceptually correct, has been largely accepted due to the computational simplicity. Finally, j_i is a flux with respect to the mass average velocity v of the system.

Initial and boundary conditions, which are necessary for solving Eq. (15) and (16), allow for the appropriate description of the experimental conditions imposed upon the drug release device. The solutions of Eqs. (15) and (16) subject to a number of boundary conditions that can be applied to various *in vitro* and *ex vivo* experiments have been obtained (Crank and Park, 1968).

In order to improve the predictive power of the Fickian diffusion theory, a concentration dependent diffusion coefficient is used in Eqs. (15) and (16). Equation (16) is then rewritten and solved with the appropriate boundary conditions:

$$\frac{\partial c_i}{\partial t} = \frac{\partial}{\partial x}\left(D_{ip}(c_i)\frac{\partial c_i}{\partial x}\right) \tag{17}$$

In Eq. (17), $D_{ip}(c_i)$ is the concentration-dependent diffusion coefficient; its form of concentration dependence is affected by the structural characteristics of the polymer carrier. A selective summary of the various forms of the diffusion coefficient is provided in Table I.

One of earliest approaches of estimating the diffusion coefficient through a polymer carrier is that of Eyring (1936). In this theory, diffusion of a solute through a medium is presented as a series of jumps instead of a continuous process. Therefore, in Eq. (18) in Table I, which comes from the Eyring analysis, λ is the diffusional jump of the drug in the polymer and v is the frequency of jumping.

TABLE I
A Selective Summary of Drug Diffusion Co-efficients

Type of carrier	Form of D_{ip}	Eq.	Ref.
Porous	$D_{ip} = \dfrac{\lambda^2 v}{6}$	(18)	Eyring, (1936)
Porous	$D_{\text{eff}} = D_{iw}K_pK_r\dfrac{\varepsilon}{\tau}$	(19)	Lightfoot, (1973)
Microporous	$\dfrac{D_{ip}}{D_b} = (1-\lambda)^2(1+\alpha\lambda+\beta\lambda^3+\gamma\lambda^5)$	(20)	Faxén, (1923)
Nonporous	$D_{ip} = D_o\exp\left\{-\dfrac{k}{v_f}\right\}$	(21)	Fujita, (1961)
Nonporous	$\dfrac{D_{2,13}}{D_{2,1}} = \varphi(q_s)\exp\left[-B\left(\dfrac{q_s}{V_{f,1}}\right)\left(\dfrac{1}{H}-1\right)\right]$	(22)	Yasuda and Lamaze, (1971)
Nonporous (highly swollen)	$\dfrac{D_{2,13}}{D_{2,1}} = k_1\left(\dfrac{\overline{M_c}-\overline{M_c^*}}{\overline{M_n}-\overline{M_c^*}}\right)\exp\left(-\dfrac{k_2r_s^2}{Q-1}\right)$	(23)	Peppas and Reinhart, (1983)

Fugita (1961) utilized the idea of free volume in polymers to estimate the drug diffusion coefficient and arrived at an exponential dependence of the drug diffusion coefficient on the free volume, v_f, which is given by Eq. (21) in Table I. Yasuda and Lamaze (1971) refined the Fujita's theory and presented molecularly based theory, which predicts the diffusion coefficients of drugs through a polymer matrix rather accurately [Eq. (22)]. In their treatment the normalized diffusion coefficient, the ratio of the diffusion coefficient of the solute in the polymer, $D_{2,13}$, to the diffusion coefficient of the solute in the pure solvent, $D_{2,1}$, is related to the degree of hydration, H, and free-volume occupied by the swelling medium, $V_{f,1}$. In addition, φ is a sieving factor which provides a limiting mesh size impermeable to drugs with cross-sectional area q_s, and B is a parameter characteristic of the polymer. In Eq. (22), the subscripts 1, 2, and 3 refer to the swelling medium, drug, and polymer, respectively.

Peppas and Reinhart (1983) also developed a theoretical model based on a free volume of the polymer matrix. In their theory they assumed the free volume of the polymer to be the same as the free volume of the solvent and they arrived at Eq. (23) in Table I. They related the normalized diffusion coefficient to the degree of swelling, Q, the solute radius, r_s, and the molecular weight of the polymer chains. More specifically, $\overline{M}_c$ is the average molecular weight of the polymer chains between adjacent crosslinks, $\overline{M}_n$ is the average molecular weight of the linear polymer chains prepared under identical conditions in the absence of the crosslinking agent, and $\overline{M}_c^*$ is the critical molecular weight between crosslinks below which a drug of size r_s could not diffuse through the polymer network. In addition, k_1 and k_2 are constants related to the polymer structure. This theory is applicable to drug transport in highly swollen, nonporous hydrogels. Equations for moderately or poorly swollen (Peppas and Moynihan, 1985) and semicrystalline (Harland and Peppas, 1989) hydrogels were also developed.

Yet another approach for the prediction of the diffusion coefficient of a drug in a controlled-release device has been adopted from the chemical engineering field (Lightfoot, 1973). More specifically, the transport phenomena in porous rocks, ion-exchange resins, and catalysis are of very similar nature to a drug diffusing through a macro- or micro-porous polymer. In these types of polymers the diffusion is assumed to be taking place predominantly through the water, or bodily fluids, filled pores. The diffusion coefficient of a drug in a polymer, D_{ip}, in Eq. (15) and (16) is replaced by an effective diffusive coefficient, D_{eff}, which is defined by Eq. (19) in Table I. In Eq. (19), ε is the porosity, or void fraction, of the polymer, which is a measure of the volume of the pores available for diffusion and τ is the tortuosity, which describes the geometric characteristics of the pores. The term K_p is the equilibrium-partitioning coefficient, which is a parameter needed when the drug is soluble in the polymer matrix. It is the ratio of the concentration inside of the pore to the concentration outside of the pore. The term K_r describes the fractional reduction in diffusivity within the pore when the solute diameter, d_s, is comparable in size to the pore diameter d_r. Equation (20) in Table I is a semiempirical relation proposed by Faxen (1923) for diffusion of spheres through porous media. In this equation, λ is the ratio of the drug radius, r_s, to the pore average radius, r_p, D and D_b are the diffusion coefficients of the sphere through the pore and in bulk, respectively; and α, β, and γ are constants. It is clear to see that as the size of the drug gets smaller with respect to the size of the pore, the ratio of D/D_b approaches the limit of one.

2. Solute Transport in Matrix-Based Systems

The drug can be either dissolved or dispersed throughout the network of the hydrogels. The drug release from these systems is modeled using Eq. (17) with concentration-dependent coefficient given by either of Eq. (21) through Eq. (23). It is clear from solutions to Eq. (17) that the fractional drug release obtained form these systems is proportional to $t^{1/2}$. This is significant in that it is impossible to obtain time independent or zero-order release in this type of system with simple geometries.

Drug can be incorporated into the gels by equilibrium partitioning, where the gel is swollen to equilibrium in concentrated drug solution, or during the polymerization reaction. Equilibrium partitioning is the favorable loading method for drug/polymer systems with large partition coefficients or for sensitive macromolecular drugs such as peptides or proteins that could be degraded during the polymerization.

In swelling-controlled release systems, the drug is dispersed within a glassy polymer. Upon contact with biological fluid, the polymer begins to swell. No drug diffusion occurs through the polymer phase. As the penetrant enters the glassy polymer, the glass transition of the polymer is lowered allowing for relaxations of the macromolecular chains. The drug is able to diffuse out of the swollen, rubbery area of the polymers. This type of system is characterized by two moving fronts; the front separating the swollen (rubbery) portion and the glassy regions which moves with velocity, v, and the polymer/fluid interface (Fig. 2). The rate of drug release is controlled by the velocity and position of the front dividing the glassy and rubbery portions of the polymer. A very important phenomenon of macromolecular relaxation takes place at the glass–rubbery interface and significantly affects the drug release.

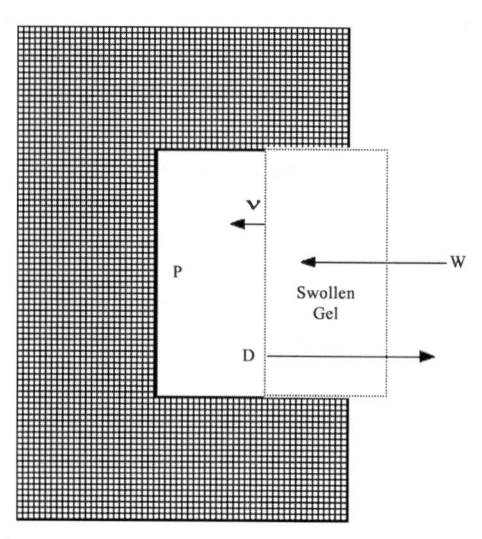

FIG. 2. Schematic representation of the behavior of a one-dimensional swelling controlled release system. The water (W) penetrates the glassy polymer (P) to form a gel. The drug (D) is released through the swollen layer.

D. ENVIRONMENTALLY RESPONSIVE HYDROGELS

Hydrogels may exhibit swelling behavior which is dependent on the conditions of the external environment. Over the last thirty years there has been a significant interest in the development and analysis of environmentally or physiologically responsive hydrogels (Peppas, 1991). Environmentally responsive materials show drastic changes in their swelling ratio due to changes in their external pH, temperature, ionic strength, nature and composition of the swelling agent, enzymatic or chemical reaction, and electrical or magnetic stimulus (Peppas, 1993). In most responsive networks, a critical point exists at which this transition occurs.

Responsive hydrogels are unique in that there are many different mechanisms for drug release and many different types of release systems based on these materials. For instance, in most cases drug release occurs when the gel is highly swollen or swelling and is typically controlled by rate of swelling, drug diffusion, or a coupling of swelling and diffusion. However, in a few instances, drug release occurs during gel synersis by a squeezing mechanism. Also, drug release can occur due to erosion of the polymer caused by environmentally responsive swelling.

Another interesting characteristic about many responsive gels is that the mechanism causing the network structural changes can be entirely reversible in nature. This behavior is depicted in Fig. 3 for a pH- or

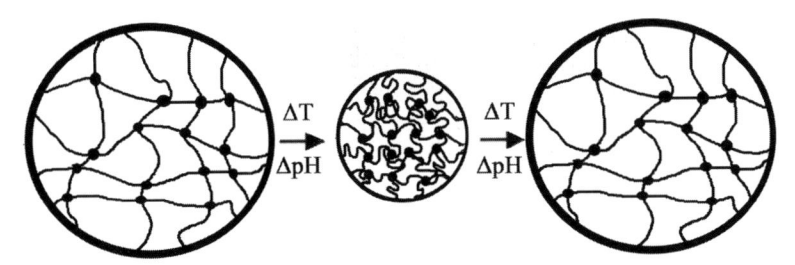

FIG. 3. Swollen temperature- and pH-sensitive hydrogels may exhibit an abrupt change from the expanded (left) to the collapsed (synresed) state (center) and then back to the expanded state (right) as temperature and pH change.

temperature-responsive gel. The ability of these materials to exhibit rapid changes in their swelling behavior and pore structure in response to changes in environmental conditions lend these materials favorable characteristics as carriers for bioactive agents, including peptides and proteins. This type of behavior may allow these materials to serve as self-regulated, pulsatile drug delivery systems. This type of behavior is shown in Fig. 4 for pH- or temperature-responsive gels. Initially, the gel is in an environment in which no swelling occurs. As a result, very little drug release occurs. However, when the environment changes and the gel swells, rapid drug release occurs (either by Fickian diffusion, anamolous transport or case II transport). When the gel collapses as the environment changes, the release can be turned off again. This can be repeated over numerous cycles. Such systems could be of extreme importance in the treatment of chronic diseases such as diabetes. Peppas (1993) and Siegel (1997) have presented detailed analyses of this type of behavior.

1. pH-Sensitive Hydrogels

One of the most widely studied types of physiologically responsive hydrogels is pH-responsive hydrogels. These hydrogels are swollen from ionic networks. These ionic networks contain either acidic or basic pendant groups. In aqueous media of appropriate pH and ionic strength, the pendant groups can ionize developing fixed charges on the gel as shown in Fig. 5 for an ionic gel. The swelling behavior of these materials has been analyzed in a previous section.

There are many advantages to using ionic materials over neutral networks. All ionic materials exhibit a pH and ionic strength sensitivity. The swelling forces developed in these systems will be increased over the nonionic materials. This increase in swelling force is due to the localization of fixed charges on the pendant groups. As a result, the mesh size of the polymeric networks can change significantly with small pH changes.

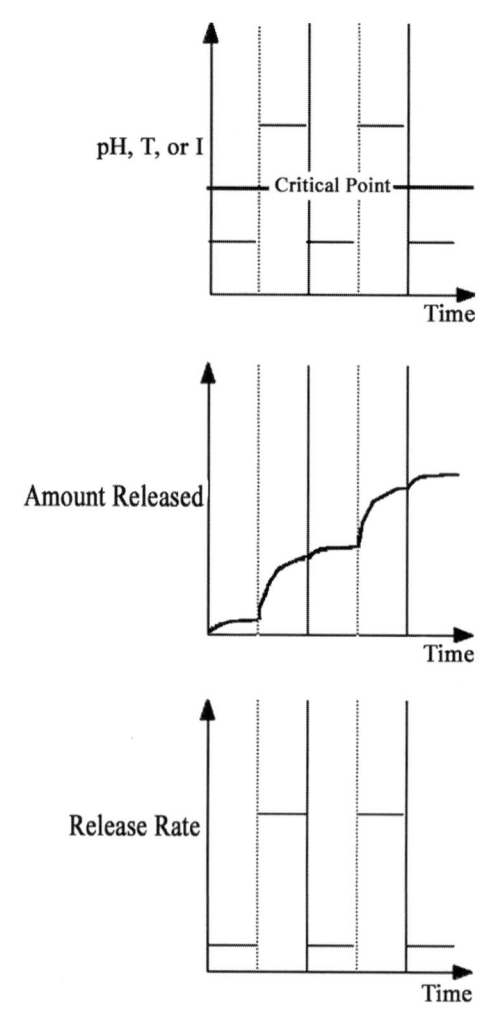

FIG. 4. Cyclic change of pH, T, or ionic strength (I) leads to abrupt changes in the drug release rates at certain time intervals in some environmentally responsive polymers.

In these materials, the drug diffusion coefficients and release rates will vary greatly with environmental pH.

2. Temperature-Sensitive Hydrogels

Another class of environmentally sensitive materials that are being targeted for use in drug delivery applications is thermally sensitive polymers. This type of hydrogel exhibits temperature-sensitive swelling behavior

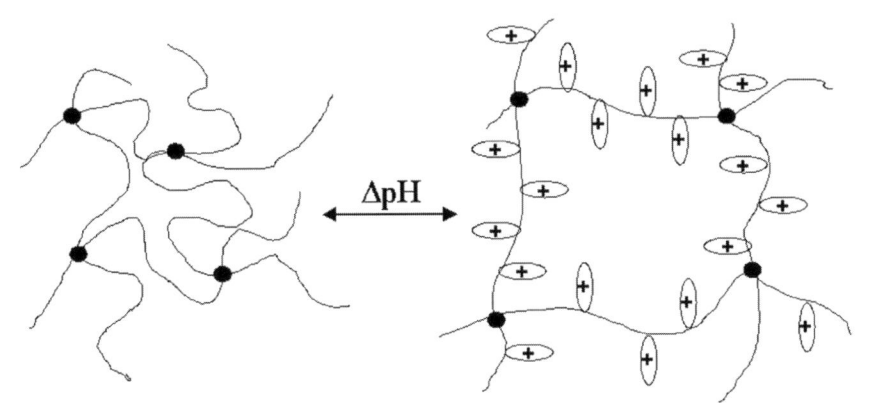

FIG. 5. Expansion (swelling) of a cationic hydrogel due to ionization of pendent groups, at specific pH values.

due to a change in the polymer/swelling agent compatibility over the temperature range of interest. Temperature-sensitive polymers typically exhibit a lower critical solution temperature (LCST), below which the polymer is soluble. Above this temperature, the polymers are typically hydrophobic and do not swell significantly in water (Kim, 1996). However, below the LCST, the crosslinked gel swell to significantly higher degrees because of the increased compatibility with water. For polymers that exhibit this sort of swelling behavior, the rate of drug release would be dependent on the temperature. The highest release rates would occur when the temperature of the environment is below the LCST of the gel.

3. Complexing Hydrogels

Some hydrogels may exhibit environmental sensitivity due to the formation of polymer complexes. Polymer complexes are insoluble, macromolecular structures formed by the noncovalent association of polymers with the affinity for one another. In this type of gel, the polymer complex behaves as a physical crosslink in the gel. As the degree of effective crosslinking is increased, the network mesh size and degree of swelling is significantly reduced. As a result, the rate of drug release in these gels will decrease dramatically upon the formation of interpolymer complexes. Since some of the more novel concepts immerging in hydrogel research involve these types of networks, the next section is devoted to a more detailed discussion on the formation and characterization of polymer complexation with an emphasis on pH sensitive complexes.

E. COMPLEXATION IN POLYMERS

1. Overview of Complexation

Interpolymer complexes possess unique physical and chemical properties which are different from those of the initial components and have found applications in technology, medicine, and other fields (Bekturov and Bimendina, 1981). The unique properties of the complexes arise due to a higher degree of molecular ordering that is a result of secondary binding forces. The resulting secondary structures are dictated primarily by the primary structure (monomer sequence), solvent, and temperature of the system. Interpolymer complexes can be classified based on the nature of the secondary binding forces as:

1. Polyelectrolyte complexes
2. Hydrogen-bonding complexes,
3. Stereocomplexes
4. Charge transfer complexes.

Polyelectrolyte complexes form due to Coulomb forces when two oppositely charged polyelectrolytes are mixed together. Mixing Lewis acids (proton donating macromolecules) with Lewis bases (proton accepting macromolecules) results in the formation of hydrogen-bonding complexes. The formation of stereocomplexes is the result of weak dispersive interactions between oriented polymer chains; for example, the van der Waals forces between isotactic and syndiotactic poly(methyl methacrylate). Charge transfer complexes arise due to charge-transfer interactions between electron-accepting and electron-donating polymers (Tsuchida and Abe, 1982). A number of experimental techniques have been applied to study interpolymer complexes: potentiometry (Bailey et al., 1964), conductometry (Bimendina et al., 1974), turbidimetry (Sato and Nakajima, 1975), viscometry (Antipina et al., 1972), calorimetry (Biros et al., 1974), sedimentation (Bimendina et al., 1977), light scattering (Liquori et al., 1966), high resolution H-nuclear magnetic resonance (NMR) spectroscopy (Spevacek and Schneider, 1974, infrared (Philippova and Starodubtzev, 1995), and electron spectroscopy (Bakeev et al., 1959).

It is the sensitivity of hydrogen bonds to their external environment that provide the pH-dependence of physical properties of hydrogen-bonding interpolymer complexes that are of interest to us.

2. Effect of PEG Chain Length on Interpolymer Complexation

Antipina et al. (1972) also investigated the complexation of poly(ethylene glycols) with linear polymethacrylic and acrylic acids of molecular weights of 100,000 and 120,000, respectively. They used potentiometry and viscometry to examine the effect of molecular weight of the PEG chain, concentration of the polymers in solution, and pH and temperature of the medium on the complex formation. By monitoring the pH levels of solutions of the polymeric acids to which PEG chains of molecular weights of 1000, 2000, 3000, 6000, 15,000 and 40,000 were added, they found that there is a critical PEG chain length that is necessary for the complexation reaction to occur. The addition of 3000 molecular weight PEG to 0.1 g/l solution of PMAA resulted in gradual increase in the solution pH. A similar effect was observed for the PAA solutions, however, the rise in the solution pH took place upon the addition of PEG 6000, and it was less profound than for the PMAA solution. The addition of higher molecular weight PEGs was accompanied by steeper increase in the solution pHs which leveled off at the polyacid/PEG molar ratio of one. These results were in complete agreement with the results obtained by viscometry. Therefore, it was concluded that the critical molecular weight of PEG needed to promote the complexation reaction with PMAA and PAA is 2000 and 6000, respectively. Additionally, the stability of the complex was suggested to be dependent on the chemical structure of the polyacid which in turn would promote hydrophobic interactions contributing to the stability of the formed complexes.

Papisov et al. (1974) performed calorimetric and potentiometric experiments to determine the thermodynamic parameters of the complex formation of PMAA and PAA with PEG. They investigated how temperature and the nature of the solvent affected the complex stability. They found that in aqueous media the enthalpy and entropy associated with the formation of the PMAA/PEG complex are positive while in an aqueous mixture of methanol both of the thermodynamic quantities become negative. The exact values are shown in Table II. The viscosities of aqueous solutions containing complexes of PMAA and PEG increase with decreasing temperature as a result of a breakdown of the complexes.

The temperature stability of the complexes seems to be dependent on the molecular weight of the PEG chain, i.e., the larger the PEG the lower the temperature at which the complex dissociates. An important observation was that the complexation/decomplexation phenomenon was reversible by changing the temperature of the system. The positive values of the thermodynamic parameters as well as the experimental observations clearly indicate the important role of hydrophobic interactions in the stabilization of the PMAA/PEG complexes. Since PAA is considerably more hydrophilic than PMAA, hydrophobic interactions do not play an important role in stabilizing the PAA/PEG complexes. This is represented by the much

TABLE II
ENTHALPY VALUES ASSOCIATED WITH THE FORMATION OF PMAA/PEG AND PAA/PEG COMPLEXES IN WATER AND WATER/METHANOL MIXTURES

Complex	M_{PEG}	Solvent	ΔH [kcal/mol]
PMAA–PEG	15,000	Water	0.30 ± 0.04
	40,000		
	6000	Water	0.26 ± 0.04
	20,000	Methanol:water (30:70 vol%)	-0.17 ± 0.04
PAA–PEG	40,000	Water	0.13 ± 0.04
	40,000	Methanol:water (30:70 vol%)	-0.18 ± 0.04

lower value of ΔH of the PAA/PEG complex and the almost nonexisting effect of temperature on the stability of the PAA/PEG complex.

Miyoshi et al. (1996, 1997) investigated interpolymer interactions, morphology and chain dynamics of the poly(acrylic acid)/poly(ethylene oxide) complex in the solid state using high-resolution solid state ^{13}C-NMR. In their study, they utilized PEO and PAA of molecular weight of 20,000 and 90,000, respectively. They concluded that there exists three hydrogen bonding forms of the carboxyl group in the PAA, namely: (1) the complex form, groups actively participating in the interpolymer hydrogen bonding with PEO chains; (2) the dimeric form, groups that form intramolecular hydrogen bonding complexes among PAA molecules; and (3) the free form, groups that are not a part of the complex nor the dimeric form.

Philippova and Starodubtzev have also extensively studied the complexation behavior of polyacids and PEG, especially, the system of crosslinked of poly(methacrylic acid) and linear poly(ethylene glycol) (Philippova and Starodubtzev, 1995; Philippova et al., 1994). They observed that decreasing the molecular weight of PEG from 6000 to 1500 resulted in its slower diffusion into the swollen network of PMAA, and a drastic decrease in both the stability and equilibrium composition of the intermacromolecular complex. Analysis of dried polymer networks of PMAA with absorbed PEG chains by FT-IR spectroscopy revealed the presence of two types of hydrogen bonded structures: (1) dimers of methacrylic acid at absorption frequency of 1700 cm^{-1} and (2) interpolymer complexes of PMAA and PEG at 1733 cm^{-1}. In addition, they also suggested as a result of their studies, that the hydrogen bonded dimer of PMAA forms preferentially to the intermacromolecular complex between the PMAA network and PEG chains.

In a more recent study, Philippova *et al.* (Skirda *et al.*, 1999) utilized the pulse field gradient (PFG)-NMR method to investigate the translational mobility of linear PEG macromolecules absorbed in loosely crosslinked PMAA hydrogels mentioned above. The goal of this study was to also explain why hydrogels of PMAA collapse when exposed to relatively low concentration of PEG (<5 wt%) and collapse and then reswell when immersed in solutions of PEG of rather high concentrations (ca. 5–10 wt%). The results of the PFG-NMR technique showed the existence of two fractions of PEG macromolecules with different chain mobilities inside the collapsed gel: (1) some PEG molecules had self-diffusion characteristics similar to those of chains of the crosslinked network, and (2) some PEG molecules exhibited free diffusion properties. In contrast, the PEG chains inside of the reswollen gels had self-diffusion coefficient independent of time indicating their absence in participating in interpolymer complexation with the PMAA network.

The formation of inter- and intrapolymer complexes has also been shown to affect the polymerization kinetics. For example, Ferguson and Shah (1968) investigated the influence of intrapolymer complexation on the kinetics of AA in the presence of copolymer matrices composed of either *N*-vinylpyrrolidone and acrylamide or *N*-vinylpyrrolidone and styrene. The polymerization rate reaches a maximum in the vicinity of AA to VP ratio equal to one for the VP/AAm matrix. This maximum in the polymerization rate is most pronounced in the presence of copolymer with the highest content of VP. When the hydrophilic acrylamide is replaced with the more hydrophobic styrene monomer in the copolymer matrix, the observed maximum in AA polymerization rate occurred at a lower than equimolar ratio of AA to VP. The hydrophilic groups of VP were interacting with the hydrophobic nucleus consisting of the styrene units in the VP/St copolymer, and were thus unable to participate in the formation of the complex unlike in the case of VP/AAm copolymer matrix.

Bajoras and Makuska investigated the effect of hydrogen bonding complexes on the reactivities of (meth)acrylic and isotonic acids in a binary mixture of dimethyl sulfoxide and water using IR spectroscopy (Bajoras and Makuska, 1986). They demonstrated that by altering the solvent composition it was possible to carry out copolymerization in the azeotropic which resulted in the production of homogeneous copolymers of definite compositions at high conversions. Furthermore, it was shown that water solvent fraction determines the rate of copolymerization and the reactivity ratios of the comonomers. This in turn determines the copolymer composition.

Verhoeven *et al.* (1989) addressed the possible effect of manufacturing conditions such as the presence of additives, namely poly(ethylene glycol), on the polymerization of 2-hydroxyethyl methacrylate (HEMA) and methacrylic acid (MAA). The suspected complexation between the additive and the methacrylic acid monomer did not have a significant effect on the reaction ratios nor the copolymer composition and tacticity as demonstrated by ^{13}C-NMR studies.

The effect of solvent on the polymerization kinetics of a system of poly(ethylene glycol) monomethacrylate and methacrylic acid was investigated by Smith and Klier (1998). In this work, a parameter of copolymer structure, namely the sequence distribution in the copolymer, was estimated by determining the reactivity ratios of the monomers using ^{1}H-NMR spectroscopy for two different solvents, D_2O and a mixture of ethanol and water. The paramount effect of the solvent on the polymerization process was exhibited by a profound change of r_1 and r_2 from 1.03 and 1.02 in the case of the D_2O solvent to 2.0 and 3.6 in the 50/50 wt% mixture of EtOH and H_2O, respectively. In the context of polymer structure, this means that while the resulting polymer would have a random structure when synthesized in D_2O it would have significantly large blocks of each co-monomer in its chains when manufactured in the EtOH/H_2O mixture. Clearly, this would significantly affect the final properties of the polymer system. Due to their potential industrial use, these polymers were the subject of a more recent publication where their molecular weight distributions and compositions were characterized (Drescher et al., 2001).

3. Infrared Spectroscopy

Infrared (IR) spectroscopy is one of the most commonly used techniques for the study and characterization of polymers (Koenig, 1992). The goal of such characterization is to relate the structure of polymers to their performance properties. IR has been used to characterize not only the resulting polymers but also the polymerization processes leading to the production of polymer systems (Scranton et al., 2003). The aim of the following sections is to summarize the use of IR in the characterization of polymer network structure with particular attention paid to intermolecular hydrogen bonding that occurs in such systems.

There are several excellent review articles and books (Coleman et al., 1991; Koenig, 1992; Scranton et al., 2003) on the use of IR in polymer systems that stand out from the rather voluminous literature on this topic. In addition to the above-mentioned monographs, there is also a number of exceptional series and articles such as the classic series by Castillo et al. (1984a,b; 1985, 1986a,b; Deng et al., 1986). IR was also employed by Ratner as one of the primary techniques to study the anomalous swelling behavior of PHEMA in urea solutions using deuterium oxide as the solvent (Ratner and Miller, 1972). In a more recent work, Perova et al. (1997) alluded to the role of and existence of different types of water present in PHEMA hydrogels using FT-IR. It was confirmed that depending upon the water concentration, there exists up to three types of water in a swollen hydrogel. At water concentrations greater than 18 wt%, loosely bound water was observed in addition to the tightly bound water molecules. When concentration of water was increased above 30 wt% some of the excess loosely bound water was shown to behave more like bulk water.

There are two major experimental techniques that can be used to analyze hydrogen bonding in noncrystalline polymer systems. The first is based on thermodynamic measurements which can be related to molecular properties by using statistical mechanics. The second, and much more powerful, way to elucidate the presence and nature of hydrogen bonds in amorphous polymers is by using spectroscopy (Coleman et al., 1991). From the present repertoire of spectroscopic techniques which includes IR, Raman, electronic absorption, fluorescence, and magnetic resonance spectroscopy, the IR is by far the most sensitive to the presence of hydrogen bonds (Coleman et al., 1991).

4. Infrared Spectroscopy and Polymer Complexation

Before discussing the details of hydrogen bonding in different polymer systems and how it affects their spectra it will be useful to review the definition of hydrogen bond. In polymer systems hydrogen bonds can be classified as:

1. self-associating
2. inter-associating

An example of self-associating hydrogen bond is a dimer of carboxylic acids while hydrogen bonding between a carboxylic acid and a nonself-associating functional group, such as ether or ester, is an example of the latter type.

Another type of classification of hydrogen bonds is based upon the relative strength of the interaction:

1. weak (PVC–Polyesters)
2. medium (self-association of –OH, Amides, Urethanes)
3. intermediate (self-association of –COOH)
4. strong (acid salts such as –COOH/NHP)

The strength of the hydrogen bonding interaction has a very profound effect on the appearance of the IR spectra and has been discussed in great detail by a number of authors (Coleman et al., 1991; Hadzi, 1965, 1976; Lee et al., 1988; Odinokov et al., 1976). In summary, weak hydrogen bonds exhibit very broad, structureless band with many submaxima centered around 3300 cm^{-1}. In spectra of hydrogen bonds of intermediate strength, such as in carboxylic acid dimers, the –OH stretching frequency is shifted lower to 3100–2800 cm^{-1} and, at the same time, "satellite" bands are observed on the lower frequency side of the broad fundamental profile. The origin of these bands was a subject of several publications and the explanation put forth by Bratoz, Hadzi, and Sheppard has been widely accepted since it satisfactorily accounts for all the observable peaks in the 3000–2500 cm^{-1} range of the spectra (Bratoz et al., 1956). The peaks are thought to arise from overtones and combinations that are intensity enhanced by Fermi resonance with the OH fundamental (Bratoz et al., 1956). IR spectra of polymer systems undergoing strong hydrogen bonding exhibit a number of peculiarities and are not commonly observed in polymer systems. One exception is that of a polyaminic model compound that complex with N-methyl pyrrolidinone (NMP). As a result of the strong hydrogen bonds formed between carboxylic acid groups present on the model compound and NMR, three broad bands are observed at 2900, 2400, and 1900 cm^{-1} in addition to various "satellite" bands (Coleman et al., 1991). These bands, typical of strong hydrogen bonds, are labeled by Hadzi as the "A," "B," and "C" bands (Hadzi, 1965, 1976).

F. TISSUE ENGINEERING ASPECTS OF NEUTRAL NETWORKS

When considering the similarity of hydrogels to soft tissue, it should come as no surprise that in the late 1960s cellularly invasive porous networks consisting of PHEMA were being designed as soft tissue replacements, such as breast augmentation and nasal cartilage replacement (Kliment et al., 1968; Simpson, 1969; Voldrich et al., 1975). However, complications with long-term calcification hindered further development. Then in the 1980s, work was done with pancreatic islet sequestering using PHEMA sponges (Klomp et al., 1983; Ronel et al., 1983). While the hydrogel sponge performed well as an immunoisolation device, long-term viability of the islets was not achieved. Although, with the rather recent advancements in scaffolding for supporting the formation of new tissue and a more developed understanding of the implant tissue response, these networks have found a revival in their utility and application. The following sections will discuss some of the key aspects of macroporous network formation, and the tissue response to these networks which is critical to the proper development of tissue supporting scaffolds.

1. Macroporous Structure of Neutral PHEMA Containing Networks

There is a significant difference in aqueous solubility of HEMA and PHEMA; the HEMA monomer is infinitely soluble in water while the polymer exhibits limited water compatibility. This dissimilar solution behavior allows for the formation of a macroporous, cellularly invasive sponge structure when reacted in dilute monomer solutions. As such, PHEMA hydrogel sponge formation is controlled by the thermodynamic phase behavior between the polymer-rich phase, and the aqueous-rich phase during polymerization. Chirila noted that the formation of the porous structure is dependant upon a kinetic competition between gel point and phase separation (Chirila et al., 1998). If gelation occurs first, the resulting material is a hydrogel with little to no macropores, but will still contain the typical hydrogel mesh size on the angstrom level. If phase separation occurs first, the resulting material contains water filled spaces that can vary in size from submicron up to 20 microns in size. The presence of the two different pore sizes present in macroporous PHEMA sponges is schematically shown in Fig. 6. Since the sponge formation is dependant upon both polymerization kinetics and solution thermodynamics, there are many variables that can be altered in order to control the pore morphology of the resulting hydrogel sponge. The following is a selection of methods that can be used to tailor PHEMA porous networks.

The amount of water added to the reaction mixture produces the most dramatic effect upon the size of the pores in a PHEMA sponge (Chirila et al., 1998; Ronel et al., 1983; Simpson, 1969). When the water content is below 45–50%, the PHEMA polymer chains remain soluble and do not form a two-phase system. When the reaction solution's water content is increased, phase separation occurs with excess water acting as the pore forming agent. Hence, as we further increase the water content, the number of water molecules excluded from the polymer phase increases creating larger voids between the polymer droplets. It is well established that networks containing 85% water or greater possess pore sizes that are large enough for cellular invasion. Unfortunately, these high water solutions result in materials with characteristically weak mechanical properties and large pore size distributions.

Since different crosslinking agents possess different solubilities in water, it was hypothesized that by altering the crosslinking agent used it should be possible to alter the networks pore morphology. Chirlia et al. (Clayton et al., 1997a,b; Lou et al., 2000) performed a rather extensive evaluation of

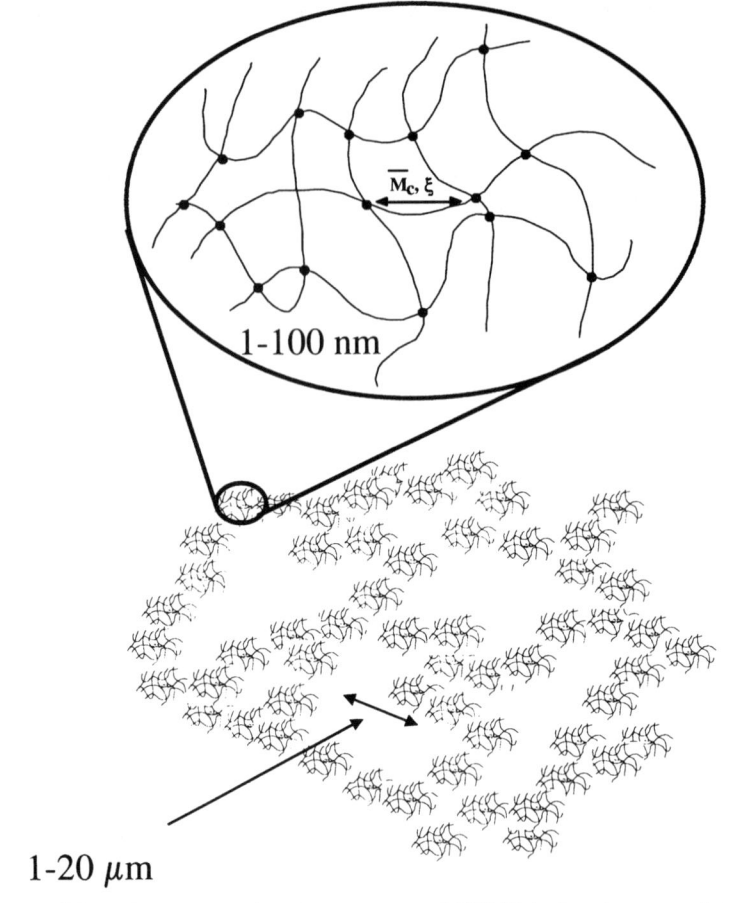

FIG. 6. Schematic representation of macroporous PHEMA hydrogel sponges. Interstitial spaces between polymer droplets create a macroporous structure 1–20 μm in size, whereas the polymer network creates a 1–100 nm mesh size in the polymer phase.

crosslinkers to determine their relative impact upon the networks ability to form large macropores. They determined that using typical concentrations of crosslinker content (0.1–2 mol%) had very little effect of the ultimate morphology and mechanical strength of the networks formed. While many studies on crosslinker selection have been performed, little work has been done on the effect of more/less hydrophilic comonomers on the formation of the macropores. The comonomers that have been attempted were more hydrophobic monomers such as methyl methacrylate (Dalton et al., 2002). This is most likely due to the commonly used hydrophilic comonomers, acrylic acid and 2,2-diethylaminomethacrylate result in transparent, homogeneous gels.

The presence of nonreacting, inert, components (porogens) can also affect the pore size of the resulting polymer sponge. A porogen is a space filling particulate that prevents polymerization in specific locations through physical hindrances (Badiger et al., 1993). Sucrose, glucose, and ice crystals have all been used as void fillers to create macroporous PHEMA hydrogels (Kang et al., 1999; Oxley et al., 1993). The porogen must be selected based on its ability to remain suspended in the reaction mixture, and provide some mechanism of being leached from the network after the sponge is formed (Carenza and Veronese, 1994).

PHEMA solubility decreases with increasing ion concentration. As a result, Mikos et al. used salt solutions of varying ionic strength to dilute the reaction mixtures (Liu et al., 2000). It was noted that increasing the ion content of the aqueous solution to $0.7M$, interconnected macropores were obtained at 60 vol% water. Surfactants may also be used to control the network pore structure. However, not much work has been done in this area, since surfactants typically work to reduce the surface repulsions between the two phases and form a uniform emulsion. These smaller emulsion droplets when gelled will create a network with an even smaller porous structure. Yet, this is still a promising area of exploration, since it may be possible to form alternate phase structures such as bicontinuous phases, which would be ideal for cellular invasion.

Isotactic PHEMA was found to possess negative temperature dependence in water (Oh and Jhon, 1989). While atactic PHEMA is not expected to have a strong negative temperature dependence, the mechanisms of this behavior can still exist over short ranges and may effect the phase behavior. As such, increased temperatures may also function to control the pore morphology by allowing the polymer to phase separate early on in the reaction.

Temperature not only plays a critical role with the thermodynamics, but also with the kinetics of the polymerization. Once phase separation occurs, the polymer phase will start to settle out of solution since it is denser than the aqueous phase. Chirlia noted this phenomenon by stating that in some reactions, a water layer was evident over the polymer sponge layer (Chirila et al., 1993). Temperature can reduce this settle-out by ramping up polymerization rate, and forcing gelation to occur sooner.

2. Tissue–Implant Interactions

a. Classic foreign body response. Implants are foreign bodies that will invoke the natural defense mechanism against such intrusions; the inflammatory response. Typically, the inflammatory response is split into two categories, acute and chronic inflammation (Anderson, 1988, 1993). During the acute phase, an influx of fluid, plasma proteins, and neutrophils enter the wound/implant site (Malech and Gallin, 1987). These neutrophils accumulate at the site of implantation and start to phagocytize any small debris/bacteria that are present. Phagocytosis is activated when the neutrophils comes into contact with activating factors called opsonins (Anderson, 1993). If an implant surface absorbs opsonins, such as the antibody immunoglobulin G (IgG), the neutrophil will try to engulf the implant. But since there is a large size disparity between the implant and neutrophils, phagocytosis cannot occur. This leads to an event known as frustrated phagocytosis, where the neutrophils dump the contents of lysosomes into the ECM (Henson, 1980). This process is highly unfavorable since it is very irritating to the surrounding tissue and leads to chronic inflammation. After the neutrophils have entered the area and cleared away any debris, granulation tissue (highly vascularized tissue) begins to form, and the natural wound healing response continues. At this point the response can split into either a chronic inflammatory response or a foreign body reaction of the acute type (Anderson, 1988). If there is a constant chemical or physical irritation (as in free movement of the implant), the chronic inflammatory response will occur (Gallin et al., 1988). If there are no negative chemical or physical signals, then classic foreign body response occurs. Typically, the foreign body response results in three characteristic layers (Anderson, 1988). A primary layer of macrophages and/or foreign body giant cell formations surrounds the implant. These cells secrete the second layer composed of dense fibrous tissue 30–100 μm in thickness. A third layer of granulation tissue surrounds this fibrous wall. This response is indefinitely stable except for a decrease in cellularity of the primary layer. The dense nature of the fibrous layer greatly impedes the diffusion of most chemical species, as a result prevents any implanted drug delivery device from functioning effectively (Scharp et al., 1984).

b. Tissue response to porous materials. The tissue response changes greatly when the implanted material has a porous morphology. Brauker et al. (1995) published a paper demonstrating the ability of porous materials to remodel the tissue response, and support vasculature up to one year postimplantation. They subcutaneously implanted several hydrophobic materials (PTFE, cellulose acetate, cellulose esters, and acrylic copolymers) with pore sizes ranging from 0.02–15 μm. It was found that materials with pores greater 5 μm were surrounded by highly vascular loose connective tissue. When the pore sizes increased further, evidence of vascular penetration was evident. The astounding part of their study was that this vasculature persisted for the entire duration of the study, one year. Shwarkawy *et al.* studied acetylized PVA with pore sizes 5, 60, and 700 μm in size (Shwarkawy *et al.*, 1997, 1998a,b). Their 5-micron pore size corroborated the results obtained by Brauker *et al.* (1995). However, they noted a very high degree of vascularization of implants with the 60 μm pore size, and when this pore size increased beyond 100 μm, the vascularity of the materials actually decreased.

Shwarkawy *et al.* (1997, 1998a,b) also demonstrated that changes in pore size not only effected vascular density but also the response to systemic uptake of drug through a vascularized implant. It was demonstrated that the 60 μm pore material delivered the drug in almost half the time it took for a subcutaneous injection to be taken up systemically. This is due to the increased vascular density as well as increased vascular permeability at these pore sizes (Shwarkawy *et al.*, 1997, 1998a,b).

There are two main theories that have been proposed to describe the dependence of vascular penetration on implant pore size. Padera and Colton have suggested that it is the macrophages degree of attachment onto the material surface that dictates the signals that they send out (Padera and Colton, 1996). When the macrophages are able to spread onto the surface of the material, they release signals that call for the deposition of the tight collagen layer. When these macrophages penetrate into a porous sample, and cannot spread fully on the surface, this signal is not released or released to a lesser extent. However, due to the macrophages being farther from a nutrient source, they release signals that initiate angiogenesis. When the macrophages penetrate into the very large pores, they are able to once again release the collagen deposition signals, and the pores become filled with the avascular collagen layer that typically surrounds a nonporous implant.

Rosengren has stated that it may be implant mobility that controls the degree of implant vascularity (Rosengren *et al.*, 1999). They suggest that smooth implants are capable of high relative motion. This motion shears the adjacent cells inducing necrosis. The degree of necrosis is the cause of the severity of the inflammatory response, hence the thickness of the fibrous capsule. They further suggest that porous materials possess little to no fibrous capsule, because the tissue that penetrates works to stabilize the relative motion. While it is still not known whether or not these hypotheses are correct or to what degree they are important, it is evident that simple morphological changes have a great effect upon the vascularization of implants.

c. Chemical and physical determinants of tissue attachment and in growth. Many of the porous implant studies compared the results of materials with varying surface chemistries. These studies looked at materials of varied hydrophilicity, such as hydrophobic PTFE, and acetylized PVA, to the more hydrophilic cellulose esters and acetates and poly(vinyl alcohol)s (Brauker et al., 1995; Lipsky, 1989; Sieminski and Gooch, 2000a; Shwarkawy et al., 1997, 1998a,b; Wake et al., 1995). It was found that the ingrowth of vascularized and loose connective tissue was dictated primarily by the pore size rather than chemical properties of the material. However, it would be wrong to assume that no control could be obtained through modifications of the implant surface chemistry.

Endothelial cells interact with the ECM through adhesion moieties called integrins (Saltzman, 1997). It is believed that cells attach onto synthetic materials through intermediary proteins, such as fibrin, which absorb onto polymer surfaces. Hence, by changing the protein absorption properties of surfaces, it is possible to alter the adhesion of endothelial cells. Moreover, it is also possible to bind specific adhesion ligands onto surfaces for a more direct control of the cellular attachment (Cook, 1997; Hubbel, 1992). Endothelial cells are able to adhere to the common attachment sequences that are found on fibrin, such as RGD and YISGR. It was found, however, that another adhesion peptide sequence, the RDEV ligand, preferentially bound endothelial cells over fibroblasts, smooth muscle cells, or activated platelets (Hubbel, 1992). Through this ligand, it may be possible to control explicitly the formation of capillaries into the implant.

Tube formation of the endothelial cells is an essential characteristic for the formation of capillaries, and is controlled by both chemical and physical properties of the material. There has been a significant lack of *in vitro* research showing the effects of synthetic biomaterials on endothelial cell's ability for tube formation (Sieminski and Gooch, 2000a). One study coated fibronectin in 10 and 30 µm stripes. They noted that tube formation occurred on the 10 µm stripes but not on 30. This study demonstrates the general trend of tube formation that the more adherent the cells are to a surface, the more they spread and the less likely they are to express phenotypes like tube formation. Also, that cells with greater spreading (attachment) exhibited increased proliferation, yet a decrease in cellular mobility. Moreover, tube formation was most prominent in surfaces that exhibited moderate adhesive characteristics (Matsuda and Kurumantani, 1990). More recently, Dziubla and Lowman (2003) demonstrated that 3D scaffolds of PEG-grafted PHEMA hydrogels were able to support EC tubule formation regardless of the adhesive characteristics. This is believed to be a result of the network pores to trap and contain the secreted ECM components of the migrating endothelial cells. There is also evidence that material stiffness also plays a part on tube formation. Ingber *et al.* showed that softer, more malleable materials exhibited an increase in cell tube formation (Ingber and Folkman, 1989).

III. Applications of Hydrogels

Hydrogels have been most extensively studied for their use in the field of controlled drug delivery. While this work is of primary importance, it is not the only biomedical application available for hydrogels. They have also been finding interesting utility in areas such as tissue engineering, biosensors, microfabrication, and cell-culturing. In this section, a more detailed summary of hydrogel applications from drug delivery to newer, novel innovations is provided.

A. Neutral Hydrogels

A major goal in drug delivery is to develop systems that deliver therapeutic agents at a constant rate over an extended period. This can be achieved by using release systems in which gel swelling is the controlling mechanism for drug release. Researchers have also attempted to develop constant-release systems by alteration of device geometry and polymer composition. One of the first researchers to use hydrogels for swelling-controlled release was Good (1976). In this work, glassy poly(2-hydroxyethyl methacrylate) containing tripelennamine-hydrochloride was swollen in water. The release rate of the solute was non-Fickian, but zero-order release was not obtained. The first such system in which zero-order release was observed was developed by Hopfenberg and Hsu (1978). In these systems, crosslinked polystyrene was used to release red dyes into hexane. Other polymers that have been used extensively in controlled release systems include poly(vinyl alcohol) (PVA), poly(*N*-vinyl-2-pyrollidone) (PNVP), poly(ethylene glycol) (PEG), poly(ethylene oxide) (PEO), and poly(ethylene vinyl *co*-acetate) (PEVAc) or copolymers thereof. In this section, we will discuss some of the applications of some of these materials.

1. Poly(2-Hydroxyethyl Methacrylate)

Poly(2-hydroxyethyl methacrylate) (PHEMA) has been the most widely used polymer in drug delivery applications. It is an extremely hydrophilic polymer and is highly stable. The permeability of these membranes is easily controlled based on the degree of crosslinking used. Researchers have studied the swelling behavior, morphology and diffusional behavior of PHEMA gels and copolymers thereof. The release of a wide range of drugs from these gels has also been studied. For example, Anderson *et al.* (1976) studied the release behavior of hydrocortisone from PHEMA gels. The release behavior was non-Fickian, but true zero order release was not achieved with these gels. Another significant study was performed by Sefton and Nishimura (1980). They investigated the diffusional behavior of insulin in PHEMA-based hydrogels. Song *et al.* (1981) developed one of the first pharmaceutically relevant zero-order release systems. They used a reservoir device consisting of a crosslinked PHEMA cylinder encapsulating a solution silicon oil and progesterone. Zero-order release was obtained with these devices for up to 10 days. Lee (1984; 1986) was able to use PHEMA to achieve zero-order release for short periods of time. In his work, oxprenolol was released from highly crosslinked PHEMA gels at constant rates for up to 3 h.

Peppas and co-workers contributed greatly to the understanding of the underlying phenomena of macromolecular relaxations in swelling controlled release systems. In particular, they studied hydrogels prepared from PHEMA and hydrophobic poly(methyl methacrylate) (PMMA). Franson and Peppas (1983) prepared crosslinked copolymer gels of P(HEMA-*co*-MAA) of varying compositions. Theophylline release was studied and it was found that near zero-order release could be achieved using copolymers containing 90% PHEMA. Further studies by Davidson and Peppas (1986) studied the effects of hydrophobicity and crosslink density on the release kinetics and diffusional properties of P(HEMA-*co*-MMA) membranes. Additionally, Korsmeyer and Peppas (1984) examined the behavior of copolymer gels consisting of PHEMA and hydrophilic PNVP (PHEMA-*co*-NVP). In this work, zero-order release of theophylline was observed for up to 5 h.

Macroporous networks of PHEMA containing hydrogels have also shown utility in long term implantable delivery devices, such as the implantable insulin pump. Typically, the functional life of the insulin pump is limited by the eventual occlusion of the catheter port. In the studies of Dziubla *et al.* (1999, 2002) it was shown that when the catheter port was coated in a hydrogel capable of supporting vascular tissue ingrowth, port occlusion is prevented even at 5 months postimplantation (typically cellular occlusion occurs after 8 weeks). Moreover, a rapid insulin uptake and systemic glucose response was noted (Fig. 7). This was assumed to be a result of the higher vascular density surrounding the catheter port.

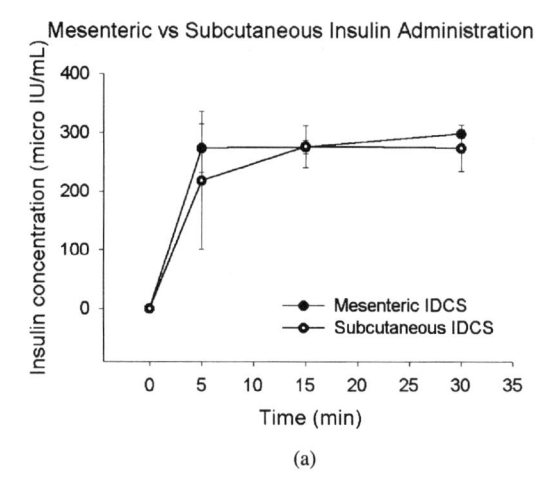

Mesenteric vs Subcutaneous Insulin Administration

(a)

Mesenteric vs Subcutaneous Glucose Concentration

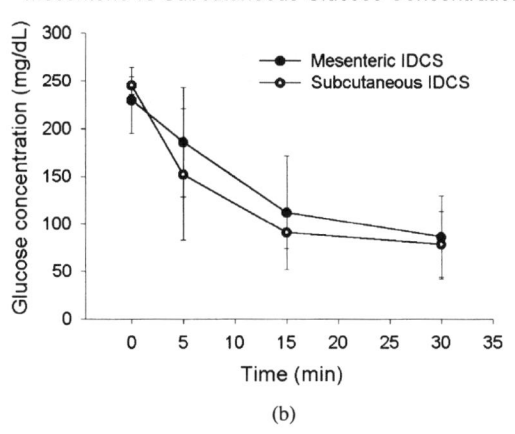

(b)

FIG. 7. Systemic (a) human insulin concentration and (b) glucose response following infusion of human insulin from external pump, 5 months postimplantation (Dziubla et al., 2002).

2. Poly(Vinyl Alcohol)

Another hydrophilic polymer that has received attention is poly(vinyl alcohol) (PVA). This material holds tremendous promise as a biological drug delivery device because it is nontoxic, hydrophilic and exhibits good mucoadhesive properties (Peppas, 1987). In one of the first applications of this material, Langer and Folkman (1976) investigated the use of copolymers of PHEMA (Hydron®) and PVA as delivery vehicles for polypeptide drugs.

Two methods exist for the preparation of PVA gels. In the first method, linear PVA chains are crosslinked using glyoxal, gluteraldehyde, or borate. In the second method, pioneered by Peppas (1975), semi-crystalline gels were prepared by exposing aqueous solutions of PVA to repeating freezing and thawing. The freezing and thawing induced crystal formation in the materials and allowed for the formation of a network structure crosslinked with the quasi-permanent crystallites. The latter method is the preferred method for preparation as it allows for the formation of an "ultrapure" network without the use of toxic crosslinking agents.

Korsmeyer and Peppas (1981) prepared PVA gels by crosslinking with borate. They studied the swelling behavior and mechanical properties of these gels. In this work, the release rate of theophylline was dependent on the degree of crosslinking. Future studies by Morimoto *et al.* (1989) examined the release behavior of a wide range of drugs. In this work, they were able to release indomethacin, glucose, insulin, heparin, and albumin from chemically crosslinked PVA gels.

Since the development of the semi-crystalline PVA gels by Peppas, significant work has been done in characterizing of these systems. Peppas and Hansen (1982) studied the kinetics of crystal formation during the freezing and thawing process. Subsequent work by Urushizaki *et al.* (1990) evaluated the effects of the number of freezing and thawing cycles on the networks properties. The gels became more rigid with increasing number of cycles. Peppas and Stauffer (1991) have also investigated the effects of crystallization conditions such as freezing temperature, number of cycles and freezing time on the structure and properties of the PVA networks.

Studies on the use of PVA prepared by the freezing/thawing technique as controlled release devices have recently been reported. Ficek and Peppas (1993) and Peppas and Scott (1992) used PVA gels for the release of bovine serum albumin. In the work of Peppas and Scott, drug release occurred by classical Fickian diffusion. Ficek and Peppas (1993) developed a method to prepare novel PVA microparticles containing BSA by a freezing/thawing technique. Here, they were able to release bovine serum albumin using these microparticles.

Other researchers have investigated the use of PVA gels as mucoadhesive delivery devices. Nagai and co-workers reported novel buccal delivery systems for ergotamine tartrate (Tsutsumi *et al.*, 1994). Peppas and Mongia (1997) have also considered PVA for mucoadhesive drug delivery applications. In their work, they investigated the mucoadhesive behavior of PVA gels prepared by the freezing/thawing technique. Additionally, they studied the release behavior of theophylline and oxprenolol from these materials. Additionally, the group of Peppas reported on the release behavior of ketanserin (Mongia et al., 1996) and metronidazole (Mallapragada and Peppas, 1997a) from these systems.

New phase erosion controlled release systems based on semicrystalline have been reported by Mallapragada and Peppas (1997a,b). These systems exhibited an unusual molecular control of the drug or protein delivery by a simple dissolution of the carrier. Hydrophilic carriers pass through a process of chain unfolding from the semicrystalline phase to the amorphous one, eventually leading to complete chain disentanglement. It has been shown that PVA and PEG are the best systems for such release behavior, and that such devices have the potential to be used for a wide range of drug delivery applications release. A detailed mathematical analysis has been developed to analyze such swellable systems (Mallapragada and Peppas, 1997b; Narasimhan and Peppas, 1997a; Peppas and Colombo, 1997).

3. Poly(Ethylene Oxide)/Poly(Ethylene Glycol)

Hydrogels of poly(ethylene oxide) (PEO) and poly(ethylene glycol) (PEG) have received significant attention in the last few years in biological drug delivery applications, especially because of their associated stealth characteristics and their protein resistance (Graham, 1992). Three major preparation techniques exist for the preparation of crosslinked PEG networks: (1) chemical crosslinking between PEG chains, (2) radiation crosslinking of PEG chains, and (3) chemical reaction of mono- and difunctional PEGs.

Some of the first chemically crosslinked PEG networks were prepared by McNeill and Graham (1984). The crosslinked linear PEG chains using diisocyanates. These gels were used as resevoir devices for the controlled delivery of smaller molecular weight drugs. McNeill and Graham (1996) have investigated the release behavior of small molecular weight solutes from PEG crosslinked with 1,2,6-hexanetriol. The release of proxyphylline from PEG spheres, slabs, and cylinders was studied. For each of the matrix devices, they observed non-Fickian release kinetics. Bromberg (1996) also studied the release of chemically crosslinked PEG networks. In this work, PEG networks were crosslinked using tris(6-isocyanatohexyl)isocyanurate. The kinetics of insulin release from PEG gels obeyed non-Fickian release kinetics.

The advantage of using radiation crosslinked PEO networks is that no toxic crosslinking agents are required. However, it is difficult to control the network structure of these materials. Stringer and Peppas (1996) have recently prepared PEO hydrogels by radiation crosslinking. The network structure was analyzed in detail, and the diffusional behavior of smaller molecular weight drugs, such as theophylline, in these gels was investigated.

Kofinas *et al.* (1996) have prepared PEO hydrogels by a similar technique. In this work, they studied the diffusional behavior of two macromolecules, cytochrome C and hemoglobin, in these gels. They noted an interesting, yet previously unreported dependence between the crosslink density and protein diffusion coefficient and the initial molecular weight of the linear PEGs.

Lowman *et al.* (Dziubla *et al.*, 1999; Lowman *et al.*, 1997) have presented an exciting new method for the preparation of PEG gels with controllable structures. Here, highly crosslinked and tethered PEG gels were prepared from PEG-dimethacrylates and -monomethacrylates. The diffusional behavior of diltiazem and theophylline in these networks was studied. The technique presented in this work is promising for the development of a new class of functionalized PEG-containing gels that may be of use in a wide variety of drug delivery applications.

B. Responsive Networks

1. pH-Sensitive Hydrogels

Hydrogels that have the ability to respond to pH changes have been studied extensively over the years. These gels typically contain side ionizable side groups such as carboxylic acids or amine groups (Oppermann, 1992; Scranton *et al.*, 1995). The most commonly studied ionic polymers include polyacrlyamide (PAAm), poly(acrylic acid) (PAA), poly(methacrylic acid) (PMAA), poly (diethylaminoethyl methacrylate) (PDEAEMA), and poly(dimethylaminoethyl methacrylate) (PDMAEMA).

Cationic copolymers based on PDEAEMA and PDMAEMA have been studied by the groups of Peppas and Siegel. Siegel and co-workers has focused on the swelling and transport behavior of hydrophobic cationic gels. Siegel and Firestone (Firestone and Siegel, 1988; Siegel and Firestone, 1988) studied the swelling behavior of hydrophobic hydrogels of PDMAEMA and poly(methyl methacrylate). Such systems were collapsed in solutions of pH greater than 6.6. However, in solutions of pH less than 6.6, such systems swelled due to protonation of the tertiary amine groups. The release of caffeine from these gels was studied (Siegel *et al.*, 1988). No caffeine was released in basic solutions, however, in neutral or slightly acidic solutions steady release of caffeine was observed for 10 days. Cornejo-Bravo and Siegel (1996) have investigated the swelling behavior of hydrophobic copolymers of PDEAEMA and PMMA. Additionally, Siegel (1990) has presented an excellent model of the dynamic behavior of ionic gels.

Peppas and co-workers has studied the swelling behavior of more hydrophilic, cationic copolymers of P(DEAEMA-co-HEMA) and P(DMAEMA-co-HEMA) Hariharan and Peppas (1996). These gels swell in solutions of pH less than 7 and collapse in basic solutions. These materials swelled to a greater degree than those prepared by Siegel (1990). Schwarte and Peppas (1997, 1998); (Schwarte et al., 1998) studied the swelling behavior of copolymers of PDEAEMA grafted with PEG. The permeability of dextrans of molecular weight 4400 and 9400 was studied. The membrane permeabilities in the swollen membranes (pH = 4.6) were two-orders of magnitude greater than permeabilities of the collapsed membranes.

Anionic copolymers have received significant attention as well. The swelling and release characteristics of anionic copolymers of PMAA and PHEMA (PHEMA-co-MAA) have been investigated. In acidic media, the gels did not swell significantly, however, in neutral or basic media, the gels swelled to a high degree due to ionization of the pendant acid group (Brannon-Peppas and Peppas, 1990; Kou et al., 1988). Brannon-Peppas and Peppas (1991b) have also studied the oscillatory swelling behavior of these gels. Copolymer gels were transferred between acidic and basic solutions at specified time intervals. In acidic solutions, the polymer swelled due to the ionization of the pendant groups. In basic solutions, rapid gel syneresis occurred. Brannon-Peppas and Peppas (1991c) modeled the time-dependent swelling response to pH changes using a Boltzman superposition-based model. The pH-dependent release behavior of theophylline and proxyphylline from these anionic gels was also studied (Bettini et al., 1995; Brannon-Peppas and Peppas, 1989). Khare and Peppas (1993, studied the pH-modulated release behavior of oxprenolol and theophyllne from copolymers of PHEMA-co-MAA and PHEMA-co-AA. In neutral or basic media, the drug release occurred rapidly by a non-Fickian mechanism. The release rate was slowed significantly in acidic media. In another study, Am Ende and Peppas (1997) examined the transport of ionic drugs of varying molecular weight in PHEMA-co-AA. They compared experimental results to a free-volume based theory and found that deviations occurred due to interactions between the ionized backbone chains and pendant acid groups. The swelling and release behavior of interpenetrating polymer networks of PVA and PAA was also investigated (Gudeman and Peppas, 1995; Peppas and Wright, 1996). These materials also exhibit strong pH-responsive swelling behavior. The permeability of these membranes was strongly dependent on the environmental pH and the size and ionic nature of the solute. New studies have used ATR–FTIR spectroscopy to characterize the interactions between polyelectrolytes and solutes (Am Ende and Peppas, 1995; Peppas and Wright, 1996).

Heller et al. (1990) studied the behavior of another type of pH-responsive hydrogel. Here, they evaluated the pH-dependent release of insulin from degradable poly(ortho esters). Other researchers have used chitosan (CS) membranes for drug delivery applications. These materials exhibited pH-dependent swelling behavior due to gelation of CS upon contact with anions (Bodmeier and Paeratakul, 1989). Interpenetrating networks of CS and PEO have been proposed as drug delivery devices due to their pH-dependent swelling behavior (Shiraishi et al., 1993; Yao et al., 1993). Calvo et al. (1997) prepared novel CS–PEO microspheres. These systems were to provide a continuous release of entrapped bovine serum albumin for one week. In another study, methotrexate, an anticancer drug, was encapsulated in microspheres of pH-sensitve CS and alginate (Narayani and Rao, 1995). Zero-order release of the drug was observed from the microspheres in pH = 1.2 buffer for greater than one week. Okano and co-workers (Kikuchi et al., 1997) studied pH-responsive calcium–alginate gel beads. In such systems, modulated release of dextran was achieved by varying the pH and ionic strength of the environmental solution. Such systems may be promising for use in protein and peptide delivery applications.

2. Temperature-Sensitive Hydrogels

Some of the earliest work with temperature-sensitve hydrogels was done by the group of Tanaka (1979). They synthesized with crosslinked poly(N-isopropylacrylimide) (PNIPAAm) and determined that the LCST of the PNIPAAm gels was 34.3°C. Below this temperature, significant gel swelling occurred. The transition about this point was reversible. They discovered that the transition temperature was raised by copolymerizing PNIPAAm with small amounts of ionic monomers. Beltran et al. (1991) also worked with PNIPAAm gels containing ionic comonomers. They observed results similar to those achieved by Tanaka (1979).

The earliest investigators studying PNIPAAm gels discovered that the response time of the materials in response to temperature changes was rather slow. Future studies focused on developing newer materials that had the ability to collapse/expand in a more rapid fashion. Dong and Hoffman (1990) prepared heterogeneous gels containing PNIPAAm that collapsed at significantly faster rates than homopolymers of PNIPAAm. Kabra and Gehrke (1991) developed new method to prepare PNIPAAM gels that resulted in significant increases in the swelling kinetics of the gels. They prepared gels below the LCST to produce a permanent phase separated microstructure in the gels. These gels expanded at rates 120 faster and collapsed at rates 3000 times faster than homogeneous PNIPAAm gels. Okano and co-workers (Kaneko et al., 1996; Yoshida et al., 1995) developed an ingenious method to prepare comb-type graft hydrogels of PNIPAAm. The main chain of the crosslinked PNIPAAm contained small molecular weight grafts of PNIPAAm. Under conditions of gel collapse (above the LCST), hydrophobic regions were developed in the pores of the gel resulting in a rapid collapse. These materials had the ability to collapse from a fully swollen conformation in less than 20 min while comparable gels that did not contain graft chains required up to a month to fully collapse. Such systems show major promise for rapid and abrupt or oscillatory release of drugs, peptides, or proteins.

Thermo-responsive polymers may be particularly useful for a wide variety of drug delivery applications (Hoffman, 1987; Kim, 1996). Okano et al. (1990) studied the temperature dependent permeability of PNIPAAm gels. They were able to use these gels as "on–off" delivery devices in response to temperature fluctuations. This type of behavior was useful for controlling the release of insulin (Bae et al., 1989) and heparin (Gutowska et al., 1992). These materials were used to modulate the release behavior of protein and peptide drugs (Gutowska et al., 1992), and were also used as "squeezing" systems (Yoshida et al., 1994). Okano et al. (Yamato et al., 2000, 2001) has pursued a novel temperature-sensitive cell culturing plate. By coating tissue culture plates with a uniformly thin coat of PNIPAAm, they have been able to create cell culture flasks with a switchable cellularly adhesive surface. This allows the growth of confluent layers of cells, which can be removed and either stacked to form multi-layered cells for *in vitro* study or *in vivo* tissue replacement (Nandkumar et al., 2002; Shimizu et al., 2003; von Recum et al., 1998).

Another promising application of these systems was explored by the Vernon et al. (1996). In this study, islets of Langerhans were entrapped by thermal gelation of PNIPAAm for use as a rechargeable artificial pancreas. Also, Fukumori et al. (Ichikawa and Fukumori, 2000; Ichikawa et al., 1998) worked with microcapsules coated in a thermosensitive layer comprised of either hydroxypropyl cellulose (HPC) or ethyl cellulose embedded with nano-particles of PNIPAAm hydrogels. These two systems result in two entirely different temperature sensitive drug release schemes. Drug release occurs readily below the LCST for the HPC coating, due to the more open mesh size present. However, above this temperature, the network collapses hindering solute transport. In the other system, the drug release occurs only at temperatures above the LCST. At these temperatures the nano-hydrogels are collapsed, leaving voids that allow for rapid release of solute. These systems were found to be fully reversible resulting in an "on/off" release behavior.

Other materials possessing a LCST near physiological conditions have also been persued. Yuk et al. (1997a,b) have proposed another temperature sensitive comonomer system comprising of DMAEMA and acrylamide (Aam). By changing the comonomer feed ratio, the LCST of these systems varied from 28°C to 50°C. They also developed a mathematical model to describe solute transport as a function of temperature and network swelling kinetics (Grassi et al., 1999). Ogata has also worked on hydrogels composed of the nucleic acid, uracil (Ogata, 1996). These hydrogels have been show to possess rapid volume changes at 35°C.

Another application of thermally sensitive hydrogels is in injectable, localized drug delivery systems. Cui and Messersmith (1998) used an aqueous solution of sodium alginate and temperature sensitive liposomes containing Ca^{2+} and drug. Once the solution is injected, the temperature of the body causes the liposomes to release the calcium ions and drug. These calcium ions then crosslink the alginate forming a hydrogel, and controlled release of the drug to the surrounding tissue is possible. Hoffman et al. (1997) created networks of chitosan grafted with Pluronic side chains. This copolymer system remains a solution until the temperature is raised to 37°C, and the side chains for hydrophobic domains that act to crosslink the network forming a hydrogel.

3. pH- and Temperature-Sensitive Hydrogels

Over the last decade, researchers have developed a novel class of hydrogels that exhibit both pH- and temperature-sensitive swelling behavior. These materials may prove to be extremely useful in enzymatic or protein drug delivery applications. Hydrogels were prepared from PNIPAAm and PAA that exhibited dual sensitivities (Dong et al., 1992; Feil et al., 1992). These gels were able to respond rapidly to both temperature and pH changes. Kim and co-workers investigated the use of such systems for carriers for insulin (Kim et al., 1994) and calcitonin (Serres et al., 1996). In general, these hydrogels only exhibited strong temperature sensitive swelling behavior with large amounts of PNIPAAm in the gel. Cationic pH- and temperature-sensitive gels were prepared using poly(amines) and PNIPAAm (Nabeshima et al., 1996). These systems were evaluated for local delivery of heparin.

Chen and Hoffman prepared new graft copolymers of PAA and PNIPAAm that responded more rapidly to external stimulus than previously studied materials (Chen and Hoffman, 1995). These materials exhibited increased temperature sensitivity due to the presence of the PNIPAAm grafts. Such systems were evaluated for use in prolonged mucosal delivery of bioactive agents, specifically peptide drugs (Hoffman et al., 1996).

Brazel and Peppas (1995) studied the pH- and temperature-responsive swelling behavior of gels containing PNIPAAm and PMAA. These materials were used to modulate the release behavior of streptokinase and heparin in response to pH and temperature changes (Brazel and Peppas, 1996). Baker and Siegel (1996) used similar hydrogels to modulate the glucose permeability. However, large amounts of PNIPAAm were needed to observe large temperature sensitivities. The group of Peppas developed novel pH- and temperature-sensitive terpolymers of PHEMA, PMAA, and PNIPAAm (Vakkalanka and Peppas, 1996). These systems were prepared to contain PNIPAAm-rich blocks and as a result, these materials were able to exhibit strong temperature sensitivity with only 10% PNIPAAm in the gel. Using these materials, they were effectively able to modulate the release kinetics of streptokinase (Vakkalanka et al., 1996).

A novel approach to pH and temperature sensitive drug release has been developed by the Ron et al. (1998). They developed a system which consists of two compartments, one which is a drug reservoir and the other contains a pH–temperature sensitive hydrogel comprised of carboxylic acid functionalized hydroxypropyl cellulose. During periods of neutral pH and low temperature, the gel is swollen preventing release of the drug from the reservoir. However, when the temperature increases, or pH decreases, the hydrogel barrier collapses, thus allowing drug release. Kaetsu et al. (1991, 1999a,b, 2000) also developed a similar technology on a silicon wafer chip. They photo etched pits into the wafer, and these pits were subsequently covered in a layer of polyethylene teraphthalate mesh filled with a polyelectrolytes gel. These gels covered the holes in the silicone wafer. Enzymes can be immobilized onto the gel, and act as the sensing mechanism. When the internal pH of the gel changes, it collapes, thus releasing the drug contained in the hole on the silicone wafer. The advantage to such a system is that a multitude of drug reservoirs can be placed onto a single chip, thus allowing for a localized complex drug delivery scheme.

4. Complexing Hydrogels

Another promising class of hydrogels that exhibit responsive behavior is complexing hydrogels. Osada studied complex formation in PMAA hydrogels (Osada, 1980). In acidic media, the PMAA membranes collapsed in the presence of linear PEG chains due to the formation of interpolymer complexes between the PMAA and PEG. The gels swelled when placed in

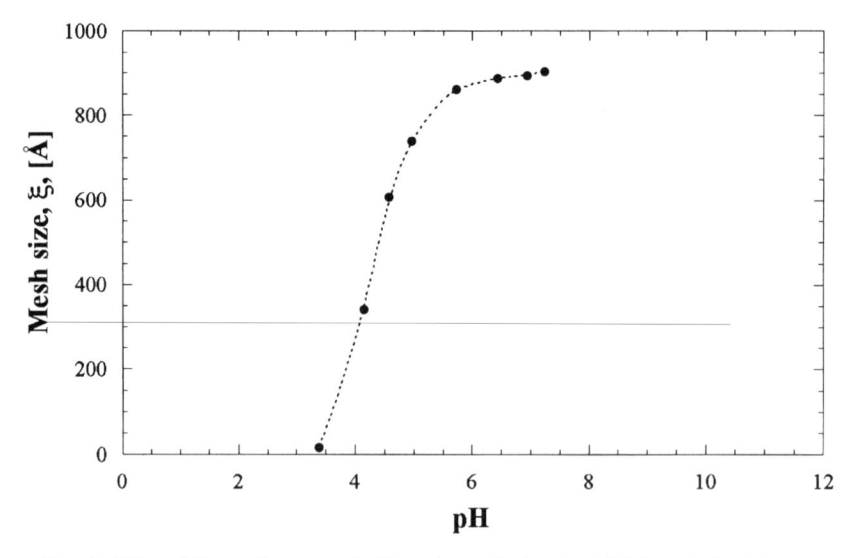

FIG. 8. Effect of the environmental pH on the mesh size, ξ, of PEG-grafted PAA polymer networks P(AA-g-PEG) of PEG molecular weight of 2000.

neutral or basic media. The permeability of these membranes was strongly dependent on the environmental pH and PEG concentration (Osada et al., 1986). Similar results were observed with hydrogels of PAA and linear PEG (Nishi and Kotaka, 1986). The significant change in permeability is directly related to the disruption of the polymer complexes, which results in gross changes in polymer mesh size (Fig. 8). Polymer complexation was also achieved in interpenetrating polymer networks of PVA and PAA (Byun et al., 1996; Shin et al., 1997). These systems, which exhibit pH and weak temperature sensitive behavior, were studied for their release behavior of indomethacin.

Peppas and co-workers has developed a class graft copolymer gels of PMAA grafted with PEG (P(MAA-g-EG)) (Bell and Peppas, 1995, 1996a,b,c; Klier et al., 1990; Lowman and Peppas, 1999a,b; Lowman et al., 1998; Peppas and Klier, 1991). These gels exhibited pH dependent swelling behavior due to the presence of acidic pendant groups and the formation of interpolymer complexes between the ether groups on the graft chains and protonated pendant groups. In these covalently crosslinked, complexing P(MAA-g-EG) hydrogels, complexation resulted in the formation of temporary physical crosslinks due to hydrogen bonding between the PEG grafts and the PMAA pendant groups. The physical crosslinks were reversible in nature and dependent on the pH and ionic strength of the environment. As a result, complexing hydrogels exhibit drastic changes in their mesh size over small changes of pH as shown in Fig. 9. One

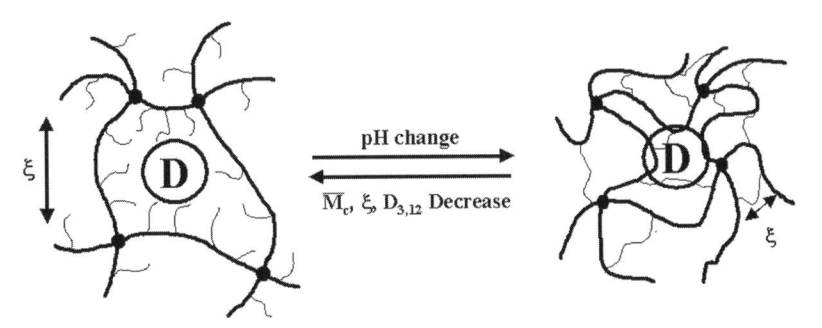

STRUCTURAL/DYNAMIC RESPONSE IN BIOMEDICAL ENVIRONMENTS 117

FIG. 9. The effect of interpolymer complexation on the correlation length, ξ, and the effective molecular weight between crosslinks, $\overline{M}_c$, in P(MAA-g-EG) graft copolymer networks with permanent, chemical crosslinks (●).

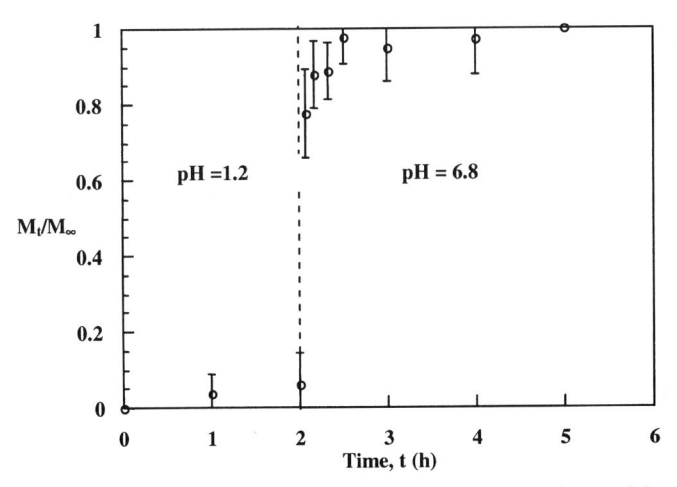

FIG. 10. Controlled release of insulin *in vitro* from P(MAA-g-EG) microparticles simulated gastric fluid (pH = 1.2) for the first two hours and phosphate buffered saline solutions (pH = 6.8) for the remaining three hours at 37°C (243).

particularly promising application for these systems is the oral delivery of protein and peptide drugs (Lowman *et al.*, 1998, 1999). As shown in Fig. 10, these copolymers severely limited the release of insulin in acidic environments like those found in the stomach. However, in conditions similar to those found in the intestines, insulin release occurred rapidly.

5. Glucose-sensitive Systems

Major developments have been reported in the utilization of environmentally responsive hydrogels as glucose-sensitive systems that could serve as self-regulated delivery devices for the treatment of diabetes. Typically, these systems have have been prepared by incorporating glucose oxidase into the hydrogel structure during the polymerization. In the presence of glucose, the glucose oxidase catalyzed the reaction between water and glucose to form gluconic acid. The gluconic acid lowered the pH of the microenvironment of the gel.

The first such systems developed by Kost et al. (1984) consisted of glucose oxidase immobilized in hydrogels based on PHEMA and PDMAEMA. These systems exhibited glucose sensitive swelling behavior. In the presence of glucose, gluconic acid was formed resulting in a decrease in the local pH. As a result, the cationic-based gel swelled to larger degrees in the presence of glucose due to the production of gluconic acid. The glucose responsive swelling behavior allowed for control over insulin permeation in these membranes by adjusting the environmental glucose concentrations (Albin et al., 1985; Ishihara et al., 1984). The kinetics of gel swelling and insulin release from cationic, glucose sensitive hydrogels was also studied (Goldraich and Kost, 1993).

Glucose responsive systems were proposed that were based on anionic hydrogels (Hassan et al., 1997; Ito et al., 1989). Ito et al. (1989) prepared systems of porous cellulose membranes containing an insulin reservoir. The pores of these devices were grafted with PAA chains functionalized with glucose oxidase. In the presence of glucose, the decrease in environmental pH caused the PAA chains to collapse opening the pores allowing for insulin release. More recently, glucose-sensitive complexation gels of P(MAA-g-EG) were developed by the group of Peppas (Hassan et al., 1997). In these gels, as the pH decreased in response to elevated glucose concentrations, interpolymer complexes formed resulting in rapid gel syneresis. The rapid collapse resulted in insulin release due to a "squeezing" phenomenon.

Other glucose responsive systems have been developed that take advantage of the formation of complexes between glucose molecules and polymeric pendant groups. Lee and Park (1994) prepared erodible hydrogels containing allyl glucose and poly(vinyl pyrrolidone). These systems were crosslinked by the noncovalent associations between concanavalin-A (Con-A) and the glucose pendant groups. In the presence of free glucose, the Con-A was bound to the free glucose and the gels dissolved due to disruption of the physical crosslinks. Newer materials developed by the group of Okano exhibited glucose responsive swelling behavior and insulin release (Aoki et al., 1996; Shiino et al., 1995, 1996). These gels were based on phenylboronic acid (PBA) and acrylamides. Another class of glucose-sensitive gels was prepared containing PBA, PNIPAAm, and PVA (Hisamitsu et al., 1997). These gels were designed to allow for the release of insulin at physiological pH and temperature.

C. Oral Insulin Delivery Systems

One of the major objectives of researchers working in the controlled release field is to design an effective, oral insulin delivery system. However, this is a difficult task due to the degradation of the drug in the upper gastrointestinal (GI) system barrier and the slow transport of insulin across the lining of the colon into the blood stream (Lee *et al.*, 1991; Saffran, 1992, 1997). Numerous attempts have been made by researchers to use hydrogels as carriers for oral delivery of insulin in order to protect the drug in the stomach and release it into more favorable regions of the GI tract.

Touitou and Rubinstein (1986) designed a reservoir system consisting of insulin encapsulated by a polyacrylate gel. The coating was designed to dissolve only in the colon. In this work, weak hypoglycemic effects were observed only with very high insulin doses and the addition of absorption enhancers. Saffran *et al.* (1986) developed a biodegradable hydrogel containing insulin. The device consisted of insulin dispersed in a terpolymer of styrene and PHEMA crosslinked with a difunctional azo-containing compound. The azo bond was cleaved by microflora present in the colon, and the polymer degraded allowing for release of insulin into the colon. In this work, a hypoglycemic effect was obtained only with addition of absorption enhancers and protease inhibitors. However, the hypoglycemic effect obtained was not affected by the initial dosing.

Morishita *et al.* (1992) administered insulin contained within Eudragit 100 gels. In these systems, the pH-responsive Eudragit® degraded in the upper small intestine allowing for insulin release. They observed strong hypoglycemic effects in healthy and diabetic rats after the addition of absorption enhancers. Platé *et al.* (1994) developed a hydrogel system containing immobilized insulin and protease inhibitors that was effective in lowering the blood glucose levels in rabbits. Mathiowitz *et al.* (1997) have developed insulin containing poly(anhydride) microspheres. These materials adhered to the walls of the small intestine and released insulin based on degradation of the polymeric carrier. They observed a 30% decrease in the blood glucose levels of healthy rats. Lowman *et al.* (1999) have developed a bioadhesive, complexation hydrogel system for oral delivery of insulin. This delivery system consisted of insulin-containing microparticles of crosslinked copolymers of P(MAA-*g*-EG). The P(MAA-*g*-EG) were more effective in delivering biologically active insulin than traditional enteric coating-type carriers because of the presence of the PEG-grafts.

The addition of PEG to the gels was critical because the PEG chains participate in the macromolecular complexes, function as a peptide stabilizer and enhance the mucoadhesive characteristics of the gels. In this work, strong dose-dependent hypoglycemic effects were observed in healthy and diabetic rats following oral administration of these gels.

D. Protein Based Hydrogels

Due to the overwhelming similarities of hydrogels and soft tissue extracellular matrices, it is not surprising to find many of its constituents being used to generate networks known as natural hydrogels. Collagen networks can be used as typical neutral hydrogels for sustained, local drug release. Moreover, collagen networks can be reabsorbed/remodeled by fibroblasts and endothelial cells, removing the need for explanting the hydrogel posttreatment (Sieminski and Gooch, 2000b). One interesting application of these networks has been the treatment of hair growth (Ozeki and Yasuhiko, 2002, 2003). In this work, they used collagen loaded with vascular endothelial growth factor or fibroblast growth factor in subcutaneous injections in order to stimulate follicle formation. In another system, Gooch et al. (Sieminski et al., 2002) used collagen gels for the support of endothelial cells genetically engineered to release human growth hormone. Here, the collagen networks allowed for the *in vitro* tubule formation of the modified EC. Then the collagen nework could be implanted, where the attachment of existing vasculature with the engineered cellular vasculature could occur.

Muzykantov et al. (Muzykantov et al., 1996, 1999; Shuvaev et al., in press) have developed a unique nanoparticle hydrogel composed entirely of crosslinked proteins. In their system, biotin–streptavidin conjugation chemistry, a strongly associating recognition pair, was used to link targeting groups, immunoglobulins (IgG), with drug. Dziubla et al. found that a simple Carathor's equation modified for nonequimolar monomer ratios and functionalities greater than 2 described the formation of the super-macromolecular structure of the conjugate (Shuvaev et al., 2003). These conjugates were capable of targeting organs with high vascular beds such as the lungs, when anti-PECAM (a unique endothelial cell adhesion molecule) was conjugated to antioxidants, such as catalase and super oxide dismutase. These conjugates were found to have a high utility in organ transplantation, where oxidative stress is one of the primary factors limiting organ storage prior to reimplantation (Kozower et al., 2003).

E. OTHER PROMISING APPLICATIONS

Promising new methods for the delivery of chemotherapeutic agents using hydrogels have been recently reported. Novel biorecognizable sugar-containing copolymers have been investigated for the use in targeted delivery of anti-cancer drugs (Peterson *et al.*, 1996; Putnam *et al.*, 1996; Rathi *et al.*, 1997). Kopecek and associates have used poly(N-2-hydroxypropyl methacrylamide) carriers for the treatment of ovarian cancer (Peterson *et al.*, 1996).

In the last few years there have been new creative methods of preparation of novel hydrophilic polymers and hydrogels that may represent the future in drug delivery applications. The focus in these studies has been the development of polymeric structures with precise molecular architectures. Stupp *et al.* (1997) synthesized self-assembled triblock copolymer, nanostructures that may have very promising applications in controlled drug delivery. Novel biodegradable polymers, such as polyrotaxanes, have been developed that have particularly exciting molecular assemblies for drug delivery (Ooya and Yui, 1997).

Dendrimers and star polymers (Dvornik and Tomalia, 1996) are exciting new materials because of the large number of functional groups available in a very small volume. Such systems could have tremendous promise in drug targeting applications. Merrill (1993) has offered an exceptional review of PEO star polymers and applications of such systems in the biomedical and pharmaceutical fields. Griffith and Lopina (1995) have prepared gels of controlled structure and large biological functionality by irradiation of PEO star polymers. Such new structures discussed in this section could have particularly promising delivery applications when combined with emerging new technologies such as molecular imprinting (Cheong *et al.*, 1997; Mosbach and Ramström, 1996).

A number of investigators have concentrated on the development of environmentally responsive gels that exhibit biodegradability. This can be achieved by a number of synthetic methods. Kopecek and co-workers (Ghandehari *et al.*, 1996) have developed biodegradable hydrogels by incorporating azo-compounds. Bae and co-workers (1989) have synthesized very promising biodegradable carriers by preparing 8-arm, star-shaped, block copolymers containing PLA and PEO. Another potentially useful biodegradable system is a photo-crosslinked polymer based on poly(L-lactic acid-*co*-L-aspartic acid) (Elisseeff *et al.*, 1996) which could be prepared *in situ* for delivery of anti-inflammatory drugs following surgery.

One of the most recent developments in the application of hydrogels have been in the field of microfluidics and microsensors. Peppas *et al.* (Bashir *et al.*, 2002; Hilt *et al.*, 2002) have successfully composed a microcantilever coated on one side with a PMAA hydrogel. Under pH changes, the equilibrium swelling of the coating changes, resulting in the deflection of the cantilever. Since this process is fully reversible, this has great implications for a rapid local pH and ionic devices. In another microfabrication application, DNA sequences have been included into poly acrylamide gels, which were photopolymerized as plugs within microfluidic channels (Seong *et al.*, 2002). These plugs can be used as microelectrophoretic gels which can hybridize with complementary DNA. Such systems may provide an enhancement over existing microchip assaying technologies due to increased mass transfer, lower sample volumes, and a potentially reusable substrate. Finally, microbioreactors have also been developed using hydrogels as the entrapment mechanism (Heo *et al.*, 2003). Here, *E. coli* were trapped within a hydrogel inside a microchannel. A nonfluorescent substrate (BCECF–am) that is converted into the fluorescent (BCECF) product by the esterase enzymes in the bacteria. Their work showed that viable bacteria can be immobilized within microchannels, and be used as either microbioreactors or sensors for the fluid flow.

REFERENCES

Albin, G., Horbett, T. A., and Ratner, B. D. *J. Control. Rel.* **2**, 153–164 (1985).
Am Ende, M. T., and Peppas, N. A. *J. Control. Rel.* **48**, 47–56 (1997).
Am Ende, M. T., and Peppas, N. A. *Pharm. Res.* **12**, 2030–2035 (1995).
Anderson, J. M. *Cardiovasc Pathol.* **2**, 33–41 (1993).
Anderson, J. M. *Trans. Am. Soc. Artif. Intern. Organs.* **19**, 101–107 (1988).
Anderson, J. M., Koinis, T., Nelson, T., Horst, M., and Love, D. S., The Slow Release of Hydrocortisone Sodium Succinate from Poly(2-Hydroxyethyl Methacrylate) Membranes, in "Hydrogels for Medical and Related Applications" (J. D. Andrade, Ed.), American Chemical Society: Washington. pp. 167–178. 1976.
Anseth, K., Bowman, C. N., and Brannon-Peppas, L. *Biomaterials* **17**, 1647–1657 (1996).
Antipina, A. D., Baranovskii, V., Papisov, I. M., and Kabanoc, V. A. *Vysokomol. Soyed.* **A14**, 941–949 (1972).
Aoki, T., Nagao, Y., Sanui, K., Ogata, N., Kikuchi, A., Sakurai, Y., Kataoka, K., and Okano, T. *Polym. J.* **28**, 371–374 (1996).
Badiger, M. V., McNeill, M. E., and Graham, N. B. *Biomaterials* **14**, 14 (1993).
Bae, Y. H., Okano, T., and Kim, S. W. *J. Control. Rel.* **9**, 271–276 (1989).
Bailey, F. E., Lundberg, R. D., and Callard, R. W. *J. Polym. Sci.* **A2**, 845–852 (1964).
Bajoras, G., and Makuska, R. *Polym. J.* **18**, 955–965 (1986).
Bakeev, N. F., Pshezhetsky, V. C., and Kargin, V. A. *Vysokomol. Soedin.*, 1812 (1959).
Baker, J. P., and Siegel, R. A. *Macromol. Rapid Commun.* **17**, 409–415 (1996).
Bashir, R., Hilt, J. Z., Elibol, O., Gupta, A., and Peppas, N. A. *Appl. Phys. Lett.* **81**, 3091–3093 (2002).
Bekturov, E. A., and Bimendina, L. A. *Adv. Polym. Sci.* **43**, 100–147 (1981).

Bell, C. L., and Peppas, N. A. *Adv. Polym. Sci.* **122**, 125–175 (1995).
Bell, C. L., and Peppas, N. A. *J. Biomater. Sci., Polym. Ed.* **7**, 671–683 (1996a).
Bell, C. L., and Peppas, N. A. *Biomaterials* **17**, 1203–1218 (1996b).
Bell, C. L., and Peppas, N. A. *J. Control. Rel.* **39**, 201–207 (1996c).
Beltran, S., Baker, J. P., Hooper, H. H., Blanch, H. W., and Prausnitz, J. M. *Macromolecules* **24**, 549–551 (1991).
Bettini, R., Colombo, P., and Peppas, N. A. *J. Control. Rel.* **37**, 105–111 (1995).
Bimendina, L. A., Roganov, V. V., and Bekturov, E. A. *J Polym. Sci. Polym. Symp.* **44**, 65–74 (1974).
Bimendina, L. A., Tleubaeva, G. S., and Bekturov, E. A. *Europ. Polym. J.* **10**, 629–632 (1977).
Biros, I., Masa, L., and Pouchly, J. *Europ. Polym. J.* **10**, 629–632 (1974).
Bodmeier, R., and Paeratakul, O. *J. Pharm. Sci.* **78**, 964–969 (1989).
Brannon-Peppas, L., and Harland, R. S. Absorbent polymer technology, *in* "Studies in Polymer Science", Vol. 8, pp. 278. Elsevier; Distributors for the United States and Canada Elsevier Science Pub., Amsterdam, New York, NY, U.S.A. (1990).
Brannon-Peppas, L., and Peppas, N. A. *J. Control. Rel.* **8**, 267–274 (1989).
Brannon-Peppas, L., and Peppas, N. A. *Biomaterials* **11**, 635–644 (1990).
Brannon-Peppas, L., and Peppas, N. A. *Chem. Eng. Sci.* **46**, 715–722 (1991a).
Brannon-Peppas, L., and Peppas, N. A. *Int. J. Pharm.* **70**, 53–57 (1991b).
Brannon-Peppas, L., and Peppas, N. A. *J. Control. Rel.* **16**, 319–329 (1991c).
Bratoz, S., Hadzi, D., and Sheppard, N. *Spectrochim. Acta.* **8**, 249–261 (1956).
Brauker, J. H., Carr-Brendel, V. E., Martinson, L. A., Crudele, J., and Johnston, W. D. *J. Bio. Mat. Res.* **29**, 1517–1524 (1995).
Brazel, C. S., and Peppas, N. A. *Macromolecules* **28**, 8016–8020 (1995).
Brazel, C. S., and Peppas, N. A. *J. Control. Rel.* **39**, 57–64 (1996).
Bromberg, L. *J. Appl. Polym. Sci.* **59**, 459–466 (1996).
Byun, J., Lee, Y. M., and Cho, C. S. *J. Appl. Polym. Sci.* **61**, 697–702 (1996).
Calvo, P., Remunán-López, C., Vila-Jato, J. L., and Alonso, M. J. *J. Appl. Polym. Sci.* **63**, 125–132 (1997).
Canal, T., and Peppas, N. A. *J. Biomed. Mater. Res.* **23**, 1183–1193 (1989).
Carenza, M., and Veronese, F. M. *J. Control. Rel.* **29**, 187–193 (1994).
Castillo, E. J., Koenig, J. L., and Anderson, J. M. *Biomaterials* **7**, 89–96 (1986a).
Castillo, E. J., Koenig, J. L., Anderson, J. M., and Jentoft, N. *Biomaterials* **7**, 9–16 (1986b).
Castillo, E. J., Koenig, J. L., Anderson, J. M., Kliment, C. K., and Lo, J. *Biomaterials* **5**, 186–193 (1984a).
Castillo, E. J., Koenig, J. L., Anderson, J. M., and Lo, J. *Biomaterials* **5**, 319–325 (1984b).
Castillo, E. J., Koenig, J. L., Anderson, J. M., and Lo, J. *Biomaterials* **6**, 338–345 (1985).
Chen, G. H., and Hoffman, A. S. *Nature* **373**, 49–52 (1995).
Cheong, S. H., McNiven, S., Rachkov, A., Levi, R., Yano, K., and Karube, I. *Macromolecules* **30**, 1317–1322 (1997).
Chirila, T. V., Constable, I. J., Crawford, G. J., Vijayasekaran, S., Thompson, D. E., Chen, Y.-C., Fletcher, W. A., and Griffen, B. J. *Biomaterials* **14**, 26–38 (1993).
Chirila, T. V., Higgins, B., and Dalton, P. D. *Cell. Polym.* **17**, 141–162 (1998).
Clayton, A. B., Chirila, T. V., and Dalton, P. D. *Polym. Int.* **42**, 45–56 (1997a).
Clayton, A. B., Chirila, T. V., and Lou, X. *Polym. Int.* **44**, 201–207 (1997b).
Coleman, M., Graf, J., and Painter, P., "Specific Interactions and the Miscibility of Polymer Blends: Practical Guides for Predicting & Designing Miscible Polymer Systems". Technomic Publishing Co., Inc, Lancaster, PA (1991).
Cook, A. *J. Biomed. Mater. Res.* **35**, 513–523 (1997).

Cornejo-Bravo, J. M., and Siegel, R. A. *Biomaterials* **17,** 1187–1193 (1996).
Crank, J., and Park, G. S., "Diffusion in Polymers", p. 452. Academic Press, London, New York, 1968.
Cui, H., and Messersmith, P. B., *ACS Symp. Ser.* 203–211 (1998).
Dalton, P. D., Flynn, L., and Shoichet, M. S. *Biomaterials* **23,** 3843–3851 (2002).
Davidson, G. W. R. III, and Peppas, N. A. *J. Control. Rel.* **3,** 243–258 (1986).
Deng, X. M., Castillo, E. J., and Anderson, J. M. *Biomaterials* **7,** 247–251 (1986).
Dong, L. C., and Hoffman, A. S. *J. Control. Rel.* **13,** 21–31 (1990).
Dong, L. C., Yan, Q., and Hoffman, A. S. *J. Control. Rel.* **19,** 171–178 (1992).
Drescher, B., Scranton, A. B., and Klier, J. *Polym.* **42,** 49–58 (2001).
Dvornik, P. R., and Tomalia, D. A. *Curr. Opin. Colloid Interf. Sci.* **1,** 221–235 (1996).
Dziubla, T. D., and Lowman Anthony, M., *J. Biomed. Mater. Res.* In Press.
Dziubla, T. D., Lowman, A. M., Torjman, M. C., and Joseph, J. I., *Biomimetic Materials and Design,* 507–531 (2002).
Dziubla, T. D., Peppas, N. A., and Lowman, A. M. *Proceedings of the International Symposium on Controlled Release of Bioactive Materials* **26,** 539–540 (1999).
Elisseeff, J., Anseth, K., Langer, R., and Hrkach, J. S. *Macromolecules* **30,** 2182–2184 (1996).
Eyring, H. *J. Chem. Phys.* **4,** 283–289 (1936).
Faxen, H. *Arkiv. Mat. Astronom. Fys.* **17,** 27 (1923).
Feil, H., Bae, Y. H., and Kim, S. W. *Macromolecules* **25,** 5528–5530 (1992).
Ferguson, J., and Shah, S. A. O. *Eur. Polym. J.* **4,** 343–354 (1968).
Ficek, B. J., and Peppas, N. A. *J. Control. Rel.* **27,** 259–264 (1993).
Firestone, B. A., and Siegel, R. A. *Polym. Comm.* **29,** 204–208 (1988).
Flory, P. J., and Rehner, J. Jr. *J. Chem. Phys.* **11,** 521–526 (1943a).
Flory, P. J., and Rehner, J. Jr. *J. Chem. Phys.* **11,** 512–520 (1943b).
Flory, P. J. "Principles of Polymer Chemistry", p. 672. Cornell Univ. Press, Ithaca, New York, 1953.
Franson, N. M., and Peppas, N. A. *J. Appl. Polym. Sci.* **28,** 1299–1310 (1983).
Fugita, H. *Fortschr. Hochpolym. Forsch.* **3,** 1–14 (1961).
Gallin, J., Goldstein, I. M., and Snyderman, R., "Inflammation: Basic Principles and Clinical Correlates". Raven Press, New York (1988).
Ghandehari, K. P., Yeh, P.Y., and Kopecek, J. *Macromol. Chem. Phys.* 197, 965–980 (1996).
Goldraich, M., and Kost, J. *Clinical Materials* **13,** 135–142 (1993).
Good, W. R., "Diffusion of Water Soluble Drugs from Initially Dry Hydrogels" (R. Kostelnik, Ed.), pp. 139–155. Gordon & Breach, New York (1976).
Graham, N. B., Poly(ethylene glycol) Gels and Drug Delivery, *in* "Poly(Ethylene Glycol) Chemistry: Biotechnical and Biomedical Applications" (J. M. Harris, Ed.), pp. 263–281. Plenum Press, New York (1992).
Grassi, M., Hong Yuk, S., and Hang Cho, S. *J. Membr. Sci.* 241–249 (1999).
Griffith, L., and Lopina, S. T. *Macromolecules* **28,** 6787–6794 (1995).
Gudeman, L. F., and Peppas, N. A. *J. Membr. Sci.* **107,** 239–248 (1995).
Gutowska, A., Bae, Y. H., Feijen, J., and Kim, S. W. *J. Control. Rel.* **22,** 95–104 (1992).
Hadzi, D. *Pure Appl. Chem.* **11,** 435–453 (1965).
Hadzi, D. *Chimia.* **26,** 7–13 (1976).
Hariharan, D., and Peppas, N. A. *Polymer* **37,** 149–161 (1996).
Harland, R. S., and Peppas, N. A. *Colloid Polym. Sci.* **267,** 218–225 (1989).
Hassan, C. M., Doyle, F. J. III, and Peppas, N. A. *Macromolecules* **30,** 6166–6173 (1997).
Heller, J., Chang, A. C., Rodd, G., and Grodsky, G. M. *J. Control. Rel.* **11,** 193–201 (1990).
Hennink, W. E., Franssen, O., and Van Dijk-Wolthuis, W. N. E. *J. Control. Rel.* **48,** 107–114 (1997).

Henson, P. *Am. J. Pathol.* **101**, 494–511 (1980).
Heo, J., Thomas, J., Seong, G. H., and Crooks, R. M. *Anal. Chem.* **75**, 22–26 (2003).
Hickey, A. S., and Peppas, N. *J. Membr. Sci.* **107**, 229–237 (1995).
Hilt, J. Z., Gupta, A. K., Bashir, R., and Peppas, N. A. *Materials Research Society Symposium Proceedings* **729**, 173–178 (2002).
Hisamitsu, K. K., Okano, T., and Sakurai, Y., *Pharm. Res.* **14**, 289–293 (1997).
Hoffman, A. S., Chen, G. H., Kaang, S. Y., Ding, Z. L., Randeri, K., and Kabra, B., Novel Bioadhesive pH- and Temperature-sensitive Graft Copolymers for Prolonged Mucosal Drug Delivery, *in* "Advanced Biomaterials in Biomedical Engineering and Drug Delivery Systems" (N. Ogata, *et al.*, Eds.), pp. 62–66. Springer, Tokyo (1996).
Hoffman, A. S., Matsura, J. E., Wu, X., and Gombotz, W. R., *Proc. Int. Symp. Controlled Release Bioact. Mater.* 126–127 (1997).
Hoffman, A. S. *J. Controlled Rel.* **6**, 297–305 (1987).
Hopfenberg, H. B., and Hsu, K. C. *Polym. Eng. Sci.* **18**, 1186 (1978).
Hubbel, J. *Ann. NY Acad. Sci.* **665**, 253–258 (1992).
Ichikawa, H. and Fukumori, Y., *J. Controlled Rel.* 107–119 (2000).
Ichikawa, H., Ohdoi, A., Fujioka, K., and Fukumori, Y. *World Congr. Part. Technol.* **3**, 1225–1234 (1998).
Ingber, D. E., and Folkman, J. *J. Cell. Bio.* **109**, 317–330 (1989).
Ishihara, K., Kobayashi, M., and Shinohara, I. *Polym. J.* **16**, 625–631 (1984).
Ito, Y., Casolaro, M., Kono, K., and Imanishi, Y. *J. Controll. Rel.* **10**, 195–203 (1989).
Kabra, B. G., and Gehrke, S. H. *Polym. Comm.* **32**, 322–323 (1991).
Kaetsu, I., Morita, Y., Takimoto, O., Yoshihara, M., Ohtori, A., and Andoh, M. *Proc. Program Int. Symp. Controlled Release Bioact. Mater., 18th.* pp. 449–450 (1991).
Kaetsu, I., Uchida, K., and Sutani, K. *Radiat. Phys. Chem.* 673–676 (1999a).
Kaetsu, I., Uchida, K., Shindo, H., Gomi, S., and Sutani, K. *Radiat. Phys. Chem.* 193–201 (1999b).
Kaetsu, I., Uchida, K., Sutani, K., and Sakata, S. *Radiat. Phys. Chem.* 465–469 (2000).
Kaneko, Y., Saki, K., Kikuchi, A., Sakurai, Y., and Okano, T. *Macromol. Symp.* **109**, 41–53 (1996).
Kang, H. W., Tabata, Y., and Ikada, Y. *Biomaterials* **20**, 1339–1344 (1999).
Katchalsky, A., and Michaeli, I. *J. Polym. Sci.* **15**, 69–86 (1955).
Khare, A. R., and Peppas, N. A. *J. Biomater. Sci. Polym. Ed.* **4**, 275–289 (1993).
Kikuchi, A., Kawabuchi, M., Sugihara, M., Sakurai, Y., and Okano, T. *J. Control. Rel.* **47**, 21–29 (1997).
Kim, S. W., Temperature Sensitive Polymers for Delivery of Macromolecular Drugs, *in* "Advanced Biomaterials in Biomedical Engineering and Drug Delivery Systems" (N. Ogata, *et al.*, Eds.), pp. 125–133. Springer, Tokyo (1996).
Kim, Y. H., Bae, Y. H., and Kim, S. W. *J. Control. Rel.* **28**, 143–152 (1994).
Klier, J., Scranton, A. B., and Peppas, N. A. *Macromolecules* **23**, 4944–4949 (1990).
Kliment, K., Stol, M., Fahoun, K., and Stockar, B. *J. Bio. Mat. Res.* **2**, 237–243 (1968).
Klomp, G. F., Hashiguchi, H., Ursell, P. C., Takeda, Y., Taguchi, T., and Dobelle, W. H. *J. Bio. Mat. Res.* **17**, 865–871 (1983).
Koenig, J. L., "Spectroscopy of Polymers". American Chemical Society, Washington, DC (1992).
Kofinas, P., Athanassiou, V., and Merrill, E. W. *Biomaterials* **17**, 1547–1550 (1996).
Korsmeyer, R. W., and Peppas, N. A. *J. Membr. Sci.* **9**, 211–227 (1981).
Korsmeyer, R. W., and Peppas, N. A. *J. Controlled Rel.* **1**, 89–98 (1984).
Kost, J., Horbett, T. A., Ratner, B. D., and Singh, M. *J. Biomed. Mater. Res.* **19**, 1133–1177 (1984).

Kou, J. H., Almindon, G. L., and Lee, P. I. *Pharm. Res.* **5**, 592–597 (1988).
Kozower, B. D., Christofidou-Solomidou, M., Sweitzer, T. D., Muro, S., Buerk, D. G., Solomides, C. C., Albelda, S. M., Patterson, G. A., and Muzykantov, V. R. *Nature Biotechnology* **21**, 392–398 (2003).
Langer, R., and Folkman, J. *Nature* **263**, 970–974 (1976).
Langer, R., and Peppas, N. *J. Macromol. Sci. Rev. Macromol. Chem. Phys.* **C23**, 61–126 (1983).
Lee, P. I. *Polymer* **25**, 973 (1984).
Lee, P. I. *J. Control. Rel.* **73**, 1344 (1986).
Lee, S. J., and Park, K. *Polym. Prepr.* **35**, 391–392 (1994).
Lee, V. H. L., Dodd-Kashi, S., Grass, G. M., and Rubas, W., Oral Route of Peptide and Protein Drug Delivery, *in* "Protein and Peptide Drug Delivery" (V. H. L. Lee Ed.), pp. 691–740. Marcel Dekker Inc., New York (1991).
Lee, J. Y., Painter, P. C., and Coleman, M. M. *Macromolecules* **21**, 954–960 (1988).
Lightfoot, E.N., Transport phenomena and living systems; biomedical aspects of momentum and mass transport, p. 495. Wiley, New York (1973).
Lipsky, M.H., Lamberton, P. *J. Bio. Mat. Res.* **23**, 1441–1452 (1989).
Liquori, A. M., De Santis, S. M., and D'alagni, M. *J. Polym. Sci.* **B4**, 943–945 (1966).
Liu, Q., Hedberg, E. L., Liu, Z., Bahulekar, R., Meszlenyi, R. K., and Mikos, A. G. *Biomaterials* **21**, 2163–2169 (2000).
Lou, X., Dalton, P. D., and Chirila, T. V. *J. Mat. Sci. Mat. Med.* **11**, 319–325 (2000).
Lowman, A. M., and Peppas, N. A. *Macromolecules* **30**, 4959–4965 (1997).
Lowman, A. M., and Peppas, N. A. *Polymer* **41**, 73–80 (1999a).
Lowman, A. M., and Peppas, N. A. *ACS Symp. Series* **728**, 30–42 (1999b).
Lowman, A. M., Dziubla, T. D., and Peppas, N. A. *Polymer Preprints (American Chemical Society Division of Polymer Chemistry)* **38**, 622–623 (1997).
Lowman, A. M., Peppas, N. A., Morishita, M., and Nagai, T. *ACS Symp. Series* **709**, 156–164 (1998).
Lowman, A. M., Morishita, M., Kajita, M., Nagai, T., and Peppas, N. A. *J. Pharm. Sci.* **88**, 933–937 (1999).
Malech, H., and Gallin, J. *N. Engl. J. Med.* **317**, 687–694 (1987).
Mallapragada, S. K., and Peppas, N. A. *J. Control. Rel.* **45**, 87–94 (1997a).
Mallapragada, S. K., and Peppas, N. A. *AIChE J.* **43**, 870–876 (1997b).
Mark, J. E. *Adv. Polym Sci.* **44**, 1–26 (1982).
Mathiowitz, Jacob, J. S., Jong, Y. S., Carino, G. P., Chickering, D. E., Chaturvedi, P., Santos, C.A., Vijayaraghavan, K., Montgomery, S., Bassett, M., and Morrell, C. *Nature* **386**, 410–414 (1997).
Matsuda, T. and Kurumantani, H. *ASAIO Trans.* 36 (1990).
McNeill, M. E., and Graham, N. B. *J. Control. Rel.* **1**, 99–107 (1984).
McNeill, M. E., and Graham, N. B. *J. Biomater. Sci. Polym. Ed.* **7**, 937–951 (1996).
Merrill, E. W. *J. Biomater. Sci. Polym. Ed.* **5**, 1–11 (1993).
Miyoshi, T., Takegoshi, K., and Hikichi, K. *Polymer* **37**, 11–18 (1996).
Miyoshi, T., Takegoshi, K., and Hikichi, K. *Polymer* **38**, 2315–2320 (1997).
Mongia, N. K., Anseth, K. S., and Peppas, N. A. *J. Biomater. Sci. Polym. Ed.* **7**, 1055–1064 (1996).
Morimoto, K., Nagayasu, A., Fukanoki, S., Morisaka, K., Hyon, S. Y., and Ikada, Y. *Pharm. Res.* **6**, 338–344 (1989).
Morishita, I., Morishita, M., Takayama, K., Machida, Y., and Nagai, T. *Int. J. Pharm.* **78**, 9–16 (1992).
Mosbach, K., and Ramström, O. *Biotechnology* **14**, 163–170 (1996).

Muzykantov, V. R., Atochina, E. N., Ischiropoulos, H., Danilov, S. M., and Fisher, A. B. *Proc. Natl. Acad. Sci. USA* **93,** 5213–5218 (1996).

Muzykantov, V. R., Christofidou-Solomidou, M., Balyasnikova, I., Harshaw, D. W., Schultz, L., Fisher, A. B., and Albelda, S. M. *Proc. Natl. Acad. Sci. USA* **96,** 2379–2384 (1999).

Nabeshima, Y., Ding, Z. L., Chen, G. H., Hoffman, A. S., Taira, H., Kataoka, K., and Tsuruta, T., Slow release of heparin from a hydrogel made from polyamine chains to a temperature-sensitive polymer backbone, *in* "Advanced Biomaterials in Biomedical Engineering and Drug Delivery Systems" (N. Ogata, *et al.*, Eds.), pp. 315–316. Springer, Tokyo (1996).

Nandkumar, M. A., Yamato, M., Kushida, A., Konno, C., Hirose, M., Kikuchi, A., and Okano, T. *Biomaterials* **23,** 1121–1130 (2002).

Narasimhan, B., and Peppas, N. A. *J. Pharm. Sci.* **86,** 297–304 (1997a).

Narasimhan, B. and Peppas, N.A. *Control. Drug Deliv.* 529–557 (1997b).

Narasimhan, B., Mallapragada, S. K., and Peppas Nicholas, A., Release Kinetics: Data Interpretation, *in* "Encyclopedia of Controlled Drug Delivery" (E. Mathiowitz Ed.), pp. 921–935. Wiley, New York (1999).

Narayani, R., and Rao, K. P. *J. Appl. Polym. Sci.* **58,** 1761–1769 (1995).

Nishi, S., and Kotaka, T. *Macromolecules* **19,** 978–984 (1986).

Odinokov, S. E., Mashkovsky, A. A., and Glazunov, V. P. *Spectrochim. Acta* **32A,** 1355–1363 (1976).

Ogata, N., in *Int. Conf. Adapt. Struct., 6th.* pp. 54–60. (1996).

Oh, S. H., and Jhon, M. S. *J. Polym. Sci. Polym. Chem.* **27,** 1731–1739 (1989).

Okano, T., Bae, Y. H., Jacobs, H., and Kim, S. W. *J. Control. Rel.* **11,** 255–265 (1990).

Ooya, T., and Yui, N. *J. Biomater. Sci. Polym. Ed.* **8,** 437–445 (1997).

Oppermann, W., Swelling Behavior and Elastic Properties of Ionic Hydrogels, *in* "Polyelectrolyte Gels: Properties, Preparation, and Applications" (R. S. Harland and R. K. Prud'homme Eds.), pp. 159–170. American Chemical Society, Washington (1992).

Osada, Y., Honda, K., and Ohta, M. *J. Membr. Sci.* **27,** 339–347 (1986).

Osada, Y. *J. Polym. Sci. Polym. Letters Ed.* **18,** 281–286 (1980).

Oxley, H., Corkhill, P. H., Fitton, J. H., and Tighe, B. J. *Biomaterials* **14,** 1064–1072 (1993).

Ozeki, M., and Yasuhiko, T. (2002).

Ozeki, M., and Yasuhiko, T. *Biomaterials* **24,** 2387–2394 (2003).

Padera, R. F., and Colton, C. K. *Biomaterials* **17,** 277–284 (1996).

Papisov, I. M., Baranovskii, V., Sergeiva, Y. I., Antipina, A. D., and Kabanov, V. A. *Vysokomol. Soyed.* **A16,** 1122–1141 (1974).

Park, K., "Controlled Release: Challenges and Strategies". ACS, Washington (1997).

Patterson, K. G., Padgett, S. J., and Peppas Nicholas, A. *Colloid Polym. Sci.* **260,** 851–858 (1982).

Peppas, N. A. *Makromol. Chem.* **176,** 3433–3440 (1975).

Peppas, N. A., Hydrogels of Poly(vinyl alcohol) and its copolymers, *in* "Hydrogels in Medicine and Pharmacy" (A. Peppas Nicholas Ed.), pp. 1–48. CRC Press, Boca Raton (1986a).

Peppas, N.A., "Hydrogels in Medicine and Pharmacy", Vol. 3. Boca Raton, Fla.: CRC Press (1986b).

Peppas, N. A., Hydrogels of poly(vinyl alcohol) and its copolymers, *in* "Hydrogels in Medicine and Pharmacy" (N. A. Peppas Ed.), pp. 1–48. CRC Press, Boca Raton, FL (1987).

Peppas, N. A. *J. Bioact. Compat. Polym.* **6,** 241–246 (1991).

Peppas, N. A., Fundamentals of pH- and temperature-sensitive delivery systems, *in* "Pulsatile Drug Delivery, Wissenschaftliche Verlagesellschaft" (R. Gurny, H.E. Junginger, and N. A. Peppas, Eds.), pp. 41–56. Stuttgart (1993).

Peppas, N. A. *Curr. Opin. Colloid Interf. Sci.* **2**, 531–537 (1997).
Peppas, N. A., and Barr-Howell, B. D., Characterization of the crosslinked structure of hydrogels, in "Hydrogels in Medince and Pharmacy" (N. A. Peppas Ed.), Vol. 1, pp. 27–56. CRC Press, Boca Raton, FL (1986).
Peppas, N. A., and Colombo, P. *J. Contr. Rel.* **45**, 35–40 (1997).
Peppas, N. A., and Hansen, P. J. *J. Appl. Polym. Sci.* **27**, 4787–4797 (1982).
Peppas, N. A., and Klier, J. *J. Control. Rel.* **16**, 203–214 (1991).
Peppas, N. A., and Langer, R. *Science* **263**, 1715–1720 (1994).
Peppas, N. A., and Merrill, E. W. *J. Polym. Sci. Polym. Chem. Ed* **14**, 441–457 (1976a).
Peppas, N. A., and Merrill, E. W. *J. Appl. Polym. Sci.* **20**, 457–1465 (1976b).
Peppas, N. A., and Merrill, E. W. *J. Appl. Polym. Sci.* **21**, 1763–1770 (1977).
Peppas, N. A., and Mikos, A. G. *Hydrogels Med. Pharm.* **1**, 1–25 (1986).
Peppas, N. A., and Mongia, N. K. *Eur. J. Pharm. Biopharm.* **43**, 51–58 (1997).
Peppas, N. A., and Moynihan, H. J. *J. Appl. Polym. Sci.* **30**, 2589–2606 (1985).
Peppas, N. A., and Reinhart, C. T. *J. Membr. Sci.* **15**, 275–287 (1983).
Peppas, N. A., and Scott, J. E. *J. Control. Rel.* **18**, 95–100 (1992).
Peppas, N. A., and Stauffer, S. R. *J. Control. Rel.* **16**, 305–310 (1991).
Peppas, N. A., and Wright, S. L. *Macromolecules* **29**, 8798–8804 (1996).
Perova, T. S., Vij, J. K., and Xu, H., *Colloid Polym. Sci.* **275**, 323–332 (1997).
Peterson, C. M., Lu, J. M., Sun, Y., Peterson, C. A., Shiah, J. G., Straight, R. C., and Kopecek, J. *Cancer Res.* **56**, 3980–3985 (1996).
Philippova, O. E., and Starodubtzev, S. G. *J Mat Sci. Pure Appl. Chem.* **A32**, 1893–1902 (1995).
Philippova, O. E., Karibyants, N. S., and Starodubtzev, S. G. *Macromolecules* **27**, 2398–2401 (1994).
Platé, N. A., Valuev, L. I., Starosel'tseva, L. K., Valueva, T. A., Vanchugova, L. V., Ul'yanova, M. V., Valuev, I. L., Sytov, G. A., Ametov, A. S., and Knyazhev, V. A. *Vysokomol. Soedin.* **36**, 1876–1879 (1994).
Putnam, D. A., Shiah, J. G., and Kopecek, J. *Biochem. Pharmac.* **52**, 957–962 (1996).
Rathi, R. C., Kopecková, P., and Kopecek, J. *Macromol. Chem. Phys.* **198**, 1–16 (1997).
Ratner, B. D. and Hoffman, A. S., Synthetic Hydrogels for Biomedical Applications, in "Hydrogels for Medical and Related Applications" (Andrade, Ed.), pp. 1–36. American Chemical Society, Washington, D.C. (1976).
Ratner, B. D., and Miller, I. F. *J Polym. Sci.* **A1, 10**, 2425 (1972).
Ricka, J., and Tanaka, T. *Macromolecules* **17** (1984).
Ron, E. S., Schiller, M. E., Roos, E., Orkisz, M., and Staples, A., *PCT Int. Appl.* (Gel Sciences, Inc., USA). WO. p. 43. (1998).
Ronel, S. H., D'Andrea, M. J., Hashiguchi, H., Klomp, G. F., and Dobelle, W. H. *J. Bio. Mat. Res.* **17**, 855–864 (1983).
Rosengren, A., Danielsen, N., and Bjursten, L. M. *J. Bio. Mat. Res.* **46**, 458–464 (1999).
Saffran, M., Kumar, G. S., Savariar, C., Burnham, J. C., Williams, F., and Neckers, D. C. *Science* **233**, 1081–1084 (1986).
Saffran, M., Oral Colon-Specific Drug Delivery With Emphasis on Insulin, in "Oral Colon-Specific Drug Delivery" (D. R. Friend Ed.), pp. 115–142. CRC Press, Boca Raton (1992).
Saffran, M., Pansky, B., Budd, G. C., and Williams, F. E. *J. Control. Rel.* **46**, 89–98 (1997).
Saltzman, W. M., Cell Interactions with polymers, in "Principles of Tissue Engineering" (R. Lanza Ed.), pp. 228–246. RG Landes Company, Austin, TX (1997).
Sato, H., and Nakajima, A. *Polym. J.* **7**, 241–247 (1975).
Scharp, D. W., Mason, N. S., and Sparks, R. E. *World J. Surg.* **8**, 221–229 (1984).
Schwarte, L. M., and Peppas, N. A. *Polymer Preprints (American Chemical Society Division of Polymer Chemistry)* **38**, 596–597 (1997).

Schwarte, L. M., and Peppas, N. A. *Polymer* **39**, 6057–6066 (1998).
Schwarte, L. M., Podual, K., and Peppas, N. A. *ACS Symp. Series* **709**, 56–66 (1998).
Scranton, A. B., Rangarajan, B., and Klier, J. *Adv. Polym. Sci.* **120**, 1–54 (1995).
Sefton, M., and Nishimura, E. *J. Pharm. Sci.* **69**, 208–213 (1980).
Seong, G. H., Zhan, W., and Crooks, R. M. *Anal. Chem.* **74**, 3372–3377 (2002).
Serres, A., Baudyš, M., and Kim, S. W. *Pharm. Res.* **13**, 196–201 (1996).
Shiino, D., Kubo, A., Murata, Y., Kim, Y. J., Koyama, Y., Kataoka, K., Kikuchi, A., Sakurai, Y., and Okano, T. *J. Biomater. Sci. Polym. Ed.* **7**, 697–705 (1996).
Shiino, D., Murata, Y., Kubo, A., Kim, Y. J., Kataoka, K., Koyama, Y., Kikuchi, A., Yokoyama, M., Sakurai, Y., and Okano, T. *J. Conrol. Rel.* **37**, 269–276 (1995).
Shimizu, T., Yamato, M., Kikuchi, A., and Okano, T. *Biomaterials* **24**, 2309–2316 (2003).
Shin, H. S., Kim, S. Y., and Lee, Y. M. *J. Appl. Polym. Sci.* **65**, 685–693 (1997).
Shiraishi, S., Imai, T., and Otagiri, M. *J. Controlled Rel.* **25**, 217–223 (1993).
Shuvaev, V., Dziubla, T. D., Rainer, W., and Muzykantov, V., Streptavidin-biotin crosslinking of therapeutic enzymes with carrier antibodies: nanoconjugates for protection against endothelial oxidative stress, *in* "Methods in Molecular biology", (C. Niemeyer, ed.), Humane Press, Louisville, KY (in press).
Shwarkawy, A. A., Klitzman, B., Truskey, G. A., and Reichert, W. M. *J. Biomed. Mater. Res.* **37**, 401–412 (1997).
Shwarkawy, A. A., Klitzman, B., Truskey, G. A., and Reichert, W. M. *J. Biomed. Mater. Res.* **40**, 586–597 (1998a).
Shwarkawy, A. A., Klitzman, B., Truskey, G. A., and Reichert, W. M. *J. Biomed. Mater. Res.* **40**, 598–605 (1998b).
Siegel, R. A., and Firestone, B. A. *Macromolecules* **21**, 3254–3259 (1988).
Siegel, R. A., Falamarzian, M., Firestone, B. A., and Moxley, B. C. *J. Control. Rel.* **8**, 179–182 (1988).
Siegel, R. A., pH-Sensitive Gels: Swelling Equilibria, Kinetics, and Applications for Drug Delivery, *in* "Pulsed and Self-Regulated Drug Delivery" (J. Kost Ed.), pp. 129–155. CRC Press, Boca Raton (1990).
Siegel, R. A., "Modeling of Self-Regulating Oscillatory Drug Delivery" (K. Park Ed.), pp. 1–27. American Chemical Society, Washington (1997).
Sieminski, A. L., and Gooch, K. J. *Biomaterials* **21**, 2233–2241 (2000a).
Sieminski, A. L., and Gooch, K. J. *Biomaterials* **21**, 2232–2241 (2000b).
Sieminski, A. L., Padera, R. F., Blunk, T., and Gooch, K. J. *Tissue Eng.* **8**, 1057–1069 (2002).
Silliman, J. E., Thesis, Massachusetts Institute of Technology: Cambridge, MA. (1972).
Simpson, B. *J. Biomed Eng.* **4**, 65–68 (1969).
Skirda, V. D., Aslanyan, I., Philippova, O. E., Karibyants, N. S., and Khokhlov, A. R. *Macromol. Chem. Phys.* **200**, 2152–2159 (1999).
Smith, B. L., and Klier, J. *J. Appl. Polym. Sci.* **68**, 1019–1025 (1998).
Song, S. Z., Cardinal, J. R., Kim, S. H., and Kim, S. W. *J. Pharm Sci.* **67**, 1352 (1981).
Spevacek, J., and Schneider, B. *Makromol. Chem.* **175**, 2939–2956 (1974).
Stauffer, S. R., and Peppas, N. A. *Polymer* **33**, 3932–3936 (1992).
Stringer, J. L., and Peppas, N. A. *J. Control. Rel.* **42**, 195–202 (1996).
Stupp, S. I., LeBonheur, V., Walker, K., Li, L. S., Huggins, K. E., Keser, M., and Amstutz, A. *Science* **276**, 384–389 (1997).
Tanaka, T. *Polymer* **20**, 1404–1412 (1979).
Touitou, E., and Rubinstein, A. *Int. J. Pharm.* **30**, 93–99 (1986).
Treloar, R. G., "The Physics of Rubber Elasticity" 2nd Edition. Oxford University Press, Oxford (1958).
Tsuchida, E., and Abe, K. *Adv. Polym. Sci.* **45**, 1–112 (1982).

Tsutsumi, K., Takayama, K., Machida, Y., Ebert, C. D., Nakatomi, I., and Nagai, T. *S.T.P. Pharma. Sci.* **4**, 230–236 (1994).
Urushizaki, F., Yamaguchi, H., Nakamura, K., and Numajiri, S. *Intern. J. Pharm.* **58**, 135–142 (1990).
Vakkalanka, S. K., and Peppas, N. A. *Polym. Bull. (Berlin)* **36**, 221–225 (1996).
Vakkalanka, S. K., Brazel, C. S., and Peppas, N. A. *J. Biomater. Sci. Polym. Ed.* **8**, 119–129 (1996).
Verhoeven, J., Peschier, L. J. C., Van Det, M. A., Bouwstra, J. A., and Junginger, H. E. *Polymer* **30**, 1942–1945 (1989).
Vernon, B., Gutowska, A., Kim, S. W., and Bae, Y. H. *Macromol. Symp.* **109**, 155–167 (1996).
Voldrich, Z., Tomanek, Z., Vacik, J., and Kopecek, J. *J. Bio. Mat. Res.* **9**, 675–685 (1975).
von Recum, H., Kikuchi, A., Okuhara, M., Sakurai, Y., Okano, T., and Kim, S. W. *J. Biomater. Sci. Polym. Ed.* **9**, 1241–1253 (1998).
Wake, M. C., Mikos, A. G., Sarakinos, G., Vacanti, J. P., and Langer, R. *Cell Transplant.* **4**, 275–279 (1995).
Wichterle, O., and Lim, D. *Nature* **185**, 117–118 (1960).
Yamato, M., Kushida, A., and Okano, T. *Tanpakushitsu Kakusan Koso.* **45**, 1766–1772 (2000).
Yamato, M., Utsumi, M., Kushida, A., Konno, C., Kikuchi, A., and Okano, T. *Tissue Eng.* **7**, 473–480 (2001).
Yao, K., Peng, T., Goosen, M. F. A., Min, J. M., and He, Y. Y. *J. Appl. Polym. Sci.* **48**, 343–348 (1993).
Yasuda, H., and Lamaze, C. E. *J. Macromol. Sci. Phys.* **B5**, 111–134 (1971).
Yoshida, R., Kaneko, Y., Sakai, K., Okano, T., Sakurai, Y., Bae, Y. H., and Kim, S. W. *J. Control. Rel.* **32**, 97–102 (1994).
Yoshida, R., Uchida, K., Kaneko, Y., Sakai, K., Kikcuhi, A., Sakurai, Y., and Okano, T. *Nature* **374**, 240–242 (1995).
Yuk, S. H., Cho, S. H., and Lee, H. B. *Temperature-sensitive drug delivery system composed of poly (N,N-dimethylaminoethyl methacrylate-co-acrylamide)* in *Proceedings of the 1997 Spring ACS Meeting.* San Francisco, CA, USA (1997); Polymeric Materials Science and Engineering, Proceedings of the ACS Division of Polymeric Materials Science and Engineering, Vol. 76. ACS, Washington, DC, USA (1997a).
Yuk, S. H., Cho, S. H., and Lee, S. H. *Macromolecules* **30**, 6856–6859 (1997b).

BIOMATERIALS AND GENE THERAPY

F. Kurtis Kasper and Antonios G. Mikos

Department of Bioengineering, Rice University, Houston, Texas 77005, USA

I. Introduction	131
A. Gene Therapy and Protein Delivery	132
B. Methods of Gene Delivery	133
II. Biomaterials for Nonviral Gene Therapy	136
A. Cationic Lipids	136
B. Cationic Polymers	138
C. Polymers for Controlled Delivery	141
III. Polymer Based Particles for Controlled DNA Release	141
A. Genetic Immunization	142
B. Advantages of Encapsulation Over Injection	143
C. PLGA for Release of DNA in Vaccination Applications	143
IV. Polymeric Scaffolds for Controlled DNA Delivery	157
A. Gene Activated Matrices	157
B. Wound Healing and Bone Regeneration	158
C. Bone Tissue Engineering	159
D. Release of DNA from Scaffolds	161
V. Conclusion	162
VI. Abbreviations	162
References	163

I. Introduction

Gene therapy seeks to alter or control the course of cellular action through the introduction of nucleic acids into a specific cell population. All gene therapy efforts to date in humans have been limited to somatic cells, such that the treatment is confined to the individual and not passed along to offspring. Gene therapy was initially conceived to treat inherited genetic disorders of a single gene, such as cystic fibrosis, adenosine deaminase deficiency associated with severe combined immunodeficiency (SCID), and hemophilia. For some conditions, the delivery of a gene encoding a protein that is pathologically absent can restore normal function. Such is the case with hemophilia, in which one of a number of blood clotting factors may be deficient, but effectively replaced through delivery of a gene encoding the factor (Connelly and Kaleko, 1997, 1998; Corr et al., 1996). In other cases, suppression of a defective gene product may be the preferred course of action. A candidate condition for such selective gene silencing is osteogenesis imperfecta, in which the production of an abnormal collagen molecule interferes with the structural integrity of connective tissue (Marini and Gerber, 1997). In either case, the original concept of gene therapy involved the delivery of nucleic acids (DNA, RNA, or oligonucleotides) into an individual to correct a genetic insufficiency.

A. Gene Therapy and Protein Delivery

Gene therapy has since evolved beyond addressing genetic disorders to include the delivery of genetic material to obtain desired cellular responses. For example, gene therapy has been employed to elicit a specific immune response or to guide tissue regeneration. Indeed, the delivery of genes encoding therapeutic proteins provides potential for overcoming the limitations associated with the delivery of the proteins themselves.

1. Limitations of Protein Delivery

Although the delivery of recombinant proteins for therapeutic purposes holds great theoretical potential, several limitations are associated with their delivery. First, the production and purification of recombinant proteins is expensive, especially on the scale that is generally required for efficacy. Second, the inclusion of large amounts of protein poses the risk of toxicity through rapid release of the factor from the carrier. Additionally, the long-term effects of a supraphysiological dose of a recombinant protein are not known (Oakes and Lieberman, 2000). Diffusion of the factor out of the local site may have an undesired effect at secondary locations. Proteins require the maintenance of complex tertiary and quaternary structure for bioactivity. In many cases, the bioactivity of these factors is diminished through exposure to the harsh conditions generally encountered in the processing of the delivery vehicle. Additionally, the half-life of the factors is often quite limited in the extracellular environment to which they are exposed upon release. Loss of protein structure may result in a reduction of bioactivity and an increase in the risk of immunogenicity. Further, proteins are subject to high rates of renal and hepatic clearance. These limitations associated with the delivery of proteins themselves have led to the exploration of gene therapy to deliver the genes encoding therapeutic proteins.

2. Advantages of Gene Delivery

The delivery of plasmid DNA containing genes encoding specific proteins presents several potential advantages over the delivery of the proteins directly. First, the chemistry of DNA grants it inherent stability and flexibility. As a result, DNA may require less complex storage and present an extended shelf-life relative to the corresponding proteins. Additionally, the stability of plasmid DNA allows for its use with traditional drug delivery routes (Goldstein and Bonadio, 1998). Plasmid DNA can be easily manufactured via bulk processes that are potentially more economically feasible than the production and purification of the related proteins (Eastman and Durland, 1998). Once cells are transfected with plasmid DNA, the encoded gene product is produced *in vivo* by the cells. The retention of the gene by the cells provides a means for prolonged expression of the desired factor. Further, the encoded proteins produced by the cells *in vivo* have the potential to retain biological activity to a greater degree than delivered factors. As the desired factor must be produced by cells *in vivo*, the risk of toxicity is lower than with outright delivery of the factor.

B. Methods of Gene Delivery

1. Ex vivo Gene Therapy

The initial approach to gene therapy involved manipulation of gene expression *ex vivo*. Toward this end, the desired target cells are identified and subsequently removed from the subject, transfected *in vitro*, then reintroduced into the patient. A number of protocols have been established for the *ex vivo* transfection of a wide variety of cell types. This method allows specific cell targeting and high transfection efficiency. However, the process is time consuming, complex, and costly. Additionally, the method is not applicable to all situations, such as those in which an immediate modification is required.

2. In vivo Gene Therapy

Alternatively, gene therapy can be performed through *in vivo* manipulation of gene expression. In this case, the desired genes must be directly delivered to the appropriate cell population in the subject *in vivo*. This strategy offers several advantages over the *ex vivo* approach. For instance, the *in vivo* approach does not require the isolation or culture of cells, thereby reducing cost, complexity, time, and donor site morbidity. Further, *in vivo* gene therapy approaches hold the potential for generating products that can be used off of the shelf. *In vivo* gene therapy, however, faces the major obstacle of identifying a safe and efficient gene delivery vehicle that can target specific cell populations (Anderson, 1998).

3. Limitations of Naked DNA Delivery

The direct injection of uncomplexed, naked plasmid DNA (pDNA) represents the simplest technique for gene transfer. Although the effectiveness of naked DNA toward inducing gene expression has been demonstrated (Wolff *et al.*, 1990), several limitations are associated with the delivery of naked DNA. A single injection of a bolus dose of pDNA typically generates expression levels that reach a maximum within one month, followed by a drop to low stable levels that can be detected for up to two years (Jiao *et al.*, 1992; Jong *et al.*, 1997; Wolff *et al.*, 1990). Some efforts to increase the efficacy of direct administration of naked DNA involve increasing the distribution of the injected DNA (Mumper *et al.*, 1996) or enhancing the level of DNA uptake by cells at the time of injection (Danko *et al.*, 1994; Vitadello *et al.*, 1994).

It has been shown that naked DNA is highly vulnerable to degradation by endonucleases, which can degrade DNA within 30 min in the extracellular spaces (Kawabata *et al.*, 1995). In addition, uncomplexed DNA introduced into the plasma via intravenous injection is quickly cleared from the circulation by scavenger receptors in the liver, which compromises its extravasasion into target tissues and organs (Pouton and Seymour, 1998; Takakura *et al.*, 1998; Yoshida *et al.*, 1996). The lymphatic system rapidly clears naked DNA that is injected directly into tissues (Choate and Khavari, 1997; Levy *et al.*, 1996; Pouton and Seymour, 1998). DNA is a large molecule with a high degree of negative charge derived from the phosphate groups of its backbone (Ledley, 1996). Indeed, plasmid DNA constructs used for gene therapy typically have a molecular weight on the order of 10^6 Da and a hydrodynamic radius greater than 100 nm (Ledley, 1996). These properties significantly impede its ability to cross biological barriers, such as the endothelium, the plasma membrane, and the nuclear membrane of cells (Ledley, 1996). The cellular plasma membrane holds a net negative charge, which likely repels large, negatively charged DNA molecules, thereby hindering the cellular uptake of DNA. Thus, entry into the cell is a major barrier faced by naked DNA, yet studies have demonstrated gene expression following introduction of naked DNA *in vivo* (Wolff *et al.*, 1990). It follows then that naked DNA can cross the plasma membrane barrier, but this likely occurs with very low efficiency. Proposed mechanisms for the cellular entry of naked DNA involve either an unidentified cell membrane transporter (Budker *et al.*, 2000) or the process of potocytosis (Wolff *et al.*, 1992).

Once the DNA enters the cell, however, several additional barriers to expression must be overcome. The DNA enters the cytosol upon crossing the plasma membrane and then migrates toward the nucleus in a process likely governed by diffusion (Luo and Saltzman, 2000a). This movement toward the nucleus is quite slow, which prolongs the duration of exposure of the DNA to the cytosol (Luo and Saltzman, 2000a). Nucleases present in the cytosol can rapidly degrade the DNA during its intracellular migration. Although finding the nucleus is a major obstacle in itself, the DNA must enter the nucleus and be expressed for the therapy to be successful. These barriers to effective expression of naked DNA have inspired the search for a gene delivery vehicle that might overcome some or all of these obstacles. In general, an optimal gene delivery system should enhance DNA stability, offer cell or tissue specificity, improve the bioavailability of the DNA, and promote cellular uptake and intracellular trafficking (Han *et al.*, 2000; Mahato *et al.*, 1999; Truong-Le *et al.*, 1998).

4. Viral Gene Therapy

Viral gene therapy takes advantage of the highly evolved and efficient transfection mechanism of viruses to transfer genetic material into a host cell. The high transfection efficiency of viral carriers has resulted in their wide exploration in gene therapy studies. Viral vectors are generated by removing a section of the viral genome, so as to render the virus replication incompetent. A gene encoding the desired product is then inserted into the void created by the removal of the viral gene segment, which is usually of very limited size. Thus, there is a limit to the amount of genetic material that can be incorporated into a viral vector (Smith, 1995). Additional limitations include safety concerns and the cost and difficulty associated with production. Just as viruses have evolved to transfect mammalian cells, mammalian cells have evolved to resist viral transfection (Verma and Somia, 1997). Thus, viral vectors are highly immunogenic, which restricts their repeated use for gene delivery (Capan *et al.*, 1999a). Additionally, some viral vectors incorporate genetic material into the host genome, thereby generating the risk of oncogenesis and mutagenesis, although this possibility is often considered to be quite small. Further, a chance exists that viral vectors will recombine *in vivo* and activate the complement immune response. The risks and limitations of viral vectors have led to the study of nonviral methods for gene delivery.

5. Nonviral Gene Therapy

The past decade has seen numerous attempts toward the development of a nonviral vector that can match the level of specificity and gene expression offered by viral vectors, while improving the safety, gene insert capacity, and immunogenicity. Although naked DNA can be introduced and has been shown to be effective *in vivo* (Wolff *et al.*, 1990, 1992), many limitations are associated with naked gene delivery. Physical methods of nonviral gene therapy have been explored including microinjection, electroporation, and biolistic delivery with the gene gun. Microinjection involves the direct injection of genes into the nuclei of individual cells one at a time. As a result, high efficiency and specificity are attained with microinjection, but the process requires a great deal of time and effort. Thus, the method is not practical for *in vivo* DNA delivery or for the transfection of large numbers of cells *in vitro*. Electroporation induces temporary pore formation in the membranes of living cells through brief exposure to high-voltage electrical pulses. Genes may enter the cells through the transient pores, which typically close on the order of minutes. Electroporation is among the most efficient methods of gene transfer, but the high mortality of cells following exposure to the high-voltage pulses limits its utility (Luo and Saltzman, 2000a). The gene gun, however, utilizes DNA-coated gold particles that are driven through the cell membrane at high velocity (Yang and Sun, 1995; Yang *et al.*, 1990). This method allows for the simultaneous introduction of DNA into many cells and has been used effectively in DNA vaccination applications (Fynan *et al.*, 1993; Qiu *et al.*, 1996). The particle bombardment approach to DNA delivery, however, requires invasive proceedures to expose tissues and organs that are not readily accessible. Delivery of DNA with polymeric materials provides an alternative method for nonviral *in vivo* gene therapy, with the potential to circumvent the limitations of physical methods for DNA delivery.

II. Biomaterials for Nonviral Gene Therapy

A. Cationic Lipids

The first use of lipid molecules with an associated positively charged head group for gene transfer was described in 1987 (Felgner *et al.*, 1987). The use of cationic lipids has since grown to become the most widely investigated method for condensing plasmid DNA for nonviral delivery (Segura and Shea, 2001). Cationic lipids are generally composed of a hydrophilic lipid anchor linked through an intermediate group to a cationic head group. The hydrophilic lipid group strongly influences the physical properties of the lipid bilayer, including the flexibility and the kinetics of lipid exchange within the bilayer (Felgner et al., 1994). A cholesterol or fatty acid group generally comprises the lipid anchor. The intermediate linker group plays a large role in determining the chemical stability and biodegradability. Additionally, the linker can affect the transfection efficiency of the cationic lipid, as it provides a site for the potential attachment of side chains to augment cellular targeting, uptake, and intracellular trafficking of the complex (Byk et al., 1998a). In general, longer linker lengths correspond to increased gene transfer (Byk et al., 1998a). The head groups vary widely in structure and charge, with multivalent groups generally having higher transfection efficiencies than the monovalent equivalents (Felgner et al., 1994; Lee et al., 1996). The generation of novel cationic lipids from libraries of components has improved understanding of the structure–activity relationships of these materials as gene carriers (Byk et al., 1998a,b; Lee et al., 1996). However, a more detailed understanding of the correlation between lipid structure, DNA complexation, and cellular interaction is required for optimization of cationic lipid gene delivery vectors.

The interaction of plasmid DNA with cationic lipids results in a tightly condensed complex (termed a lipoplex), in which the cationic lipids completely or partially cover the DNA. This interaction is driven by the entropy increase derived from the release of water molecules and counter ions associated with the surfaces of the DNA and lipid molecules (Radler et al., 1997). The formulations of cationic lipids used for gene delivery typically include a zwitterionic or neutral lipid in addition to the cationic lipid group to enhance transfection (Ferrari et al., 2002). Properties such as the size and stability of the lipoplexes are influenced by the charge ratio of the amines on the cationic lipid to the phosphates groups on the DNA more so than the composition of the lipids (Xu et al., 1999). Large aggregates (greater than one micrometer) are formed from the complexation of DNA and cationic lipids at a neutral, or one-to-one, charge ratio (Xu et al., 1999), hence positive or negative charge ratios are typically used for gene delivery. As cell membranes carry a net negative charge, lipoplexes with a positive charge ratio are generally used to delivery DNA for *in vitro* studies, as they promote electrostatic interaction with the cell membrane. It has been proposed, however, that *in vivo* studies may require different charge ratios for efficacy due to possible interactions with components of the physiological environment (Mahato et al., 1999). Indeed, DNA can be released from complexes due to the binding to the lipid of polyanionic species with a sufficient charge density, such as heparin (Xu and Szoka, 1996). Thus, DNA may be prematurely released from cationic lipids and subject to nuclease degradation before reaching cells *in vivo*. Conjugation of poly(ethylene glycol) (PEG) to the lipid has been shown to reduce the extent of protein binding and complement activation of the lipoplexes, however gene expression of the modified complexes is significantly reduced (Filion and Phillips, 1998).

Initial theories proposed that lipoplexes enter the cytoplasm after fusing directly with the plasma membrane (Felgner *et al.*, 1987; Smith *et al.*, 1993). Current thought, however, suggests that complex entry follows endocytosis, which can be enhanced with the use of endosomolytic agents such as chloroquine (Zuhorn *et al.*, 2002; Zabner *et al.*, 1995). Although the mechanism of cellular entry is not well understood, high efficiency of delivery has been demonstrated with several cell types *in vitro* (Bebok *et al.*, 1996; Zabner *et al.*, 1995). Following cellular entry of the lipoplex, the next important barrier is the release of the plasmid DNA from the lipid (Xu and Szoka, 1996). The final obstacle is nuclear entry of the DNA for expression. Indeed, it has been proposed that the dissociation of DNA from the lipid and subsequent entry into the nucleus represent the most significant hurdles for gene expression with cationic lipid carriers (Zabner *et al.*, 1995).

Despite their current wide use in nonviral gene therapy, cationic lipids present several limitations. First, the structure and transfection mechanism of cationic lipoplexes are not well characterized. Second, although the lipoplexes are able to enter cells efficiently, they exhibit poor cell targeting and gene expression. Additionally, cationic lipoplexes are highly toxic upon repeated use (Han *et al.*, 2000), and induce a strong anti-inflammatory response *in vivo* (Filion and Phillips, 1997; Tan and Huang, 2002). As a result of these limitations, interest in polymeric gene carriers has grown in recent years.

B. Cationic Polymers

Another nonviral approach to gene delivery is the use of polycationic polymers to form electrostatic complexes with plasmid DNA. The polycationic polymers have a high density of primary amines, which endow the molecules with a large quantity of positive charge in the physiologic pH range. As a result, DNA is able to electrostatically complex with the polymers and condense into small particles capable of entering cells. The primary amines on the polymer chain also provide a site for chemical modification with peptides or ligands through which enhanced cell targeting and transfection may be achieved via receptor-mediated endocytosis (Erbacher *et al.*, 1999; Gottschalk *et al.*, 1994; Wagner *et al.*, 1990). Many different cationic polymers have been investigated for use in gene delivery, and they range in structure from linear to highly branched. The most widely investigated cationic polymers for gene delivery are poly(L-lysine) (PLL), poly(ethylenimine) (PEI), and poly(amidoamine) dendrimers.

Poly(L-lysine) has been used to complex with DNA in a variety of salt conditions and has demonstrated gene transfer both *in vitro* and *in vivo* (Duguid *et al.*, 1998; Gonsho *et al.*, 1994). PLL is typically synthesized on a solid support through a series of protecting/deprotecting steps to generate fairly monodisperse polypeptides. Charge ratios of amine groups on PLL to phosphate groups on DNA between 3:1 and 6:1 are typically used to generate complexes. High molecular weight PLL forms smaller complexes with DNA than lower molecular weight PLL. These smaller, tighter complexes offer greater protection of DNA from the effects of sonication and salt concentration (Adami *et al.*, 1998), yet have a higher associated cytotoxicity relative to the larger complexes (Duguid *et al.*, 1998). Complexes of PLL and DNA are subject to aggregation under physiological conditions. Chemical modification of PLL with such molecules as dextran (Maruyama *et al.*, 1998), poly(ethylene glycol) (Choi *et al.*, 1998; Lee *et al.*, 2002), and poly[N-(2-hydroxypropyl)methacrylamide] (Oupicky *et al.*, 2000) has been shown to reduce aggregation of the complexes without compromising the ability of the complex to form. The modification of PLL with PEG has also been shown to decrease the high degree of cytotoxicity associated with PLL alone (Choi *et al.*, 1998; Lee *et al.*, 2002).

Another cationic polymer that has been investigated for gene delivery applications is poly(ethylenimine) (PEI). It presents a high density of positive charge, as nitrogen represents every third atom along its backbone. Both linear and branched forms of PEI exist, but only two-thirds of the backbone nitrogens can carry a charge in the branched form, whereas all of the nitrogens can be charged in the linear form (Garnett, 1999). In either form, the effectiveness of PEI in complexing and transferring DNA into a variety of cell types has been demonstrated both *in vitro* and *in vivo* (Boussif *et al.*, 1995). The PEI/DNA complexes have been shown to attach to the cell surface and aggregate into clumps, which are subsequently endocytosed (Godbey *et al.*, 1999b). The endocytosed PEI enters the nucleus in an ordered structure, whether or not it is complexed with DNA (Godbey *et al.*, 1999b). It has been proposed that PEI may protect DNA from nuclease degradation in and enhance release of the complex from the lysosome through buffering action and swelling, which leads to lysosomal rupture (Boussif *et al.*, 1995). In this process, termed the proton sponge effect, the previously uncharged amines of the PEI are protonated by an influx of positively charged protons. The resulting charge gradient leads to the entry of negative ions, such as Cl^-, into the endosome. The accumulation of ions within the endosome leads to osmotic swelling and rupture of the endosome, allowing release of the PEI/DNA complexes into the cytosol. A study by Godbey *et al.* (2000), however, challenged the proton sponge hypothesis for PEI transfection. This study demonstrated that the pH in the lysosome remained constant over the time frame needed for nuclear entry of the DNA, and endosome–lysosome fusion was not observed. Thus, it was suggested that PEI/DNA complexes escape from the endosomes before the pH drops to acidic coniditons (Godbey *et al.*, 2000). Further, the molecular weight of PEI affects gene transfer, with transfection efficiency increasing with the molecular weight of PEI (Godbey *et al.*, 1999a). However, complexes of PEI and DNA are cytotoxic and prone to aggregation.

Dendrimers of poly(amidoamine) (PAMAM) have also received attention as polycationic nonviral gene delivery vehicles. The diameter and surface charge of the starburst PAMAM dendrimers is a function of the number of synthetic cycles, also known as generations, used in the synthesis (Haensler and Szoka, 1993). Higher transfection efficiencies have been observed for DNA complexed with fifth- and sixth-generation PAMAM dendrimers when compared to lower generations (Haensler and Szoka, 1993). PAMAM dendrimers are generally synthesized from core molecules of ammonia or ethylenediamine to which methyl acrylate and ethylenediamine are successively added (Tomalia *et al.*, 2002). The core molecules from which the synthesis originates determine the shape, density, and surface charge of the resulting dendrimer, which can be either "fractured" or "intact," depending on the number of branch arms extending from every branch point. Fractured dendrimers may have as few as zero and as many as two arms extending from each branch point; while intact dendrimers extend two arms from every branch point (Tang *et al.*, 1996). Electrostatic interaction between the phosphate groups of plasmid DNA and the terminal primary amines of the PAMAM dendrimers generates condense complexes that are capable of mediating gene delivery (Bielinska *et al.*, 1997; Haensler and Szoka, 1993; Qin *et al.*, 1998). This gene transfer, however, has generally lacked cell specificity.

Although cationic lipids and cationic polymers present several advantages over viral techniques and the administration of naked DNA for gene therapy, a number of limitations are generally associated with these materials. In contrast to viral vectors, virtually any size of plasmid DNA can be delivered with cationic complexes. The complexed DNA is partially protected from degradation by endonucleases and sonication, yet dissociation of the DNA from the carrier can be difficult. Additionally, these complexes are highly efficient at entering cells in a nonspecific manner, yet the delivered genes are not efficiently expressed. A complete understanding of the cellular entry, trafficking, and expression of these vectors has not been developed. Further, cationic DNA carriers generally exhibit significant cytotoxicity. These limitations have led to the investigation of controlled release from polymer constructs.

C. Polymers for Controlled Delivery

The nonviral methods for gene therapy discussed above present a short period of time during which the DNA is available for cellular entry, which is adequate for some applications. However, other applications require a long-term or sustained presence of the transfection agent for efficacy. As a result, technology for the controlled release of proteins from biocompatible polymers has recently been applied to the delivery of DNA. In this method, plasmid DNA is entrapped within a biocompatible polymeric material. The polymer construct may then either hold the DNA *in situ* while cells migrate into the scaffold to encounter the DNA, or the DNA may be released from the scaffold in a controlled manner. The polymer entrapment method for controlled DNA delivery offers several potential advantages over the other nonviral gene transfer techniques. To begin, physical entrapment may protect DNA from degradation until its release or cellular uptake. Second, long-term localized release may be achieved through the polymeric constructs without need for repeated administration, or the construct may be tailored to deliver the DNA in a rapid, bolus fashion depending upon the particular application. Additionally, cellular or tissue specific targeting may be achieved through introduction of the polymer at the desired site. The localization of the DNA within the scaffold provides a safety mechanism for ending the therapy as the implant could be easily retrieved. Although the potential applications of controlled release of plasmid DNA from polymer constructs are expansive, the majority of work to date has focused on the application of the technology toward genetic vaccination and tissue engineering. Indeed, polymeric microparticle delivery systems have been widely studied for DNA vaccines, while large constructs have been developed for tissue engineering or guided tissue regeneration applications. The current discussion will focus on the development of polymeric materials for the entrapment and controlled delivery of plasmid DNA toward these applications.

III. Polymer Based Particles for Controlled DNA Release

Polymeric-based particles have been utilized for the encapsulation and release of proteins and peptides for numerous applications. Recently, however, attention has been granted to the use of polymeric particles for the encapsulation and release of genetic material. The search for a nonviral delivery method for genetic immunization has prompted much of the investigation of microparticles for gene delivery. Microparticles and nanoparticles have been fabricated from both natural and synthetic materials, including, chitosan, gelatin, and poly(D,L-lactic-*co*-glycolic) acid (PLGA) for the encapsulation and release of plasmid DNA.

A. GENETIC IMMUNIZATION

Direct introduction of naked plasmid DNA has been explored as a novel and effective method of vaccination (Donnelly *et al.*, 1997; Hassett and Whitton, 1996; Shiver *et al.*, 1996). DNA vaccinations, in opposition to conventional protein immunization, provide a means for extended expression of antigens and the elicitation of both humoral and cellular immune responses (Donnelly *et al.*, 1997). This strategy emerged following reports that direct injection of naked plasmid DNA into muscle cells could induce gene expression (Wolff *et al.*, 1990). The approach for genetic immunization involves the direct introduction of plasmid DNA into host cells, such that the encoded antigenic protein is expressed and induces a desired immune response (Wang *et al.*, 1999). Indeed, an initial report of genetic immunization demonstrated the generation of cytotoxic T lymphocytes and protective immunity in mice following intramuscular injection of plasmid DNA encoding the influenza A nucleoprotein (Ulmer *et al.*, 1993). Since that report in 1993, protective immunity following DNA immunization has been demonstrated in numerous independent studies (Donnelly *et al.*, 1997). Indeed, the effectiveness of DNA vaccines has been demonstrated in both small and large animals, including porcine, bovine and equine models (Donnelly *et al.*, 1995; Porgador *et al.*, 1998; Singh *et al.*, 2000). Recent studies in humans and nonhuman primates, however, have required large doses (milligrams) of plasmid DNA to induce antibody and cytotoxic T lymphocyte responses (Calarota *et al.*, 1998; Letvin *et al.*, 1997; MacGregor *et al.*, 1998; Wang *et al.*, 1998). Although the demonstrated effectiveness of genetic immunization is promising, the use of milligram quantities of DNA is not appealing from an economic perspective, especially if multiple administrations are required.

The activation of a T-cell response and subsequent efficacy of DNA vaccines is ultimately determined by professional antigen presenting cells, such as macrophages, dendritic cells, and Langerhans cells (Corr *et al.*, 1996; Doe *et al.*, 1996; Iwasaki *et al.*, 1997; Ulmer *et al.*, 1996). It follows that successful DNA vaccination strategies should seek to target DNA delivery to these cells or to tissue rich in these cells, such as the lymph nodes, spleen, skin, and sub-mucosal tissues (Lunsford et al., 2000). It has been shown that naked DNA introduced through intramuscular and intradermal injection remains localized at the site of injection (Lunsford et al., 2000; Nichols et al., 1995; Parker et al., 1999; Winegar et al., 1996). Delivery of DNA encapsulated in polymer particles may facilitate the selective transfection of phagocytotic cells, such as macrophages, by size exclusion, as microspheres between 1 and 10 μm in diameter are too large to enter cells by endocytosis, but small enough to be phagocytosed (Eldridge et al., 1989; Tabata and Ikada, 1990).

B. Advantages of Encapsulation Over Injection

The use of biodegradable polymeric microparticles presents several potential advantages for the delivery of plasmid DNA (pDNA). First, encapsulation of pDNA within or adsorption to the surface of microparticles offers increased resistance to degradation via endonucleases (Capan et al., 1999a). Additionally, biodegradable microparticles provide a means for sustained, localized delivery of pDNA in a controlled manner, which may increase the level of pDNA retention in the tissue (Davis et al., 1993a). High concentrations of pDNA retained within the tissue may enhance the transfection efficiency of the local cells by increasing the physical concentration of pDNA at the cell surface (Luo and Saltzman, 2000b). Another advantage of microparticle delivery is the potential for minimally invasive administration of the carrier by means such as direct injection or oral delivery.

C. PLGA for Release of DNA in Vaccination Applications

The majority of work toward the development of microparticles for DNA encapsulation and release has involved the polymer poly(D,L-lactic-co-glycolic) acid (PLGA). Since the FDA approved its use as a suture material, PLGA has been widely investigated for medical applications ranging from implant fabrication to drug release systems. Indeed, the biocompatibility of PLGA is generally accepted as the material degrades in the body via hydrolysis to yield lactic acid and glycolic acid, both of which are metabolized by natural pathways. The degradation of PLGA can be controlled through varying the ratio of lactic to glycolic acid in the polymer and varying the molecular weight of the polymer chains. An increase in the ratio of glycolic acid in the copolymer results in a decrease in the hydrophobicity of the polymer and an increase in the degradation rate

(Heller *et al.*, 1987), with a 50:50 ratio of lactic to glycolic acid degrading most rapidly (Gupta *et al.*, 1998). Similarly, a decrease in the molecular weight of the polymer chains results in an increase in the rate of degradation (Gupta *et al.*, 1998). Exposure of the polymer to water results in hydrolytic cleavage of the ester bonds via a bulk process, such that the polymer chains become successively smaller until they are soluble in the aqueous environment (Hausberger and DeLuca, 1995). This controllable, steady degradation mechanism has led to the application of PLGA for drug encapsulation and delivery (Mehta *et al.*, 1994). In recent years, investigators have explored the use of PLGA based nano- and microparticles for the encapsulation and release of plasmid DNA.

The initial investigation of PLGA microparticles for delivery of encapsulated plasmid DNA was conducted by Jones *et al.* (1997). This report demonstrated that encapsulated DNA was effectively protected from degradation following parenteral and oral administration and that cellular uptake was facilitated so that systemic and mucosal antibody responses were invoked. It was shown that the antigen was effectively presented so as to elicit IgM, IgG, and IgA antibody responses. Although this study demonstrated proof of principle, the encapsulation efficiency was limited to about 25%, and released DNA retained only about 25% of its bioactivity when compared to unencapsulated controls following *in vitro* gene expression assays. Further, the DNA, which was initially in a super-coiled isoform, was converted predominately to an open circular form. This pilot study promoted further investigation into the mechanism behind and control of DNA release from PLGA nano- and microspheres.

Luo *et al.* (1999) investigated the effects of adjusting the polymer molecular weight and the composition of poly(L-lactic acid) (PLA)/PLGA in the fabrication of microspheres upon the release of encapsulated DNA. A bi-phasic release profile was observed, with an initial burst of DNA followed by a slow release for all microsphere formulations. Three polymer formulations were examined for DNA release, namely PLA of low molecular weight (2 kDa), PLA of high molecular weight (300 kDa), and PLGA (50:50 ratio of lactide to glycolide). Microspheres fabricated from the lower molecular weight PLA were observed to release a greater amount of the loaded DNA than the lower molecular weight PLA. The microspheres made from PLGA, however, demonstrated the most rapid release, as 95% of the loaded DNA was released within two days. It was suggested that the inclusion of the glycolic acid into the material increased the hydrophilicity and, subsequently, degradation rate of the PLGA relative to PLA, which would accelerate the release of DNA. It was concluded that the release of DNA from PLGA microspheres depends on both polymer degradation and DNA diffusion. Indeed, a number of factors can influence the release of

DNA from polymeric microspheres, including the chemical characteristics and molecular weight of the material, the size and morphology of the microspheres, as well as the amount of DNA loaded into the microspheres (Luo et al., 1999).

Several processing techniques have been successfully employed in the encapsulation of plasmid DNA within PLGA nano- and microspheres, including double-emulsion (water-oil-water) solvent-evaporation (Ando et al., 1999; Barman et al., 2000; Cohen et al., 2000; Hao et al., 2000; Lunsford et al., 2000; Tinsley-Bown et al., 2000; Wang et al., 1999) and spray drying (Walter et al., 1999, 2001). In the double-emulsion solvent-evaporation technique, the DNA is suspended in an aqueous solution, while the PLGA is dissolved in a partially water-miscible organic solvent, usually methylene chloride or ethyl acetate. An emulsion is then generated between the two phases through either sonication or homogenization. Polymers such as poly(vinyl alcohol) (PVA) and poly(vinylpyrrolidone) (PVP) may be used as emulsion stabilizers in the double-emulsion process and are deposited on the surface of the microspheres to prevent coalescence. The first emulsion is subsequently added to a much larger volume of aqueous solution and mixed in a similar manner to create the double-emulsion. The organic solvent is then evaporated from the double-emulsion, allowing the solidification of the polymer rich droplets into nano- or microspheres. The remaining aqueous solution may be either centrifuged or filtered to isolate the polymer spheres. Finally, the microspheres are lyophilized to remove the water from the interior aqueous phase, leaving the DNA within the PLGA matrix.

A study by Wang et al. (1999) investigated the effect of PLGA molecular weight upon the entrapment efficiency and release kinetics of plasmid DNA in microspheres created with the double-emulsion solvent-evaporation technique. The DNA entrapment efficiency increased as the PLGA molecular weight increased, ranging from 22.5% for 6000 Da PLGA to 53.3% for 50,000 Da PLGA. The microspheres fabricated from the low molecular weight PLGA, however, displayed the fastest and highest total amount of DNA release, with 20% of the encapsulated DNA being released over the course of 28 days in vitro. The microspheres made from PLGA of 30,000 Da or higher released less than 5% of the encapsulated DNA over the course of 28 days. The release profile in all cases was bi-phasic, with an initial burst followed by little subsequent release. The polymer particles ranged in size from 400 nm to 2 μm, with no observed effect from the molecular weight of the PLGA. The DNA extracted from microspheres was found to have a higher fraction of open circular and lower fraction of super-coiled DNA than unencapsulated controls. This indicates that degradation of the DNA was induced in the encapsulation process.

The low entrapment efficiencies for microparticles that released appreciable amounts of DNA and the observed denaturation of DNA following encapsulation prompted Tinsley-Bown et al. (2000) to optimize some of the processing parameters in the double-emulsion solvent-evaporation technique. The double-emulsion process was conducted with the use of ethyl acetate as the organic solvent, rather than methylene chloride, which had typically been used. Additionally, the temperatures and volume ratios of the reagents were adjusted from typical values. Further, emulsification was induced with a blender on low speed rather than through sonication or homogenization. It was concluded that the optimized processing parameters resulted in higher entrapment efficiencies than previous reports from their group (Jones and Farrar, 1995; Jones et al., 1997) and others (Wang et al., 1999) using the double-emulsion technique. The observed DNA incorporation in this study, however, ranged from only 19 to 54%, depending upon the PLGA formulation used and the total polymer concentration in solution. A trade-off effect for the blending speed was observed between particle size and the structural integrity of the encapsulated DNA. The optimized blender process resulted in approximately 30–40% of the DNA retaining its super-coiled structure in comparison to about 10% when a homogenizer was used in a previous study by the same group (Jones and Farrar, 1995; Jones et al., 1997). The structural integrity of encapsulated DNA was shown to decrease significantly with time upon release *in vitro* relative to unencapsulated controls. The control DNA was only partially degraded to the open circular form after six weeks, whereas little of the encapsulated DNA was detected at the fifth week. It was suggested that the loss of DNA integrity may be a result of degradation induced by the low pH in the microenviroment within the PLGA matrix during degradation (Ando et al., 1999; Walter et al., 1999; 2001). Thus, this study proposed that DNA degradation may occur both in the encapsulation process and during the degradation of the polymer matrix.

A study by Ando et al. sought to determine the mechanism of degradation during the double-emulsion solvent-evaporation technique and to develop methods to counteract it (Ando et al., 1999). They hypothesized that DNA was damaged by (1) exposure to sheer stresses in the homogenization or sonication steps of processing and (2) the formation of crystals of the buffer salts during lyophilization. A cryopreparation process was introduced to address the first hypothesis. Cryopreparation involves lowering the temperature of the primary emulsion below the freezing point of the aqueous phase, such that a solid particulate suspension is produced. They proposed that the shear stresses encountered by the DNA in the frozen phase should be minimal during the homogenization step to form the secondary emulsion. As a result, the DNA should retain its super-coiled isoform. Additionally, it was suggested that freezing the inner phase should prevent diffusion of DNA from the microspheres during homogenization, thereby increasing the entrapment efficiency. The second hypothesis was addressed by including saccharides in the primary emulsion to hinder the formation of salt crystals during lyophilization. Increasing rates of homogenization were found to increase the degree of degradation of DNA. However, the cryopreparation technique preserved the super-coiled structure of DNA at all homogenization rates relative to samples made without the cryopreparation step. Additionally, it was found that the inclusion of ethylenediaminetetraacetic acid (EDTA) and lactose in the DNA solution was an important factor in maintaining the super-coiled structure of DNA during cryopreparation. When microspheres were prepared using optimized conditions, the average particle diameter was 4.8 µm, 88% of the DNA retained its super-coiled isoform, and the encapsulation efficiency was 89%, versus values of 4.5 µm, 39% and 29%, respectively for microspheres fabricated with the standard double-emulsion method. The inclusion of saccharides into the primary emulsion was adopted by other studies for the encapsulation of DNA in PLGA microparticles (Barman et al., 2000; Hao et al., 2000). Although this study addressed the problems associated with DNA degradation during microparticle fabrication, the issue of protection against DNA degradation during polymer degradation remains to be addressed.

Other studies have sought to encapsulate plasmid DNA that has been complexed with another polymer, such as PLL, within PLGA nano- and microspheres by the double-emulsion solvent-evaporation technique (Capan et al., 1999a,b). The first of the studies demonstrated that PLL-complexed DNA encapsulated within PLGA microspheres retained a significantly higher percentage of its super-coiled form relative to encapsulated, uncomplexed control DNA (76.7–85.6% vs 16.6%, respectively) (Capan et al., 1999a). The encapsulation efficiency and total percentage of the loaded DNA released was lower for encapsulated, PLL-complexed DNA than for encapsulated, uncomplexed controls. It was also observed that the encapsulated, PLL-complexed DNA was protected from enzymatic degradation in vitro. The second study investigated the influence of various formulation parameters on the size of the microparticles, the degradation of DNA, the loading efficiency, and the in vitro release kinetics (Capan et al., 1999b). A complex ratio of DNA to PLL of 1:0.33 (w/w) was encapsulated in all formulations. The hydrophobic PLGA resulted in a higher entrapment efficiency (46.2%) and maintenance of super-coiled structure (64.9%) of DNA than microspheres fabricated from either a lower molecular weight PLGA (26.1 and 45.1%, respectively) or a more hydrophilic formulation of PLGA (15.9 and 58.7%, respectively). The hydrophobic PLGA, however, demonstrated lower cumulative release of the encapsulated DNA over 38 days *in vitro* (54.2%), relative to the low molecular weight and hydrophilic PLGA formulations (95.9 and 84.9%, respectively). The release profiles for all formulations were bi-phasic, with an initial burst release. A decrease in particle size (6.6 to 2.2 µm) was observed as the concentration of PVA was increased from 1 to 7%, however, the fraction of super-coiled DNA was significantly reduced. Additionally, microspheres stabilized with PVA demonstrated a higher DNA–PLL entrapment efficiency than those stabilized with PVP at the same concentration (46.2 vs 24.1%). It was shown that the encapsulated, PLL-complexed DNA was protected from degradation by DNase I *in vitro*, yet a loss of super-coiled isoform was observed. This study suggests that the type and concentration of the surfactant, as well as the properties of the PLGA, can affect the encapsulation and release of PLL-complexed DNA. Although these studies demonstrated that the entrapment of PLL-complexed DNA protected the DNA from enzymatic degradation and reduced the conversion of super-coiled DNA to open circular and linear isoforms, the entrapment efficiencies were low, relative to those obtained with cryopreparation (Ando *et al.*, 1999) and optimized double-emulsion solvent-evaporation processing parameters (Tinsley-Bown *et al.*, 2000).

Following the general concept introduced by Capan *et al.* (1999a,b), another group investigated the encapsulation of DNA in PLGA nanospheres fabricated through the double-emulsion solvent-evaporation technique, but with the inclusion of calcium in the surfactant phase (Cohen *et al.*, 2000). This approach resulted in a high encapsulation efficiency of approximately 70%. It was suggested that the inclusion of calcium in the surfactant phase electrostatically hindered the diffusional escape of DNA from the primary aqueous phase during the processing, thereby increasing the encapsulation efficiency. The typical bi-phasic release pattern was observed with the calcium modified nanospheres in this study. The nanospheres released approximately 80% of the encapsulated DNA over the course of 28 days *in vitro*, and a loss of super-coiled isoform was observed with time. Despite the loss of super-coiled structure, however, the *in vitro* bioactivity of the DNA was not significantly affected. It was proposed that some of the DNA was exposed on the surface during the emulsification process, and that the immediate release of this exposed, soluble DNA accounted for the observed initial burst release, with the remainder of the release being controlled by polymer degradation. The use of calcium may provide protection of the encapsulated DNA from degradation, in a similar fashion to PLL, yet circumvent the toxicity commonly associated with PLL. This was the first study to demonstrate the direct transfection of cells *in vitro* with DNA released from nanoparticle carriers.

Higher expression levels were associated with the encapsulated DNA than with the administration of naked DNA *in vitro*, but standard liposomal transfection yielded the highest level of gene expression. *In vivo*, however, the encapsulated DNA exhibited higher levels of sustained expression of a marker gene at 28 days, than that associated with naked DNA or DNA delivered with liposomes. Thus, this study indicated the potential for DNA encapsulated in degradable nanospheres to elicit sustained gene expression *in vivo*.

An alternative approach to PLGA microsphere fabrication for DNA encapsulation was explored by Walter *et al.* (1999, 2001). They proposed the use of a spray-drying technique. In this method, a primary emulsion is generated much as in the double-emulsion technique, with an aqueous solution of DNA dispersed in an organic phase of PLGA and solvent. The dispersion is then spray-dried, and the resulting particles are washed, filtered, and vacuum dried. The initial study (Walter *et al.*, 1999) examined the integrity and functionality of three types of DNA (plasmid DNA, high molecular weight linear DNA, and low molecular weight linear DNA) during fabrication, after encapsulation, and after *in vitro* release. As ultrasonication is employed to generate the primary emulsion in the spray-drying technique, the effect of ultrasonication on each of the DNA types was investigated. It was found that both plasmid and high molecular weight linear DNA were degraded by ultrasonication. However, the inclusion of the buffer $NaHCO_3$ or of phosphate buffered saline solution prevented the conversion of plasmid DNA to the open circular form and significantly improved transfection activity relative to DNA in water alone. Additionally, exposure of plasmid DNA to an acidic environment (pH 3.5) resulted in a conversion from the super-coiled to the open circular isoform. Further, a significant reduction in biological activity was observed following exposure of the DNA to pH values of 3 or lower. A reduction in the duration of ultrasonication reduced the degree of DNA degradation, but decreased the encapsulation efficiency and increased the initial burst release *in vitro*. Increased nominal loading of DNA resulted in a reduction in the encapsulation efficiency, but an increase in the DNA stability. Comparison of DNA extracted from microspheres following fabrication with the DNA released in the initial burst phase indicated that the structural integrity of the DNA is independent of its location within the microparticle. A bi-phasic release pattern was typically observed in this study, with an initial burst phase followed by a sustained release governed by polymer degradation. Only negligible amounts of double-stranded DNA (dsDNA) were detected in the second release phase, according to analysis with the PicoGreen® dye, which specifically binds to dsDNA. A complete loss of bioactivity was associated with plasmid DNA released from day 16 onward *in vitro*, indicating a high degree of DNA degradation in the second release phase. It was proposed that the acidic microenvironment created in the degradation of the PLGA results in a significant degradation of the entrapped plasmid DNA. This study demonstrated the ability to protect DNA from degradation during microsphere fabrication, yet demonstrated the need for a method to stabilize DNA against acidic degradation as the PLGA is hydrolyzed.

The second study using the spray-drying fabrication technique (Walter *et al.*, 2001) investigated the effect of PLGA properties, such as molecular weight and hydrophilicity, upon the encapsulation efficiency and release kinetics of DNA *in vitro*. Additionally, the delivery of the microspheres to phagocytotic cells, namely human-derived macrophages and dendritic cells was examined *in vitro*. The molecular weight and the hydrophobicity of the PLGA had a marked effect on the encapsulation efficiency and *in vitro* release of plasmid DNA. Higher encapsulation efficiency and faster release of intact DNA were associated with the hydrophilic formulations in relation to the more hydrophobic formulations. Although all formulations displayed similar release in the burst phase, the hydrophilic formulations released DNA more rapidly in the second phase than the hydrophobic formulations. This faster release was shown to result in higher amounts of dsDNA in the second release phase. In addition, the *in vitro* release kinetics were examined under various pH values, ranging from 5.4 to 7.4. The initial burst phase of release was similar at all pH values, as 10–12% of the encapsulated DNA was released in the first 2.5 h. The release of DNA in the second phase was enhanced by acidic conditions. The DNA was found to lose its super-coiled structure and biological activity with time at all pH values. Additionally, this study demonstrated that the hydrophilic PLGA microspheres were phagocytosed with almost the same efficiency as the hydrophobic formulations in dendritic cells. The macrophages showed a slightly higher uptake of the hydrophobic microparticles, but still phagocytosed the hydrophilic microspheres. It was concluded, then, that all of the formulations held a degree of hydrophobicity that fell within the optimal range for cellular uptake. Once inside the cells, the hydrophilic microspheres were completely degraded within 9 days with a dispersion of the fluorescently marked DNA throughout the cell. Thus, the hydrophilic formulations were able to release the DNA within 2 weeks, a time frame compatible with the life span of the cells. The hydrophobic microspheres, however, were still intact after 13 days, having released little DNA at that time point. The degradation of the microspheres and subsequent release of plasmid DNA within the cell occurred more rapidly than in PBS. Indeed, the acidic environment encountered by the particles in the lysosomes may accelerate PLGA hydrolysis in a manner consistent with that observed in the acidic *in vitro* release component of this study. The phagocytosed microparticles did not induce significant necrosis or apoptosis in either cell type. Although this study demonstrated that PLGA microparticles can be phagocytosed by cells to release their encoded plasmid DNA, the activity of the reporter gene could not be monitored once the cells were transfected. Thus, further investigation is warranted to elucidate the barriers to gene expression encountered by the released DNA.

Hirosue *et al.* (2001) employed a third processing technique to encapsulate plasmid DNA in PLGA nanospheres. They explored the use of a modified phase inversion/solvent diffusion method, in which the cationic lipid dimethyl dioctadecyl ammonium bromide (DDAB) was used as an excipient. This process allowed for particles to be formed without exposure to the shear stresses commonly employed in the double-emulsion and spray-drying techniques. The phase inversion/solvent diffusion involved the addition of a solution of the condensing agent (DDAB) in a solvent (trifluoroethanol, TFE) to a solution of the PLGA in TFE. This resulting solution was mixed by inversion. Subsequently, a solution of DNA in water was slowly introduced to the mixture with a pipette. The nanospheres were formed upon rapid addition of ethanol (50% v/v) to the resulting mixture, thereby allowing phase inversion to occur. The suspension was then diluted with water, and the solvents were removed under reduced pressure. This process resulted in nanospheres that were less than 150 nm in diameter, regardless of the molecular weight of the PLGA used. Free DNA and DNA/DDAB complexes were separated from the nanospheres through use of a density separation method. In contrast to the bi-phasic release characteristic of previous studies, the release of DNA from the phase inversion nanospheres was approximately zero-order, with no burst effect observed. The nanospheres released up to approximately 20% of the encapsulated DNA after 30 days *in vitro*. Although the released DNA retained some bioactivity, it was significantly less than unencapsulated plasmid control DNA. It was suggested that the manner of entrapment likely governs the release kinetics. In contrast to the double-emulsion method, the phase inversion process likely results in the formation of a uniform matrix of polymer, lipid, and DNA, from which release would be expected to be near constant with no initial burst effect (Hirosue *et al.*, 2001). Although this study presented an extended, zero-order release, the structural integrity and bioactivity of the DNA may significantly decrease with time. Additionally, the extended release is likely not practical for DNA vaccination applications, in which a need for rapid release of DNA has been suggested (Tinsley-Bown *et al.*, 2000; Walter *et al.* 1999, 2001).

A subsequent study by Perez *et al.* (2001) investigated the use of poly (ethylene glycol)-(D,L-lactide) (PEG–PLA) nanospheres for encapsulation and release of plasmid DNA. They proposed that the use of nanospheres over microspheres might preserve the stability of encapsulated DNA, as acidic oligomers created in the degradation of the polymer could potentially diffuse out of the smaller construct with greater ease. They encapsulated plasmid DNA alone or with either PVA or PVP through one of two methods: double-emulsion solvent-evaporation or water-in-oil (w/o) solvent diffusion. The w/o solvent diffusion method involved the creation of an emulsion of aqueous DNA solution in an organic polymer solution by sonication. Subsequently, the emulsion was poured into ethanol under stirring to precipitate the polymer particles. The solution was diluted with water, and the solvents were removed through reduced pressure. Finally, the nanoparticles were collected by centrifugation. The nanospheres had negative ζ potential and were in the range of 150–300 nm in diameter, and the processing method influenced both of these parameters. High encapsulation efficiencies were obtained (60–90%), independent of the presence of PVA or PVP. The w/o solvent diffusion technique resulted in slightly higher encapsulation efficiencies than the double-emulsion (80–90% vs 60–80%). The encapsulation efficiencies of the nanospheres fabricated through double-emulsion were higher than generally observed. Indeed, it was proposed that high encapsulation efficiencies were the result of an interaction between plasmid DNA and the PEG chains of the polymer. The preparation technique was found to significantly affect the release kinetics: w/o solvent-diffusion nanospheres released the DNA rapidly (within an hour), whereas double-emulsion nanospheres followed the typical bi-phasic release over the course of 28 days *in vitro*. Thus, this study demonstrated high encapsulation efficiency through the interaction of DNA with PEG chains of the polymer. Further, in accord with previous studies, it was concluded that the preparation technique strongly influences the DNA release kinetics (Hirosue *et al.*, 2001).

A debate exists in the literature regarding whether DNA should be adsorbed to the surfaces of synthetic polymeric particles or be encapsulated within them. The studies discussed to this point have involved the encapsulation of the plasmid DNA within the particle, which has been proposed to promote DNA stability and allow for possible surface modification of the carriers (Hirosue *et al.*, 2001). Other studies, however, have investigated the adsorption of plasmid DNA to the surface of the particle (Maruyama *et al.*, 1997; Singh *et al.*, 2000). It has been suggested that surface adsorption could reduce the exposure of the DNA to the harsh conditions typically involved in the encapsulation process and increase the amount of DNA available for early release (Singh *et al.*, 2000). Indeed, Singh *et al.* fabricated PLGA microparticles with a cationic surface, through the inclusion of either dimethyl dioctadecyl ammonium bromide (DDAB) or

1,2-dioleoyl-1,3-trimethylammonio-propane (DOTAP) in the polymer phase or the addition of cetyltrimethylammonium bromide (CTAB) to the primary emulsion of the double-emulsion process. It was found that the inclusion of any of these cationic surfactants resulted in a positive ζ potential, with CTAB generating particles with the highest positive surface charge. Additionally, a high loading efficiency was observed for particles containing CTAB over those with DDAB or DOTAP (92, 68 and 62%, respectively). The DNA was released from PLGA–CTAB microspheres with an initial burst effect (35% released at day 1), followed by a slower release rate (75% of adsorbed DNA was released by day 14). The released DNA was shown to lose super-coiled structure with time. It was shown that DNA released from PLGA–CTAB nanospheres following intramuscular injection into a rat model resulted in an enhanced seroconversion relative to naked DNA controls. Additionally, a size effect of the particles was observed, with DNA released from 300 nm spheres generating a significantly higher Ig titer than from 1 μm to 30 μm spheres (10,000, 4000, and 0 titers, respectively). Although this study demonstrated that DNA adsorbed to particle surfaces can elicit an immune response in DNA vaccination applications, the system requires further characterization.

1. Natural Polymers for Release of DNA in Vaccination Applications

Some of the initial studies toward the investigation of polymeric nano- and microparticles involved the complex coacervation of DNA with natural polymers such as gelatin and chitosan (Leong et al., 1998; Mao et al., 2001; Roy et al., 1999; Truong-Le et al., 1998, 1999). Complex coacervation is a process in which oppositely charged macromolecular species are mixed in aqueous solution. The electrostatic interaction between the macromolecules drives a spontaneous phase separation to yield a phase rich in polymer (termed the coacervate) and a supernatant. The complex coacervation of gelatin and chondroitin sulfate has been used to encapsulate a variety of proteins and pharmaceuticals. Investigators have also explored the use of DNA as a polyanionic species for producing microspheres by complex coacervation with cationic macromolecules such as gelatin and chitosan (Leong et al., 1998).

Gelatin is a natural material derived from the denaturation of collagen, and it has been widely applied in the food and pharmaceutical industries. It has the ability to act as an acid in the presence of a strong acid or a base in the presence of a strong base. Gelatin carries a net positive charge at pH values below 5, thus it can form a coacervate with DNA through electrostatic complexation in these conditions (Leong et al., 1998).

The gelatin can subsequently be crosslinked to stabilize the complex. The crosslinked gelatin matrices are enzymatically degraded to release the DNA (Fukunaka et al., 2002; Truong-Le et al., 1998). An initial study by Truong-Le et al. (1998) investigated the release of plasmid DNA from DNA–gelatin microspheres generated through complex coacervation. Sodium sulfate was used in the process to facilitate the formation of coacervates through inducing desolvation in the water environment surrounding the polyelectrolytes (Leong et al., 1998). They obtained nanospheres in the size range of 200–700 nm with 25–30% (w/w) DNA loading. The higher molecular weight gelatin resulted in higher entrapment efficiency (~98%), likely through chain entanglement of the polyelectrolytes (Truong-Le et al., 1998). Although there was no evidence of DNA crosslinking to itself or to gelatin, increased crosslinking densities resulted in lower amounts of DNA released over the course of one hour *in vitro* (PBS with trypsin). It was found that the nanoparticles enhanced protection of DNA for up to 4 h in serum, but it was completely degraded by 12 h. Naked DNA incubated under the same conditions was completely degraded within half an hour. The release medium was found to affect the release kinetics, with enhanced cumulative release observed in serum versus PBS or water over the course of one week *in vitro*. For *in vitro* transfection analysis, an endosomolytic agent, chloroquine, was coencapsulated with the DNA, and human transferrin was conjugated to the nanosphere surface. The expression of a marker gene was greater and more prolonged over three weeks following intramuscular injection of the nanospheres into a mouse model, relative to controls of either naked DNA or DNA complexed with the cationic lipid Lipofectamine. This study demonstrated the encapsulation of DNA within gelatin nanospheres and subsequent gene expression following administration *in vivo*. Further, it was shown that other molecules could be coencapsulated with the DNA and that molecules could be conjugated onto the surface of the nanospheres to enhance DNA stability and cellular uptake.

A subsequent study by the same group sought to further characterize the gelatin–DNA nanosphere system through examination of the reaction conditions for particle formation, the protection offered to the DNA through encapsulation, and the effect of adding calcium as an additional coencapsulant on transfection (Truong-Le et al., 1999). The particle size was influenced by the temperature of the reaction, the size of the plasmid DNA, the concentration of sodium sulfate, and the speed of mixing employed. The encapsulated DNA was partially protected from DNase I induced damage at low concentrations. The optimal formulation for transfection included the coencapsulation of choloroquine and calcium with the DNA, as well as conjugation of transferrin on the nanosphere surface. Over 50% of cultured cells transfected with the nanospheres exhibited expression of a model gene for a transporter protein. Further, the cells demonstrated effective transport through the generated transporter protein.

The use of chitosan–DNA nanoparticles as DNA carriers has also been explored (Aral *et al.*, 2000; Leong *et al.*, 1998; Mao *et al.*, 2001; Roy *et al.*, 1999). Chitosan is a natural material derived from the shells of crustaceans. The biodegradability and nontoxicity of chitosan has led to the wide application of this polysaccharide in medical and pharmaceutical applications. Recent studies have demonstrated the ability of chitosan to effectively complex with and partially protect DNA (MacLaughlin *et al.*, 1998; Richardson *et al.*, 1999). An initial study by Leong *et al.* (1998) examined the encapsulation of DNA in chitosan nanospheres generated through complex coacervation. This study demonstrated that transferrin could be conjugated to the surface of the chitosan–DNA nanospheres and that chloroquine could be coencapsulated with the DNA, however, unmodified chitosan–DNA nanospheres were as effective at transfecting cells *in vitro* as nanospheres with transferrin and nanospheres with transferrin and chloroquine. The *in vitro* transfection efficiency of the nanopsheres was less efficient than observed with Lipofectamine. This study, however, did not examine the *in vitro* release kinetics of DNA or *in vivo* gene expression. A subsequent study by the same group evaluated the efficacy of the chitosan–DNA nanoparticles in delivering DNA to a mucosal surface (Roy *et al.*, 1999). A murine peanut allergy model was used, and plasmid DNA encoding an anaphylaxis-inducing antigen was delivered orally via chitosan–DNA nanospheres. The DNA was delivered effectively to the small intestine of the mice through oral administration and elicited a high IgG2a response, which protected the sensitized mice from challenge with the peanut allergen. A third study by this group sought to further examine the preparation parameters for the chitosan–DNA nanospheres and characterize the physico-chemical properties (Mao *et al.*, 2001). In this study, several processing parameters were examined and optimized for nanoparticle production. It was found that the processing of the nanospheres has a negligible effect on the conformation of the DNA. Further, this study suggested that encapsulation within the nanospheres offered protection of the DNA from degradation. The *in vitro* transfection efficiency of the nanospheres was shown to depend on the cell type, yet was several times lower than that obtained with Lipofectamine–DNA complexes. This result corresponded with results from a previous study (Leong *et al.*, 1998). As in the previous study (Leong *et al.*, 1998), the enhancement of transfection through co-encapsulating chloroquine or conjugating transferrin to the surface was limited. Conjugation of the viral

KNOB protein, however, was shown to improve gene expression markedly (130-fold in HeLa cells). Additionally, it was shown that PEG could be conjugated to the surface of the nanospheres to prevent aggregation during lyophilization without a loss of bioactivity following one month in storage. The PEGylated particles, however, were cleared from mice at a slower rate than unmodified controls and were found to accumulate in the kidney and liver at 15 min after intravenous administration. There was no difference after one hour, however.

Another study by an independent group examined the effect of various processing parameters on the *in vivo* transfection efficiency of chitosan–DNA microspheres (Aral *et al.*, 2000). Additionally, this study investigated the effect of plasmid size on the *in vitro* release kinetics and transfection properties. An initial burst phase was observed with all chitosan–DNA microsphere formulations, which was likely due to release of DNA from the surface of the microspheres (Aral *et al.*, 2000). The effect of chitosan concentration on the release of DNA seemed to be dependent on the size of the incorporated plasmid. Plasmid adsorbed to the surface of the microspheres was released more rapidly *in vitro* than DNA entrapped within the microspheres. Further, larger plasmids were released more rapidly *in vitro* than smaller plasmids (7.2 vs 2.69 kilobases). Although the released DNA showed some conversion from super-coiled to open circular and linear conformations upon release, the entrapment was shown to protect the DNA from nuclease degradation *in vitro*. The DNA delivered with chitosan–DNA microspheres demonstrated significantly higher expression *in vivo* than naked DNA, with the highest expression associated with the low-dose chitosan–DNA formulation. The effect of plasmid size on transfection was not clear. The studies with chitosan–DNA microspheres demonstrate its ability to enhance transfection *in vitro* and *in vivo*, to protect DNA from degradation, and to allow for conjugation of cell-targeting moieties on the surface of the microspheres.

The use of polymeric nano- and microparticles for DNA entrapment and release has demonstrated promise for use in DNA vaccination applications. Several materials have been investigated, each with their own set of advantages and limitations. In general, the release kinetics of the DNA can be controlled through manipulation of the formulation parameters in fabrication of the carrier particles. PLGA particles demonstrate a degree of control over the release kinetics, and processing techniques have been introduced to reduce the extent of DNA damage during fabrication. However, protection of the DNA from the acidic microenvironment during particle degradation remains an issue. Further, there appears to be a trade-off between entrapment efficiency and release kinetics with the PLGA carriers. The natural materials, such as gelatin and chitosan, offer the potential for less damage to the DNA during fabrication and allow for conjugation of cell-targeting moieties to the surface of the spheres. The use of natural materials, however, has an associated risk of potential immunogenecity of the material, as it is derived from a natural source. Additionally, the characterization and control of release from the natural materials requires further investigation.

The entrapment and release of plasmid DNA from polymeric nano- and microparticles has not been limited to DNA vaccination applications. Indeed, the delivery of DNA from nano- and microparticles for application in guided tissue regeneration applications has been explored. Labhasetwar *et al.* (1998) demonstrated effective expression of a marker gene in a rat osteotomy model following delivery of DNA-loaded PLGA nanospheres generated with a double-emulsion solvent-evaporation technique. This study demonstrated the potential for DNA delivery from a polymeric material introduced into a wound site. Another study demonstrated that tissue engineering scaffolds can be fabricated from DNA-loaded PLGA microspheres through either compression molding or a gas-foaming process (Nof and Shea, 2002). Additionally, it was shown that porous scaffolds could be fabricated with these techniques in conjunction with a salt-leaching method (Nof and Shea, 2002). This study evaluated the *in vitro* release of the incorporated plasmid DNA. The release from the scaffolds showed minimal burst effect in the initial phase of release when compared to the microspheres from which they were fabricated. This study demonstrated the potential for fabricating tissue engineering scaffolds from DNA loaded microspheres and the ability to control the release of DNA from the scaffold through manipulation of processing parameters. Indeed, these studies have led to the investigation of release of plasmid DNA from polymeric scaffolds to augment guided tissue regeneration in tissue engineering applications.

IV. Polymeric Scaffolds for Controlled DNA Delivery

A. Gene Activated Matrices

A method was recently developed to deliver plasmid DNA locally to cells involved in wound repair (Bonadio *et al.*, 1999; Fang *et al.*, 1996; Shea *et al.*, 1999). The technique involves the introduction of a porous, biodegradable polymer matrix into the wound site (Bonadio *et al.*, 1998). The scaffold (a gene activated matrix, or GAM), in its simplest form comprises plasmid DNA and the polymer matrix (Bonadio, 2000). Naked plasmid DNA is physically entrapped into the polymer network during scaffold fabrication. It has been proposed that the matrix holds the plasmid DNA *in situ* as wound healing cells, mainly fibroblasts, infiltrate the construct from the periphery (Fang *et al.*, 1996). The cells incorporate the DNA as they encounter it and begin to produce the encoded factor (Fang *et al.*, 1996; Martin, 1997). The transfected fibroblasts then serve as local bioreactors, producing the encoded gene product at physiological levels in the wound site. This factor can, in turn, influence the course of events at the wound site (Fang *et al.*, 1996). The ability of GAMs to transfect wound healing fibroblasts has opened the technology to application in a wide range of tissues, including bone (Bonadio *et al.*, 1999; Fang *et al.*, 1996; Patil *et al.*, 2000), skin (Chandler *et al.*, 2000; Shea *et al.*, 1999), arteries (Klugherz *et al.*, 2000), cardiac and skeletal muscle (Labhasetwar *et al.*, 1998), tendon (Zhu *et al.*, 1994), and cartilage (Samuel *et al.*, 2002). The application of GAM technology in bone regeneration, however, will serve as the focus for the current discussion.

B. WOUND HEALING AND BONE REGENERATION

The wound healing response involves a complex cascade of events, yet is a conserved process between tissues and among mammals (Martin, 1997). A wide variety of cells participate in wound healing, including platelets, lymphocytes, macrophages, fibroblasts, endothelial cells, and various progenitor cells (Bonadio, 2000). The migration, proliferation, and differentiation of these cells are coordinated through the local action of cytokines and growth factors. The complex signal cascade and subsequent cellular response depends upon the nature of the tissue injury. The initial response to acute injury typically involves hemostasis and clearing of cellular debris from the site as part of an acute inflammatory response (Bonadio, 2000; Park and Lakes, 1992). Subsequently, granulation tissue appears from which either a scar is formed or tissue regeneration occurs. Tissue engineering strategies seek to guide the wound healing process toward the path of tissue regeneration.

The regenerative capacity of bone is robust and effective at addressing wounds under normal conditions. A proportion of fractures, however, present conditions that are not conducive to regeneration and place the fracture at high risk for nonunion or delayed union. For example, fractures located at sites of marginal vascularity and those associated with a large area of bone loss repair with difficulty if at all. As a result, a great deal of effort has been invested in the development of treatment methods for fractures and defects at risk of nonunion, as they would not likely heal unaided. The treatment options range from fixation of the fracture coupled with pain management to attempts to augment bone regeneration.

The surgical transfer of autologous bone tissue to the defect site is the "gold standard" for augmentation of bone regeneration. The procedure is generally successful, however, the amount of autologous bone tissue available for transfer is limited, and often not of the desired shape. Additionally, the recruitment of distal bone from the patient requires the introduction of a second defect and creates a risk of donor site morbidity. The employment of allogenic bone tissue provides an alternative method to autografts. Although allograft material is more plentiful than autologous bone for grafting, processing of the allogenic tissue limits its osteoinductive properties and does not eliminate the risk of pathogen transmission.

C. BONE TISSUE ENGINEERING

The limitations associated with bone grafting techniques have led researchers to seek additional methods to augment bone repair. As a result, tissue engineering strategies have been developed to enhance bone formation in large defects. Such methods generally involve the employment of biocompatible materials with osteoinductive properties. Three general tissue engineering strategies for bone exist: (1) implantation of a scaffold that is conducive to bone tissue infiltration, (2) inclusion of bioactive molecules within a conductive scaffold, and (3) *in vitro* seeding of cells on a conductive scaffold prior to implantation (Murphy and Mooney, 1999). In some cases, combinations of the various strategies are employed to regenerate bone tissue.

1. Bioactive Factor Delivery

The approach of bioactive factor delivery for bone tissue engineering is of particular interest for the current discussion. The wound repair cascade in bone involves the generation of numerous factors, which influence and direct cellular migration, proliferation, and differentiation. Isolation of these factors and identification of their specific roles in the regeneration response has led to their implementation in bone tissue engineering scaffolds. Indeed, numerous studies have shown the *in vivo* osteoinductive potential of various recombinant growth factors including bone morphogenetic proteins (BMPs), transforming growth factor beta (TGF-β), and insulin-like growth factor (IGF) [see Babensee *et al.* (2000) and Linkhart *et al.* (1996) for a review]. The limitations associated with the direct delivery of growth factors and cytokines has led to the exploration of growth factor delivery via gene therapy. Although many methods of gene therapy exist, the delivery of uncomplexed, nonviral plasmid DNA is of particular interest in the current discussion.

2. GAMs and Bone: Small Animals

The first study to investigate the feasibility of GAMs for bone repair utilized a rat model (Fang *et al.*, 1996). In that study, collagen sponge GAMs were introduced into 5-mm segmental defects in rat femurs with external fixation. The first portion of the study involved the implantation of GAMs containing plasmids for the marker genes β-galactasidase and luciferase in order to assess the *in vivo* transfection of wound healing cells. The marker gene GAMs were implanted into 23 animals at various dosages. The study demonstrated the infiltration of fibroblasts into the GAM, uptake of the plasmid DNA by these cells, and functional expression of the encoded markers. The remainder of the study focused on the ability of GAMs containing plasmid genes encoding osteoinductive factors to augment bone regeneration. GAMs in this portion of the study contained either a BMP-4 plasmid or a plasmid encoding for the first 34 amino acids of parathyroid hormone alone, or both plasmids together. Each GAM resulted in new bone filling the gap. Interestingly, the GAMs containing both plasmids, which act synergistically *in vitro*, led to a faster regeneration response than either plasmid alone. It is important to note that control defects containing collagen matrices alone or collagen matrices with marker gene plasmids demonstrated no new bone formation. This work was the first to demonstrate that bone formation is augmented through the *in vivo* delivery of osteoinductive plasmid genes from GAMs. Additionally, this study demonstrated the feasibility of delivering two plasmid genes at once from a GAM to elicit a synergistic biological effect.

3. GAMs and Bone: Larger Animals

Another study was conducted to investigate the potential for GAM technology to be scaled-up to augment bone regeneration in larger animals (Bonadio *et al.*, 1999). Two canine models were used in this study. In the first model, GAMs were implanted into 8-mm diameter by 8-mm deep cylindrical defects drilled into the distal femurs and proximal tibias of large mongrel dogs. GAMs in the first portion of the study contained either a plasmid for β-galactasidase or no plasmid at all (control), in order to assess *in vivo* transfection and functional protein expression. The control defects were negative for β-galactasidase staining, whereas the defects receiving plasmid GAMs were positive. The authors estimated that the staining marked 30–50% of the available granulation tissue cells. Further, based upon morphological criteria, the authors found most of the transfected cells to be fibroblasts.

A final portion of the study utilized the second model to examine the effects of plasmid dose and defect size on the regeneration of bone. A beagle tibia critical defect model (2-cm) with external fixation was used in this portion of the study. Collagen GAMs were formulated with and without (control) the inclusion of the plasmid for hPTH$_{1-34}$. Bone regeneration was not induced in defects receiving doses of 1.0–20.0 mg of plasmid. Defects receiving doses of 40.0 and 100.0 mg of plasmid, however, demonstrated significant bone formation relative to controls over the course of 12 weeks, yet no complete filling of the gap was observed. Smaller defects (1.6 and 1.0 cm) receiving GAMs with 100.0 mg of plasmid demonstrated new bone formation and complete filling of the gap over the course of six months. Control defects in all cases produced little or no new bone. This study demonstrated that bone regeneration can be substantially and reproducibly augmented in large defects through the use of GAMs. Further, the bone formation appeared to be dose dependent and to follow a predictable time course.

4. GAMs and Bone: Summary

These initial studies demonstrated the feasibility of nonviral DNA delivery via a porous, degradable matrix (GAM) for the regeneration of bone in small and large animals. Although these studies demonstrated functional results in various bone defect models, they have not examined in detail dose response or transfection efficiency. Additionally, the GAMs in these studies were fabricated using collagen sponges. It has been demonstrated, however, that other materials may be used as matrix carriers of plasmid DNA, including alginate (Ho and Neufeld, 2001; Quong *et al.*, 1996), poly(ethylene vinyl *co*-acetate) (Jong *et al.*, 1997), poly(lactide-*co*-glycolide) (PLGA) (Klugherz *et al.*, 2000; Shea *et al.*, 1999), and poly(vinyl alcohol) (Chandler *et al.*, 2000). Indeed, it has been proposed that GAMs may be optimized through the choice of the matrix material and the choice of the gene or genes required to propel the desired biological effect (Goldstein, 2000).

D. RELEASE OF DNA FROM SCAFFOLDS

Scaffolds have also been investigated for the controlled release of plasmid DNA rather than holding the DNA *in situ* as with GAMs. Fukunaka *et al.* (2002) investigated the controlled release of plasmid DNA from cationized gelatin hydrogels. They demonstrated that the release was controlled by the enzymatic degradation of the gelatin, which could be controlled by manipulating the degree of crosslinking or the water content of the gels. Another group demonstrated *in vivo* expression and controlled release of DNA from a collagen minipellet (Ochiya *et al.*, 1999). Park *et al.*, (2002) investigated the controlled release of plasmid DNA from mucoadhesive poloxamers (poly(carbophil) or poly(ethylene glycol)) in intranasal applications. The controlled release of plasmid DNA from nondegradable EVAc matrices was demonstrated by Jong *et al.*, (1997). An additional development involved the incorporation of plasmid containing collagen within the pores of a PVA matrix for tissue engineering to regulate angiogenesis (Kyriakides *et al.*, 2001). Regardless of the material of choice, polymeric scaffolds have been shown to be effective in the controlled delivery of plasmid DNA, so as to guide tissue formation in tissue engineering applications.

V. Conclusion

The concept of gene therapy has evolved in recent years to include the application of gene delivery to DNA vaccinations and guided tissue regeneration. Although several methods of gene therapy exist, the use of polymeric biomaterials for nonviral gene therapy has been a major area of focus in recent years. Methods have been developed for the controlled delivery of plasmid DNA from polymer nano- and microspheres as well as from tissue engineering scaffolds. Entrapment of DNA within polymeric carriers has been shown to enhance DNA stability, improve bioavailability, and promote cellular uptake. However, further investigation is warranted to improve the transfection efficiency and cell or tissue targeting.

VI. Abbreviations

DOTAP	1,2-dioleoyl-1,3-trimethylammonio-propane
BMP	bone morphogeneic protein
CTAB	cetyltrimethylammonium bromide
DNA	deoxyribonucleic acid
DDAB	dimethyl dioctadecyl ammonium bromide
dsDNA	double-stranded DNA
EDTA	ethylenediaminetetraacetic acid
hPTH$_{1-34}$	first 34 amino acids of human parathyroid hormone
FDA	Food and Drug Administration

GAM	gene activated matrix
IGF	insulin-like growth factor
PBS	phosphate buffered saline
pDNA	plasmid DNA
PAMAM	poly(amidoamine)
PLGA	poly(D,L-lactic-*co*-glycolic) acid
PEG	poly(ethylene glycol)
PEI	poly(ethylenimine)
PLA	poly(L-lactic acid)
PLL	poly(L-lysine)
PVP	poly(vinylpyrrolidone)
RNA	ribonucleic acid
SCID	severe combined immunodeficiency
TGF-β	transforming growth factor β
TFE	trifluoroethanol

ACKNOWLEDGMENTS

This work was partially supported by NSF-IGERT Grant DGE-0114264.

REFERENCES

Adami, R. C., Collard, W. T., Gupta, S. A., Kwok, K. Y., Bonadio, J., and Rice, K. G. *J. Pharm. Sci.* **87,** 678 (1998).
Anderson, W. F. *Nature* **392,** 25 (1998).
Ando, S., Putnam, D., Pack, D. W., and Langer, R. *J. Pharm. Sci.* **88,** 126 (1999).
Aral, C., Ozbas-Turan, S., Kabasakal, L., Keyer-Uysal, M., and Akbuga, J. *Stp. Pharma. Sci.* **10,** 83 (2000).
Babensee, J. E., McIntire, L. V., and Mikos, A. G. *Pharm. Res.* **17,** 497 (2000).
Barman, S. P., Lunsford, L., Chambers, P., and Hedley, M. L. *J. Control. Rel.* **69,** 337 (2000).
Bebok, Z., Abai, A. M., Dong, J. Y., King, S. A., Kirk, K. L., Berta, G., Hughes, B. W., Kraft, A. S., Burgess, S. W., Shaw, W., Felgner, P. L., and Sorscher, E. J. *J. Pharmacol. Exp. Ther.* **279,** 1462 (1996).
Bielinska, A. U., Kukowska-Latallo, J. F., and Baker, J. R. Jr. *Biochim. Biophys. Acta* **1353,** 180 (1997).
Bonadio, J. *J. Mol. Med.* **78,** 303 (2000).
Bonadio, J., Goldstein, S. A., and Levy, R. J. *Adv. Drug. Deliv. Rev.* **33,** 53 (1998).
Bonadio, J., Smiley, E., Patil, P., and Goldstein, S. *Nat. Med.* **5,** 753 (1999).
Boussif, O., Lezoualc'h, F., Zanta, M. A., Mergny, M. D., Scherman, D., Demeneix, B., and Behr, J. P. *Proc. Natl. Acad. Sci. USA* **92,** 7297 (1995).

Budker, V., Budker, T., Zhang, G., Subbotin, V., Loomis, A., and Wolff, J. A. *J. Gene. Med.* **2**, 76 (2000).
Byk, G., Dubertret, C., Escriou, V., Frederic, M., Jaslin, G., Rangara, R., Pitard, B., Crouzet, J., Wils, P., Schwartz, B., and Scherman, D. *J. Med. Chem.* **41**, 229 (1998a).
Byk, G., Soto, J., Mattler, C., Frederic, M., and Scherman, D. *Biotechnol. Bioeng.* **61**, 81 (1998b).
Calarota, S., Bratt, G., Nordlund, S., Hinkula, J., Leandersson, A. C., Sandstrom, E., and Wahren, B. *Lancet* **351**, 1320 (1998).
Capan, Y., Woo, B. H., Gebrekidan, S., Ahmed, S., and DeLuca, P. P. *Pharm. Res.* **16**, 509 (1999a).
Capan, Y., Woo, B. H., Gebrekidan, S., Ahmed, S., and DeLuca, P. P. *J. Control. Rel.* **60**, 279 (1999b).
Chandler, L. A., Gu, D. L., Ma, C., Gonzalez, A. M., Doukas, J., Nguyen, T., Pierce, G. F., and Phillips, M. L. *Wound Repair Regen.* **8**, 473 (2000).
Choate, K. A., and Khavari, P. A. *Hum. Gene. Ther.* **8**, 1659 (1997).
Choi, Y. H., Liu, F., Kim, J. S., Choi, Y. K., Park, J. S., and Kim, S. W. *J. Control. Rel.* **54**, 39 (1998).
Cohen, H., Levy, R. J., Gao, J., Fishbein, I., Kousaev, V., Sosnowski, S., Slomkowski, S., and Golomb, G. *Gene. Ther.* **7**, 2000 (1896).
Connelly, S., and Kaleko, M. *Thromb. Haemost.* **78**, 31 (1997).
Connelly, S., and Kaleko, M. *Haemophilia* **4**, 380 (1998).
Corr, M., Lee, D. J., Carson, D. A., and Tighe, H. *J. Exp. Med.* **184**, 1555 (1996).
Danko, I., Fritz, J. D., Jiao, S., Hogan, K., Latendresse, J. S., and Wolff, J. A. *Gene. Ther.* **1**, 114 (1994).
Davis, H. L., Demeneix, B. A., Quantin, B., Coulombe, J., and Whalen, R. G. *Hum. Gene. Ther.* **4**, 733 (1993a).
Doe, B., Selby, M., Barnett, S., Baenziger, J., and Walker, C. M. *Proc. Natl. Acad. Sci. USA* **93**, 8578 (1996).
Donnelly, J. J., Friedman, A., Martinez, D., Montgomery, D. L., Shiver, J. W., Motzel, S. L., Ulmer, J. B., and Liu, M. A. *Nat. Med.* **1**, 583 (1995).
Donnelly, J. J., Ulmer, J. B., and Liu, M. A. *Life. Sci.* **60**, 163 (1997).
Duguid, J. G., Li, C., Shi, M., Logan, M. J., Alila, H., Rolland, A., Tomlinson, E., Sparrow, J. T., and Smith, L. C. *Biophys. J.* **74**, 2802 (1998).
Eastman, E. M., and Durland, R. H. *Adv. Drug. Deliv. Rev.* **30**, 33 (1998).
Eldridge, J. H., Gilley, R. M., Staas, J. K., Moldoveanu, Z., Meulbroek, J. A., and Tice, T. R. *Curr. Top. Microbiol. Immunol.* **146**, 59 (1989).
Erbacher, P., Remy, J. S., and Behr, J. P. *Gene. Ther.* **6**, 138 (1999).
Fang, J., Zhu, Y. Y., Smiley, E., Bonadio, J., Rouleau, J. P., Goldstein, S. A., McCauley, L. K., Davidson, B. L., and Roessler, B. J. *Proc. Natl. Acad. Sci. USA* **93**, 5753 (1996).
Felgner, P. L., Gadek, T. R., Holm, M., Roman, R., Chan, H. W., Wenz, M., Northrop, J. P., Ringold, G. M., and Danielsen, M. *Proc. Natl. Acad. Sci. USA* **84**, 7413 (1987).
Felgner, J. H., Kumar, R., Sridhar, C. N., Wheeler, C. J., Tsai, Y. J., Border, R., Ramsey, P., Martin, M., and Felgner, P. L. *J. Biol. Chem.* **269**, 2550 (1994).
Ferrari, M. E., Rusalov, D., Enas, J., and Wheeler, C. J. *Nucleic. Acids. Res.* **30**, 1808 (2000).
Filion, M. C., and Phillips, N. C. *Br. J. Pharmacol.* **122**, 551 (1997).
Filion, M. C., and Phillips, N. C. *Int. J. Pharm.* **162**, 159 (1998).
Fukunaka, Y., Iwanaga, K., Morimoto, K., Kakemi, M., and Tabata, Y. *J. Control. Rel.* **80**, 333 (2002).

Fynan, E. F., Webster, R. G., Fuller, D. H., Haynes, J. R., Santoro, J. C., and Robinson, H. L. *Proc. Natl. Acad. Sci. USA* **90,** 11478 (1993).
Garnett, M. C. *Crit. Rev. Ther. Drug. Carrier. Syst.* **16,** 147 (1999).
Godbey, W. T., Barry, M. A., Saggau, P., Wu, K. K., and Mikos, A. G. *J. Biomed. Mater. Res.* **51,** 321 (2000).
Godbey, W. T., Wu, K. K., and Mikos, A. G. *J. Biomed. Mater. Res.* **45,** 268 (1999a).
Godbey, W. T., Wu, K. K., and Mikos, A. G. *Proc. Natl. Acad. Sci. USA* **96,** 5177 (1999b).
Goldstein, S. A., and Bonadio, J. *Clin. Orthop.* S154 (1998).
Goldstein, S. A. *Clin. Orthop.* S113 (2000).
Gonsho, A., Irie, K., Susaki, H., Iwasawa, H., Okuno, S., and Sugawara, T. *Biol. Pharm. Bull.* **17,** 275 (1994).
Gottschalk, S., Cristiano, R. J., Smith, L. C., and Woo, S. L. *Gene. Ther.* **1,** 185 (1994).
Gupta, R. K., Singh, M., and O'Hagan, D. T. *Adv. Drug. Deliv. Rev.* **32,** 225 (1998).
Haensler, J., and Szoka, F. C. Jr. *Bioconjug. Chem.* **4,** 372 (1993).
Han, S., Mahato, R. I., Sung, Y. K., and Kim, S. W. *Mol. Ther.* **2,** 302 (2000).
Hao, T., McKeever, U., and Hedley, M. L. *J. Control. Rel.* **69,** 249 (2000).
Hassett, D. E., and Whitton, J. L. *Trends. Microbiol.* **4,** 307 (1996).
Hausberger, A. G., and DeLuca, P. P. *J. Pharm. Biomed. Anal.* **13,** 747 (1995).
Heller, J., Penhale, D. W., Fritzinger, B. K., and Ng, S. Y. *J. Control. Rel.* **5,** 173 (1987).
Hirosue, S., Muller, B. G., Mulligan, R. C., and Langer, R. *J. Control. Rel.* **70,** 231 (2001).
Ho, J., and Neufeld, R. J. *Stp. Pharma. Sci.* **11,** 109 (2001).
Iwasaki, A., Stiernholm, B. J., Chan, A. K., Berinstein, N. L., and Barber, B. H. *J. Immunol.* **158,** 4591 (1997).
Jiao, S., Williams, P., Berg, R. K., Hodgeman, B. A., Liu, L., Repetto, G., and Wolff, J. A. *Hum. Gene. Ther.* **3,** 21 (1992).
Jones, D.H., and Farrar, G. H., PCT/GB205/23019 (1995).
Jones, D. H., Corris, S., McDonald, S., Clegg, J. C., and Farrar, G. H. *Vaccine* **15,** 814 (1997).
Jong, Y. S., Jacob, J. S., Yip, K., Gardner, G., Seitelman, E., Whitney, M., Montgomery, S., and Mathiowitz, E. *J. Control. Rel.* **47,** 123 (1997).
Kawabata, K., Takakura, Y., and Hashida, M. *Pharm. Res.* **12,** 825 (1995).
Klugherz, B. D., Jones, P. L., Cui, X., Chen, W., Meneveau, N. F., DeFelice, S., Connolly, J., Wilensky, R. L., and Levy, R. J. *Nat. Biotechnol.* **18,** 1181 (2000).
Kyriakides, T. R., Hartzel, T., Huynh, G., and Bornstein, P. *Mol. Ther.* **3,** 842 (2001).
Labhasetwar, V., Bonadio, J., Goldstein, S., Chen, W., and Levy, R. J. *J. Pharm. Sci.* **87,** 1347 (1998).
Ledley, F. D. *Pharm. Res.* **13,** 1595 (1996).
Lee, H., Jeong, J. H., and Park, T. G. *J. Control. Rel.* **79,** 283 (2002).
Lee, E. R., Marshall, J., Siegel, C. S., Jiang, C., Yew, N. S., Nichols, M. R., Nietupski, J. B., Ziegler, R. J., Lane, M. B., Wang, K. X., Wan, N. C., Scheule, R. K., Harris, D. J., Smith, A. E., and Cheng, S. H. *Hum. Gene. Ther.* **7,** 1701 (1996).
Leong, K. W., Mao, H. Q., Truong-Le, V. L., Roy, K., Walsh, S. M., and August, J. T. *J. Control. Rel.* **53,** 183 (1998).
Letvin, N. L., Montefiori, D. C., Yasutomi, Y., Perry, H. C., Davies, M. E., Lekutis, C., Alroy, M., Freed, D. C., Lord, C. I., Handt, L. K., Liu, M. A., and Shiver, J. W. *Proc. Natl. Acad. Sci. USA* **94,** 9378 (1997).
Levy, M. Y., Barron, L. G., Meyer, K. B., and Szoka, F. C. Jr. *Gene. Ther.* **3,** 201 (1996).
Linkhart, T. A., Mohan, S., and Baylink, D. J. *Bone* **19,** 1S (1996).
Lunsford, L., McKeever, U., Eckstein, V., and Hedley, M. L. *J. Drug. Target.* **8,** 39 (2000).
Luo, D., and Saltzman, W. M. *Nat. Biotechnol.* **18,** 33 (2000a).
Luo, D., and Saltzman, W. M. *Nat. Biotechnol.* **18,** 893 (2000b).

Luo, D., Woodrow-Mumford, K., Belcheva, N., and Saltzman, W. M. *Pharm. Res.* **16,** 1300 (1999).
MacGregor, R. R., Boyer, J. D., Ugen, K. E., Lacy, K. E., Gluckman, S. J., Bagarazzi, M. L., Chattergoon, M. A., Baine, Y., Higgins, T. J., Ciccarelli, R. B., Coney, L. R., Ginsberg, R. S., and Weiner, D. B. *J. Infect. Dis.* **178,** 92 (1998).
MacLaughlin, F. C., Mumper, R. J., Wang, J., Tagliaferri, J. M., Gill, I., Hinchcliffe, M., and Rolland, A. P. *J Control Rel.* **56,** 259 (1998).
Mahato, R. I., Smith, L. C., and Rolland, A. *Adv. Genet.* **41,** 95 (1999).
Mao, H. Q., Roy, K., Troung-Le, V. L., Janes, K. A., Lin, K. Y., Wang, Y., August, J. T., and Leong, K. W. *J. Control. Rel.* **70,** 399 (2001).
Marini, J. C., and Gerber, N. L. *JAMA.* **277,** 746 (1997).
Martin, P. *Science* **276,** 75 (1997).
Maruyama, A., Ishihara, T., Kim, J. S., Kim, S. W., and Akaike, T. *Bioconjug. Chem.* **8,** 735 (1997).
Maruyama, A., Watanabe, H., Ferdous, A., Katoh, M., Ishihara, T., and Akaike, T. *Bioconjug. Chem.* **9,** 292 (1998).
Mehta, R. C., Jeyanthi, R., Calis, S., Thanoo, B. C., Burton, K. W., and Deluca, P. P. *J. Control. Rel.* **29,** 375 (1994).
Mumper, R. J., Duguid, J. G., Anwer, K., Barron, M. K., Nitta, H., and Rolland, A. P. *Pharm. Res.* **13,** 701 (1996).
Murphy, W. L., and Mooney, D. J. *J. Periodontal. Res.* **34,** 413 (1999).
Nichols, W. W., Ledwith, B. J., Manam, S. V., and Troilo, P. J. *Ann. NY. Acad. Sci.* **772,** 30 (1995).
Nof, M., and Shea, L. D. *J. Biomed. Mater. Res.* **59,** 349 (2002).
Oakes, D. A., and Lieberman, J. R. *Clin Orthop.* S101 (2000).
Ochiya, T., Takahama, Y., Nagahara, S., Sumita, Y., Hisada, A., Itoh, H., Nagai, Y., and Terada, M. *Nat. Med.* **5,** 707 (1999).
Oupicky, D., Howard, K. A., Konak, C., Dash, P. R., Ulbrich, K., and Seymour, L. W. *Bioconjug. Chem.* **11,** 492 (2000).
Park, J. S., and Lakes, R. S., "Biomaterials: An Introduction", p. 225. Plenum Press, New York (1992).
Park, J. S., Oh, Y. K., Yoon, H., Kim, J. M., and Kim, C. K. *J. Biomed. Mater. Res.* **59,** 144 (2002).
Parker, S. E., Borellini, F., Wenk, M. L., Hobart, P., Hoffman, S. L., Hedstrom, R., Le, T., and Norman, J. A. *Hum. Gene. Ther.* **10,** 741 (1999).
Patil, P. V., Graziano, G. P., and Bonadio, J. *Trans. Ortho. Res. Soc.* **25,** 360 (2000).
Perez, C., Sanchez, A., Putnam, D., Ting, D., Langer, R., and Alonso, M. J. *J. Control. Rel.* **75,** 211 (2001).
Porgador, A., Irvine, K. R., Iwasaki, A., Barber, B. H., Restifo, N. P., and Germain, R. N. *J. Exp. Med.* **188,** 1075 (1998).
Pouton, C. W., and Seymour, L. W. *Adv. Drug. Deliv. Rev.* **34,** 3 (1998).
Qin, L., Pahud, D. R., Ding, Y., Bielinska, A. U., Kukowska-Latallo, J. F., Baker, J. R. Jr., and Bromberg, J. S. *Hum. Gene. Ther.* **9,** 553 (1998).
Qiu, P., Ziegelhoffer, P., Sun, J., and Yang, N. S. *Gene. Ther.* **3,** 262 (1996).
Quong, D., O'Neill, I. K., Poncelet, D., and Neufeld, R. J., Immobilized Cells: Basics and Applications, *in* "Gastro-Intestinal Protection of Cellular Component DNA within an Artificial Cell System for Environmental Carcinogen Biomonitoring" (R. G. Wijffels, R. M. Buitelaar, H. S. Wessels, C. Bucke, and J. Tramper Eds.), , p. 814. Elsevier Science, Amsterdam (1996).
Radler, J. O., Koltover, I., Salditt, T., and Safinya, C. R. *Science* **275,** 810 (1997).

Richardson, S. C., Kolbe, H. V., and Duncan, R. *Int. J. Pharm.* **178,** 231 (1999).
Roy, K., Mao, H. Q., Huang, S. K., and Leong, K. W. *Nat. Med.* **5,** 387 (1999).
Samuel, R. E., Lee, C. R., Ghivizzani, S. C., Evans, C. H., Yannas, I. V., Olsen, B. R., and Spector, M. *Hum. Gene. Ther.* **13,** 791 (2002).
Segura, T., and Shea, L. D. *Annu. Rev. Mater. Res.* **31,** 25 (2001).
Shea, L. D., Smiley, E., Bonadio, J., and Mooney, D. J. *Nat. Biotechnol.* **17,** 551 (1999).
Shiver, J. W., Davies, M. E., Perry, H. C., Freed, D. C., and Liu, M. A. *J. Pharm. Sci.* **85,** 1317 (1996).
Singh, M., Briones, M., Ott, G., and O'Hagan, D. *Proc. Natl. Acad. Sci. USA* **97,** 811 (2000).
Smith, A. E. *Annu. Rev. Microbiol.* **49,** 807 (1995).
Smith, J. G., Walzem, R. L., and German, J. B. *Biochim. Biophys. Acta.* **1154,** 327 (1993).
Tabata, Y., and Ikada, Y. *Adv. Polymer. Sci.* **94,** 107 (1990).
Takakura, Y., Mahato, R. I., and Hashida, M. *Adv. Drug. Deliv. Rev.* **34,** 93 (1998).
Tan, Y., and Huang, L. *J. Drug. Target.* **10,** 153 (2002).
Tang, M. X., Redemann, C. T., and Szoka, F. C. Jr. *Bioconjug. Chem.* **7,** 703 (1996).
Tinsley-Bown, A. M., Fretwell, R., Dowsett, A. B., Davis, S. L., and Farrar, G. H. *J. Control. Rel.* **66,** 229 (2000).
Tomalia, D. A., Brothers, H. M. 2nd, Piehler, L. T., Durst, H. D., and Swanson, D. R. *Proc. Natl. Acad. Sci. USA* **99,** 5081 (2002).
Truong-Le, V. L., August, J. T., and Leong, K. W. *Hum. Gene. Ther.* **9,** 1709 (1998).
Truong-Le, V. L., Walsh, S. M., Schweibert, E., Mao, H. Q., Guggino, W. B., August, J. T., and Leong, K. W. *Arch. Biochem. Biophys.* **361,** 47 (1999).
Ulmer, J. B., Deck, R. R., Dewitt, C. M., Donnhly, J. I., and Liu, M. A. *Immunology* **89,** 59 (1996).
Ulmer, J. B., Donnelly, J. J., Parker, S. E., Rhodes, G. H., Felgner, P. L., Dwarki, V. J., Gromkowski, S. H., Deck, R. R., DeWitt, C. M., Friedman, A., et al. *Science* **259,** 1745 (1993).
Verma, I. M., and Somia, N. *Nature* **389,** 239 (1997).
Vitadello, M., Schiaffino, M. V., Picard, A., Scarpa, M., and Schiaffino, S. *Hum. Gene. Ther.* **5,** 11 (1994).
Wagner, E., Zenke, M., Cotten, M., Beug, H., and Birnstiel, M. L. *Proc. Natl. Acad. Sci. USA* **87,** 3410 (1990).
Walter, E., Dreher, D., Kok, M., Thiele, L., Kiama, S. G., Gehr, P., and Merkle, H. P. *J. Control. Rel.* **76,** 149 (2001).
Walter, E., Moelling, K., Pavlovic, J., and Merkle, H. P. *J. Control. Rel.* **61,** 361 (1999).
Wang, R., Doolan, D. L., Le, T. P., Hedstrom, R. C., Coonan, K. M., Charoenvit, Y., Jones, T. R., Hobart, P., Margalith, M., Ng, J., Weiss, W. R., Sedegah, M., de Taisne, C., Norman, J. A., and Hoffman, S. L. *Science* **282,** 476 (1998).
Wang, D., Robinson, D. R., Kwon, G. S., and Samuel, J. *J. Control. Rel.* **57,** 9 (1999).
Winegar, R. A., Monforte, J. A., Suing, K. D., O'Loughlin, K. G., Rudd, C. J., and Macgregor, J. T. *Hum. Gene. Ther.* **7,** 2185 (1996).
Wolff, J. A., Dowty, M. E., Jiao, S., Repetto, G., Berg, R. K., Ludtke, J. J., Williams, P., and Slautterback, D. B. *J. Cell. Sci.* **103**(Pt 4), 1249 (1992).
Wolff, J. A., Malone, R. W., Williams, P., Chong, W., Acsadi, G., Jani, A., and Felgner, P. L. *Science* **247,** 1465 (1990).
Xu, Y., and Szoka, F. C. Jr. *Biochemistry* **35,** 5616 (1996).
Xu, Y., Hui, S. W., Frederik, P., and Szoka, F. C. Jr. *Biophys. J.* **77,** 341 (1999).
Yang, N. S., and Sun, W. H. *Nat. Med.* **1,** 481 (1995).
Yang, N. S., Burkholder, J., Roberts, B., Martinell, B., and McCabe, D. *Proc. Natl. Acad. Sci. USA* **87,** 9568 (1990).

Yoshida, M., Mahato, R. I., Kawabata, K., Takakura, Y., and Hashida, M. *Pharm. Res.* **13,** 599 (1996).
Zabner, J., Fasbender, A. J., Moninger, T., Poellinger, K. A., and Welsh, M. J. *J. Biol. Chem.* **270,** 18,997 (1995).
Zhu, Y. Y., Voytik, S. L., Badylak, S. F., and Bonadio, J. *Trans. Ortho. Res. Soc.* **19,** 223 (1994).
Zuhorn, I. S., Kalicharan, R., and Hoekstra, D. *J. Biol. Chem.* **277,** 18021 (2002).

SURFACE-ERODIBLE BIOMATERIALS FOR DRUG DELIVERY

Balaji Narasimhan and Matt J. Kipper

Department of Chemical Engineering, Iowa State University, Ames, IA 50011, USA

I. Introduction	169
II. Chemistry and Synthesis	172
A. Early Synthesis of Polyanhydrides	172
B. Synthesis of Polyanhydrides for Drug Delivery	173
C. Chemistries of Polyanhydrides Used in Drug Delivery	176
III. Polyanhydride Characterization	189
A. Chemical Characterization of Polyanhydrides	189
B. Characterization of Thermal Properties, Crystallinity, and Phase Behavior of Polyanhydrides	192
C. Biocompatibility of Polyanhydrides	199
IV. Degradation, Erosion, and Drug Release Kinetics	200
A. Experiments	200
B. Modeling Degradation, Erosion, and Drug Release Kinetics	207
V. Design of Polyanhydride Carriers for Controlled Release	209
A. Implantable Systems	210
B. Injectable Systems	211
C. Aerosols and Systems Designed for Mucosal Delivery	212
VI. Conclusions and Future Opportunities	213
References	214

I. Introduction

Bioerodible polymers offer a unique combination of properties that can be tailored to suit nearly any controlled drug delivery application. By far the most common bioerodible polymers employed for biomedical applications are polyesters and polyethers (e.g., poly(ethylene glycol), polylactide, polyglycolide and their copolymers). These polymers are biocompatible, have good mechanical properties, and have been used in many controlled release applications. However, their chemistries are limited, thereby restricting structural modifications resulting in tailored properties. Over the past two decades, researchers have begun investigating alternative biodegradable polymers, resulting in a vast body of literature on both the synthesis of, and mechanisms of drug release from, biodegradable polymers.

Drug release may be controlled by several mechanisms including diffusion of the drug through a matrix, dissolution of the polymer matrix, and degradation of the polymer. The chemistry of the polymer matrix may be tailored to facilitate drug stabilization, target delivery to specific tissues, or alter the release kinetics. Bioerodible polymers erode *in vivo*, thus obviating the need for surgical removal after the useful lifetime of the device has expired. The erosion may actually determine the drug release kinetics, or may occur on a time scale much slower than that of drug release.

It is important to distinguish between erosion and degradation. Erosion is mass loss from a bioerodible polymer and may be a consequence of polymer dissolution or degradation of the polymer backbone, followed by dissolution of the degradation products. Degradation typically occurs by hydrolysis of the polymer backbone, the kinetics of which is a function of the polymer chemistry. Thus, erosion is the sum of several elementary processes, one of which may be polymer degradation.

Some biodegradable chemistries are listed in Table I (Pierre and Chiellini, 1986; Siepmann and Goepferich, 2001; Staubli *et al.*, 1990; Weinberg *et al.*, 1998). Pierre and Chiellini (1986) have summarized hydrolysis mechanisms for many biomedically relevant systems. Degradation half-lives range from millennia (for amides, carbonates, and urethanes) to minutes (for the fastest degrading anhydrides) (Pierre and Chiellini, 1986). Though all of these chemistries are hydrolyzable, hydrolysis rates vary depending not only on the functional group (Albertsson, 1995; Pierre and Chiellini, 1986), but also what lies between the functional groups. Polyanhydrides, for example, are one of the most labile classes, and their hydrolysis is shown in Scheme 1.

Erosion is typically characterized by either occurring on the surface or in the bulk. Surface erosion is controlled by the chemical reaction and/or dissolution kinetics, while bulk erosion is controlled by diffusion and transport processes such as polymer swelling, diffusion of water through the polymer matrix, and the diffusion of degradation products from the swollen polymer matrix. The processes of surface and bulk erosion are compared schematically in Fig. 1. These two processes are idealized descriptions. In real systems, the tendency towards surface versus bulk erosion behavior is a function of the particular chemistry and device geometry (Tamada and Langer, 1993). Surface erosion may permit the

TABLE I
FUNCTIONAL GROUPS FOUND IN BIOERODIBLE POLYMERS

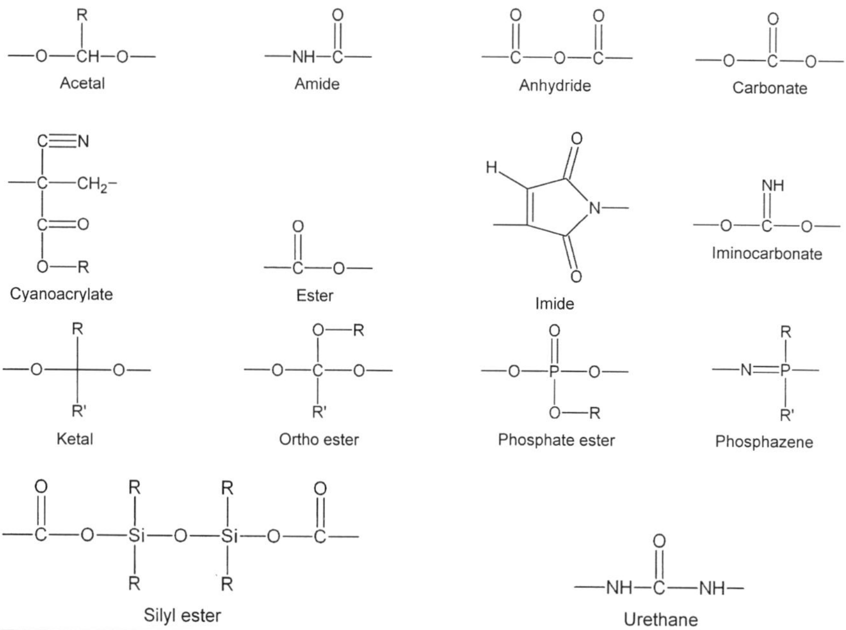

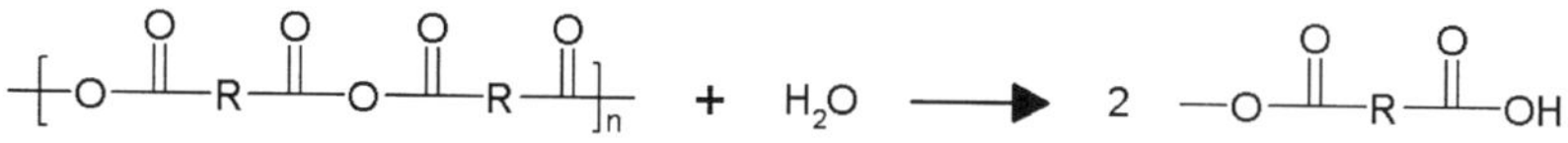

Structure	Name
—O—CHR—O—	Acetal
—NH—C(=O)—	Amide
—C(=O)—O—C(=O)—	Anhydride
—O—C(=O)—O—	Carbonate
—C(C≡N)(CH₂—)(C(=O)O—R)—	Cyanoacrylate
—C(=O)—O—	Ester
Maleimide ring	Imide
—O—C(=NH)—O—	Iminocarbonate
—O—C(R)(R')—O—	Ketal
—O—C(OR)(R')—O—	Ortho ester
—O—P(=O)(OR)—O—	Phosphate ester
—N=P(R)(R')—	Phosphazene
—C(=O)—O—Si(R)(R)—O—Si(R)(R)—O—C(=O)—	Silyl ester
—NH—C(=O)—NH—	Urethane

SCHEME 1. Hydrolysis of polyanhydrides to carboxylic acids.

stabilization of macromolecular drugs and offers the potential to tailor release profiles by tailoring the composition and drug distribution.

Polyanhydrides are typically characterized as surface eroding because the anhydride bond itself is quite reactive with respect to hydrolysis, but the structure of the dicarboxylic acid monomer can render the polymer very hydrophobic, thereby limiting water ingress. These materials are interesting for controlled drug delivery due to the wide range over which the degradation kinetics can be varied. Thus, polyanhydrides have emerged as an extremely diverse and promising class of polymers for drug delivery and other biomedical applications. This review will discuss the novel chemistries and synthesis, characterization, and applications of polyanhydrides as surface erodible biomaterials for drug delivery.

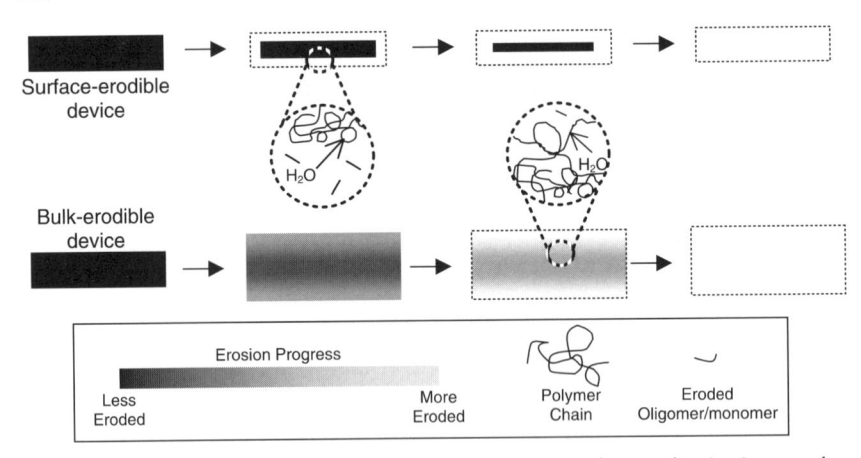

FIG. 1. Schematic comparing surface and bulk erosion. In surface erosion (top), water does not penetrate far into the bulk, but hydrolyzes functional groups on the surface. The resulting monomers dissolve and diffuse away from the device. In bulk erosion (bottom), water penetrates into the bulk, polymer may dissolve, and is ultimately hydrolyzed into monomer.

Several synthesis routes have been investigated to design polyanhydrides, and these are discussed in Section II. Section III reviews the microstructural characterization of homopolymers, blends, and copolymers of polyanhydrides. Section IV discusses the important features that affect erosion and drug release kinetics and reviews some of the modeling efforts that have been undertaken to predict erosion and drug release. Section V discusses the design of polyanhydride drug carriers with respect to delivery routes, mechanisms of release, and factors affecting release profiles. Finally, Section VI presents some of the future directions for polyanhydride research. Polyanhydrides have a variety of microstructural characteristics that affect the release profiles of encapsulated drugs. It is important to accurately describe the microstructure to predict and tailor drug release profiles. If the effects of these microstructural characteristics can be accurately understood, they can be exploited to control drug release profiles and effectively design controlled release formulations.

II. Chemistry and Synthesis

A. Early Synthesis of Polyanhydrides

Synthesis of polyanhydrides from the aromatic dicarboxylic acids (isophthalic and terephthalic acids) by melt polycondensation was first reported by Bucher and Slade in 1909. In the early 1930s, Hill and Carothers explored the synthesis of aliphatic polyanhydrides for use as fibers for the textile industry. Hill (1930) reported the polymerization of the aliphatic adipic acid, and later, Hill and Carothers (1932) reported the polymerization of sebacic acid, both by melt polycondensation and dehydrochlorination. The melting points of these polymers were too low and hydrolysis was too fast for them to be of use as fibers, and the study of anhydrides was abandoned.

In the late 1950s through the mid 1960s Conix (1957, 1958, 1966) reported the synthesis of the poly[α,ω-bis(p-carboxyphenoxy)alkanes], improving the fiber and film forming properties of polyanhydrides. From 1959 to 1962, Yoda (1959; Yoda and Akihisa, 1959), being encouraged by the work of Conix, synthesized random copolymers by melt polycondensation and alternating copolymers by dehydrochlorination, from a variety of aliphatic and aromatic monomers in attempts to improve the fiber and film properties of polyanhydrides. Windholz (1965) later patented a similar process for producing polyanhydrides as intermediates in the production of polyesters. Polyanhydride homopolymers and copolymers containing heterocyclic rings (Yoda, 1962a,b), and aliphatic and aromatic thioethers (Yoda, 1962c) were also synthesized by Yoda. Despite these efforts, polyanhydrides remained inferior to polyesters and other classes of polymers, never gaining prominence in the textile industry.

B. Synthesis of Polyanhydrides for Drug Delivery

Interest in polyanhydrides waned until the 1980s when Langer and coworkers (Rosen et al., 1983) suggested that their biodegradability would make them suitable for controlled drug delivery applications. Their initial study was conducted with poly[bis(p-carboxyphenoxy)methane] (PCPM) made by melt polycondensation and they showed near zero order release kinetics of a model drug (cholic acid) from compression-molded PCPM slabs (Rosen et al., 1983). These first results on drug release from polyanhydrides initiated what has now been two decades of extensive research. The same group studied additional chemistries (Leong et al., 1985) as well as alternate synthetic routes (Leong et al., 1987). The melt polycondensation and dehydrochlorination syntheses discussed in Section II.A were explored, along with a third route, dehydrative coupling (Chasin et al., 1988; Leong et al., 1987). An alternative solution technique for the polymerization of poly(terephthalic acid) (PTA) is offered by Subramanyam and Pinkus (1985). Domb et al. (1993) reviewed several polymerization methods including melt polycondensation, ring opening

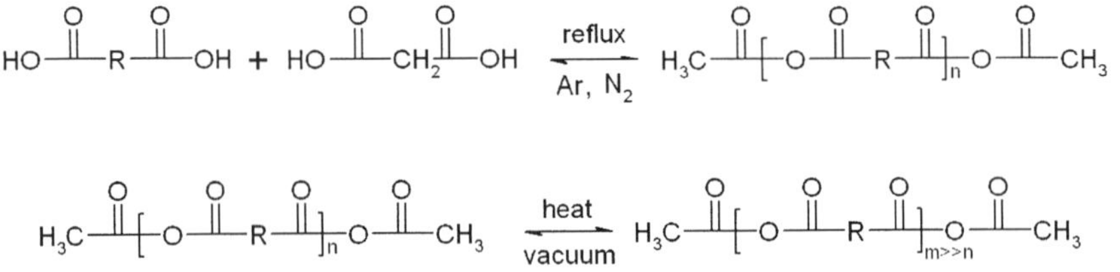

SCHEME 2. Polyanhydride synthesis via melt polycondensation involves first the formation of oligomeric acetylated prepolymers, followed by condensation under vacuum. Acetic acid is formed as a byproduct of the second reaction.

polymerization, solution polymerization (dehydrohalogenation and dehydrative coupling), and interfacial polymerization (dehydrohalogenation). A review of the important polyanhydride synthesis routes follows.

1. Melt Polycondensation

Melt polycondensation is performed by first acetylating the dicarboxylic acids by refluxing in excess acetic anhydride in a dry atmosphere, and then melting under vacuum to remove the condensation byproduct. This procedure is represented in Scheme 2. Domb and Langer (1987) improved upon the melt polycondensation technique (Scheme 2) to obtain higher molecular weight homopolymers and copolymers of aliphatic and aromatic dicarboxylic acids. They obtained weight average molecular weights of up to 137,300, for poly(sebacic acid) (PSA). In the same study (Domb and Langer, 1987), the synthesis of poly[1,3-bis(p-carboxyphenoxy)propane] (PCPP), poly[1,6-bis(p-carboxyphenoxy)hexane] (PCPH), poly(1,4-phenylenedipropionic acid) (PPDP), and poly(dodecanedioic acid) (PDDA), as well as the copolymers P(CPP–SA), P(CPP–DDA), and the copolymer of sebacic acid with isophthalic acid P(IPA–SA) was reported. A method for copolymer synthesis was patented by the same authors (Domb and Langer, 1988a). Methods employing a variety of coordination catalysts were also reported (Domb and Langer, 1987). The anhydride interchange reaction mechanism for the melt polycondensation (Scheme 3) has been proposed by Albertsson and Lundmark (1990a). This mechanism may also result in the formation of lower molecular weight cyclic macromers and contribute to the high polydispersity characteristic of the resulting polymers (Domb and Langer, 1987). Gupta (1989) patented a melt polycondensation procedure from a bis(trimethylsilyl)ester of a dicarboxylic acid and a diacid chloride that produces alternating copolymers. The majority of recent work with polyanhydrides has been conducted using the polycondensation

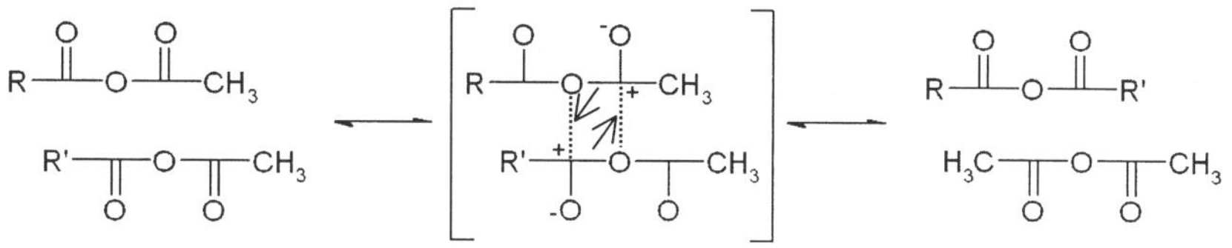

SCHEME 3. Anhydride interchange mechanism proposed for polymerization. The same mechanism may be responsible for cyclization.

synthesis originated by Conix (1966) and later improved upon by Domb and Langer (1987).

2. Dehydrochlorination

In the dehydrochlorination synthesis developed by Yoda (1959; Yoda and Akihisa, 1959) diacid chlorides are first formed by either reacting dicarboxylic acids with phosphorous pentachloride or refluxing dicarboxylic acids in thionyl chloride. Reaction is then carried out in the presence of pyridine. Dehydrochlorination (Schotten-Baumann condensation), offers two main advantages over melt polycondensation. First, it can be performed at much milder temperatures. Second, the copolymer sequence can be precisely controlled to form alternating copolymers. Leong et al. (1987) studied this route both as a solution technique, and at aqueous and non-aqueous interfaces. In general, somewhat lower molecular weights are obtained by this method than by the melt polycondensation (Leong et al., 1987).

3. Dehydrative Coupling

The third synthesis mechanism studied by Leong et al. (1987) is an extension of a technique used by previous researchers (Cabré-Castellví et al., 1981; Mestres, 1981) to form monomeric anhydrides, employing strong dehydration agents (e.g., organophosphorous compounds) such as those employed in peptide synthesis. A variety of dehydration agents were studied. Of the three synthesis methods studied by Leong et al. (1987), this one yielded the lowest molecular weight, and presented the most difficulties with respect to product purification.

To address purification, Domb and Langer (1988b) developed two techniques involving phosgene or diphosgene as coupling agents, both of which are single step polymerizations yielding pure product, by selective dissolution of either the polymer or the byproducts. A variety of polymers were synthesized including PSA, PCPP, PTA, PAA, PDDA, though only with PSA was a weight-average molecular weight above 15,000 (16,300) obtained. Most of the polymers had weight-average molecular weights less than 10,000. The advantages of this method are that relatively pure polymers are obtained without the exposure to extreme temperatures (Domb and Langer, 1988b).

4. Ring Opening Polymerization

Dicarboxylic acid monomers that form monomeric anhydride rings, such as adipic anhydride (oxepane-2,7-dione), can be polymerized by ring-opening polymerization (Albertsson and Lundmark, 1988). A catalyst such as tin 2-ethylhexanoate, tin octanoate, aluminum isopropoxide, or *n*-butyl lithium is added and the reaction proceeds via an insertion mechanism (Albertsson and Lundmark, 1990b; Edlund and Albertsson, 1999). Ring opening can be performed both in solution and in the melt (Albertsson and Lundmark, 1988, 1990b). Ropson *et al.* (1997) reported a mechanism for insertion in living polymerizations of adipic anhydride using aluminum alkoxides as initiators. Ring opening polymerizations are limited to chemistries capable of forming rings, but offer the capability of easily forming block copolymers via living polymerizations. Block copolymers of adipic anhydride with ε-caprolactone (Ropson *et al.*, 1997) and trimethylene carbonate (Edlund and Albertsson, 1999) have been formed by this synthetic route. Deng *et al.* (2003) have cleverly surmounted the chemistry limitation by using potassium poly(ethylene glycol)ate as a macro-initiator, thereby synthesizing a poly(adipic acid-*block*-ethylene glycol) copolymer. The same group has also recently studied the use of dibutylmagnesium as an alternative initiator (Li *et al.*, 2003).

5. Polymerization with Ketene

In an attempt to avoid the polymerization/depolymerization equilibrium that occurs during melt polycondensation, Albertsson and Lundmark (1988) also studied the irreversible reaction of adipic anhydride with ketene. However, they reported very little difference in molecular weights when two ketene syntheses were compared to melt polycondensation and ring-opening polymerization using a zinc catalyst (Albertsson and Lundmark, 1988).

C. CHEMISTRIES OF POLYANHYDRIDES USED IN DRUG DELIVERY

We have already mentioned a few of the polyanhydride chemistries that have been studied in drug delivery applications. Tables II through VII present some of the polyanhydrides that have been explored for drug

TABLE II
Aliphatic Polyanhydrides

Structure	Name	
![structure 1]	$x=4$ Poly(adipic acid)	PAA
	$x=5$ Poly(pimelic acid)	PPA
	$x=6$ Poly(suberic acid)	PSA
	$x=7$ Poly(azalaic acid)	PAZ
	$x=8$ Poly(sebacic acid)	PSA
	$x=10$ Poly(dodecanedioic acid)	PDDA
	$x=12$ Poly(dodecanedicarboxylic acid)	PDX
![structure 2]	Poly(1,4-cyclohexane dicarboxylic acid)	PCDA

delivery applications and we briefly discuss the literature on each one. Copolymers are discussed separately.

1. Aliphatic Polyanhydrides

Aliphatic polyanhydrides (Table II) together with the α,ω-bis(*p*-carboxyphenoxy)alkanes are the most commonly studied polyanhydrides for drug delivery applications. Poly(sebacic acid) (PSA) was first suggested as a polymer for drug delivery by Langer and coworkers in 1987 and was among the monomers on which they studied alternative synthesis methods (Domb and Langer, 1987; Leong *et al.*, 1987). Poly(dodecanedioic acid) (PDDA) is also synthesized by melt polycondensation and yields similar molecular weights (Domb and Langer, 1987). The synthesis of poly(adipic acid) (PAA) by multiple methods was discussed in Section II.B. Poly(1,4-cyclohexyldicarboxylic acid) (PCDA) was first synthesized via melt polycondensation by Zhang *et al.* (2000, 2001). Domb and Nudelman (1995) reported the synthesis of the series of aliphatic polyanhydrides from PAA to poly(dodecanedicarboxylic acid) (PDX).

2. Polyanhydrides from Unsaturated and Fatty Acid-derived Monomers

Polyanhydrides based on unsaturated and fatty acid-derived monomers are shown in Table III. Poly(fumaric acid) (PFA) was fist synthesized by Domb *et al.* (1991) by both melt polycondensation and solution polymerization. The copolymer of fumaric acid and sebacic acid (P(FA–SA)) has been synthesized and characterized (Domb *et al.*, 1991; Mathiowitz *et al.*, 1990b). The mucoadhesive properties of this polymer

TABLE III
POLYANHYDRIDES FROM UNSATURATED AND FATTY ACID DERIVED MONOMERS

Structure	Name	
	Poly(fumaric acid)	PFA
	Poly(Fatty acid dimer) (erucic acid)	PFAD
	Poly(Dimer acid)	PDA

have been shown to aid in increasing the bioavailability of encapsulated model drugs in oral delivery experiments (Chickering et al., 1995, 1996).

Fatty acids have also been converted to difunctional monomers for polyanhydride synthesis by dimerizing the unsaturated erucic or oleic acid to form branched monomers. These monomers are collectively referred to as fatty acid dimers and the polymers are referred to as poly(fatty acid dimer) (PFAD). PFAD (erucic acid dimer) was synthesized by Domb and Maniar (1993) via melt polycondensation and was a liquid at room temperature. Desiring to increase the hydrophobicity of aliphatic polyanhydrides such as PSA without adding aromaticity to the monomers (and thereby increasing the melting point), Teomim and Domb (1999) and Krasko et al. (2002) have synthesized fatty acid terminated PSA. Octanoic, lauric, myristic, stearic, ricinoleic, oleic, linoleic, and lithocholic acid acetate anhydrides were added to the melt polycondensation reactions to obtain the desired terminations. As desired, a dramatic reduction in the erosion rate was obtained (Krasko et al., 2002; Teomim and Domb, 1999).

Teomim and Domb (2001) report the termination of PSA with monoesters of ricinoleic acid (i.e., *cis*-12-hydroxyoctadeca-9-enoic acid) and fatty acids. The fatty acids used in this study range in length from C10 to C18. The combination of PSA with FAD is not limited to terminal modification. P(FAD–SA) and P(fatty acid trimer–SA) (P(FAT–SA)) copolymers have been synthesized (Domb and Maniar, 1993) and their release properties have been studied (Shieh et al., 1994; Tabata and Langer, 1993; Tabata et al., 1993, 1994).

Xu et al. (2001) synthesized the copolymers of a dimer fatty acid (dimer of oleic and linoleic acids) and sebacic acid (P(DA–SA)) by melt polycondensation of acetylated prepolymers. Degradation and drug release kinetics showed that increasing dimer acid content decreased the release rate (Xu et al., 2001).

Another class of PSA–fatty acid-based copolymers has been synthesized from the ricinoleic acid and ricinoleic half-esters with maleic and succinic anhydride, poly(sebacic-co-ricinoleic acid maleate), poly(sebacic-co-ricinoleic acid succinate), and poly(sebacic-co-12-hydroxystearic acid succinate) (P(SA–RAM), P(SA–RAS), and P(SA–HSAS)) (Krasko et al., 2003; Teomim et al., 1999). These syntheses result in poly(anhydride-co-esters).

3. Aromatic Polyanhydrides

Aromatic polyanhydrides (Table IV) are typically characterized by slow degradation rates, high melting temperatures, brittle mechanical properties, and low solubility in organic solvents compared to the aliphatic polyanhydrides. PCPM was the first aromatic polyanhydride to be synthesized as a candidate for controlled drug delivery (Rosen et al., 1983). Other polymers in the family of poly[α,ω-(p-carboxyphenoxy)alkanes] that had originally been synthesized by Conix (1957, 1958, 1966) soon followed including PCPP, poly(terephthalic acid) (PTA) (Leong et al., 1985), and PCPH (Leong et al., 1987). Also included in the later study were poly(terephthalic-alt-sebacic acid) (P(SA-alt-TA)), poly(1,4-phenylene dipropionic acid) (PPDP) and poly[2,2'-(p-xylylenedithio)diacetic acid] (PXDA) (Leong et al., 1987). Domb et al. (1989) synthesized several polyanhydrides based on ω-carboxyphenoxyalkonoic acids including poly(carboxyphenoxy acetic acid) (PCPA), poly[5-(p-carboxyphenoxy)-valeric acid] (PCPV), and poly[8-(p-carboxyphenoxy)octanoic acid] (PCPO) by melt polycondensation and studied the release of model drugs from them. Domb (1992) also synthesized poly(isophthalic acid) (PIPA) and poly(terephthalic acid) (PTPA) by melt polycondensation.

Campo et al. (1999) synthesized the ortho-isomers of PCPP and PCPH, poly[1,3-bis(o-carboxyphenoxy)propane] (Po-CPP) and poly[1,6-bis(o-carboxyphenoxy)hexane] (Po-CPH), in an attempt to improve the solubility and processability of these two polymers. Solubility was improved

TABLE IV
Aromatic Polyanhydrides

Structure	Name	
	$x = 1$ Poly[bis(p-carboxyphenoxy)methane] $x = 3$ Poly[1,3-bis(p-carboxyphenoxy)propane] $x = 6$ Poly[1,6-bis(p-carboxyphenoxy)hexane]	PCPM PCPP PCPH
	Poly(Terephthalic acid)	PTA
	Poly(Isophthalic acid)	PIPA
	Poly(Phenylene dipropionic acid)	PPDP
	Poly[2,2'-(p-xylenedithio)diacetic acid]	PXDA

$x = 1$ Poly[2-(p-carboxyphenoxy)acetic acid]	PCPA
$x = 4$ Poly[5-(p-carboxyphenoxy)valeric acid]	PCPV
$x = 7$ Poly[8-(p-carboxyphenoxy)octanoic]	PCPO
$x = 3$ Poly[1,3-bis(o-carboxyphenoxy)propane]	Po-CPP
$x = 6$ Poly[1,6-bis(o-carboxyphenoxy)hexane]	Po-CPP
Poly[o-bis(p-carboxyphenoxy)xylene]	Po-p-CPX
Poly[m-bis(p-carboxyphenoxy)xylene]	Pm-p-CPX
Poly[o-bis(o-carboxyphenoxy)xylene]	Po-o-CPX
Poly[m-bis(o-carboxyphenoxy)xylene]	Pm-o-CPX
Poly[p-bis(o-carboxyphenoxy)xylene]	Pp-o-CPX
Poly[4,4′-(hexafluoroisopropylidine)bis-benzoic acid]	PHFB

and crystallinity reduced, but T_gs were also lowered to below physiological temperature, which may limit their applicability as biomaterials.

In an attempt to increase T_g of the poly[bis(o-carboxyphenoxy)alkanes], Anastasiou and Uhrich (2000a) replaced the alkane moiety by *ortho-*, *meta-*, and *para*-xylenes producing poly[o-/m-bis(p-carboxyphenoxy)xylene]s (P*o-p*-CPX, and P*m-p*-CPX) and poly[o-/m-/p-bis(o-carboxyphenoxy)xylene]s (P*o-o*-CPX, P*m-o*-CPX, and P*p-o*-CPX). They found P*o-p*-CPX to be relatively insoluble and were unable to synthesize poly[p-bis(p-carboxyphenoxy)xylene] because of the insolubility of the dicarboxylic acid (Anastasiou and Uhrich, 2000a). P*o-o*-CPX and P*m-o*-CPX demonstrated the most favorable solubility and neither exhibited a melting temperature. All of the polymers synthesized had T_gs between 71 and 101°C (Anastasiou and Uhrich, 2000a).

4. Copolymers of Aliphatic and Aromatic Polyanhydrides

Researchers interested in polyanhydrides as candidates for drug delivery realized the value of co-polymerizing aliphatic and aromatic residues. In this way, a large number of polymers could be made from only a handful of chemistries and chemical and physical properties could be tailored by combination. Initially, the goal was to obtain a variety of release times by making simple changes to the copolymer composition. The first such copolymer was P(CPP–SA) synthesized via melt polycondensation by Leong *et al.* (1985). The alternating copolymers of adipic acid, sebacic acid, and dodecanedioic acid with terephthaloyl chloride (P(AA-*alt*-TA), P(SA-*alt*-TA), and P(DDA-*alt*-TA)) and sebacic acid with isophthaloyl chloride and P(IPA-*alt*-SA)) were produced by dehydrochlorination and the random copolymers P(CPM–SA) and P(CPH–SA) were produced by melt polycondensation for the first time in the extensive study by Leong *et al.* (1987). The copolymers P(IPA–SA) and P(CPP–DDA) via melt polycondensation were added to the repertoire of copolymers by Domb and Langer (1987). Domb (1992) later synthesized the copolymers P(CPP–IPA), P(IPA–TA), P(IPA–FA), P(CPP–FA), P(FA–TA), P(SA–TA), and P(IPA–SA).

Sanders *et al.* (1999) attempted to lower the melting points of aromatic polyanhydrides by substituting branched alkyl groups in place of the linear alkyls of P(CPP–SA). They synthesized poly[1,2-bis(p-carboxyphenoxy)-propane-*co*-sebacic acid] (P(1,2-CPP-SA)), poly[1,3-bis(p-carboxyphenoxy)-2-methyl propane-*co*-sebacic anhydride] (P(CPMP-SA)), and poly[1,3-bis (p-carboxyphenoxy)-2,2-dimethyl propane-*co*-sebacic anhydride] (P(CPDP-SA)), all of which had melting points below 165°C.

TABLE V
POLY(ANHYDRIDE-co-IMIDE)S

Structure	Name	
	Poly(trimellitylimido glycine)	PTMAgly
	Poly(pyromellitylimido alanine)	PMAala
	Poly(trimellitylimido tyrosine)	PTMAtyr

5. Poly(anhydride-co-imide)s

Another important class of polyanhydrides is the poly(anhydride-co-imide)s (Table V). This class of polymers was first synthesized by Fontán and co-workers (De Abajo *et al.*, 1971; González *et al.*, 1976) as potential candidates for fiber forming polymers. Staubli *et al.* (1990) developed a technique for incorporating amino acids into polyanhydrides by first reacting them with N-trimellitic acid. Uhrich *et al.* (1995) synthesized copolymers of trimellitylimido glycine, pyromellitylimido alanine and the monomers of PSA and PCPH by melt polycondensation and proposed the use of (P(TMAgly–SA), P(TMAgly–CPH), P(PMAala–SA), and P(PMAala–CPH)) as potential candidates to improve the mechanical properties of polyanhydrides. Hanes *et al.* (1996) later synthesized the copolymer of trimellitylimido L-tyrosine with PSA and PCPP (P(TMAtyr–CPP–SA)) as a candidate polymer for vaccine delivery.

6. Poly(anhydride-co-ester)s and Poly(anhydride-co-ether)s

Poly(anhydride-co-ester)s (Table VI) were suggested as potential polymers for drug delivery and synthesized by Pinther and Hartmann (1990),

TABLE VI
POLY(ANHYDRIDE-*co*-ESTER)S

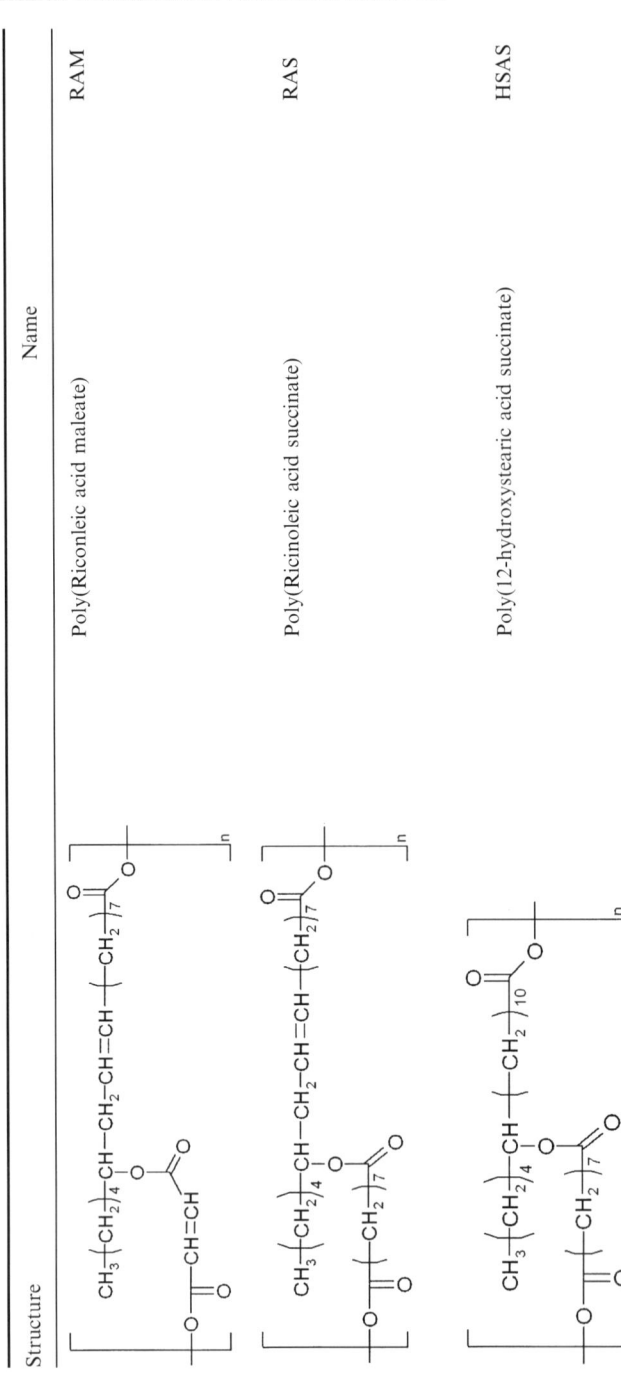

Structure	Name	
(structure)	Poly(Riconleic acid maleate)	RAM
(structure)	Poly(Ricinoleic acid succinate)	RAS
(structure)	Poly(12-hydroxystearic acid succinate)	HSAS

Structure	Abbreviation	Name
	PCPS	Poly[bis(*o*-carboxyphenoxy) sebacate]
	PCPSM / CPAM	$x = 2$ poly(*p*-carboxyphenoxy) succinic monoester anhydride $x = 4$ poly(*p*-carboxyphenoxy) adipic monoester anhydride

and Kricheldorf and Jürgens (1994). Other poly(anhydride-*co*-ester)s already mentioned in Section II.B.4 include poly(adipic acid-*block*-ε-caprolactone) (P(AA-*block*-ε-CL)), poly(adipic acid-*block*-trimethylene carbonate) (P(AA-*block*-TMC)), and poly(adipic acid-*block*-ethylene glycol) (P(PAA-*block*-EG). Others have synthesized poly(anhydride-*block*-ethylene glycol) copolymers. Jiang and Zhu (1999) synthesized and characterized poly(sebacic acid-*block*-ethylene glycol) (P(SA-*block*-EG)) and poly[(sebacic acid-*co*-trimellitylimidoglycine)-*block*-ethylene glycol] (P[(SA-*co*-TMA)-*block*-EG]) by melt polycondensation. The ethylene glycol segments were added by first acetylating polyoxyethylene dicarboxylic acid and then adding it to the PSA polymerization (Jiang and Zhu, 1999). Qiu and Zhu (2001) proposed the use of this material in laminated devices for pulsed release. P(SA-*co*-TMA-*block*-EG) and PSA were also used by Qiu and Zhu (2000) to make blends of poly[bis(glycine ethyl ester)phosphazene] in order to regulate the degradation rate of the phosphazene as well as to decrease its cost. The *in vitro* and *in vivo* erosion kinetics of the P[(SA-*co*-TMA)-*block*-EG] containing blend was later studied in detail by Qiu (2002).

Wu *et al.* (2000) showed the formation of self-assembled nanoparticles of P(SA-*block*-EG) in an aqueous environment and studied their degradation as a function of pH and temperature. Fu *et al.* (2002) repeated the synthesis of P(SA-*block*-EG) and studied the morphology and erosion kinetics of microspheres which they propose as vehicles for mucosal drug delivery.

Poly(lactic acid) (PLA) has also been added to poly(SA) via melt polycondensation to produce the triblock copolymers poly(lactic acid-*block*-sebacic acid-*block*-lactic acid) (P(LA-*block*-SA-*block*-LA)) by Slivniak and Domb (2002). The PLA (D-, L-, and DL-) was incorporated by acetylation and addition to the PSA synthesis. They showed the formation of stable stereocomplexed particles with increased melting points and reduced solubility, and studied the degradation and drug release characteristics of the same (Slivniak and Domb, 2002). The stereocomplexes self-assemble as a consequence of the chirality in the PLA portions of the chains (Slivniak and Domb, 2002).

Erdmann and Uhrich (2000; Erdmann *et al.*, 2000) recently synthesized novel poly(anhydride-*co*-ester)s containing salicylic acid in the backbone, by melt polycondensation of the disalicylic acid ester of sebacic acid, poly[bis(*o*-carboxyphenoxy)sebacate] (PCPS) and the copolymer P(CPH–CPS). The release of salicylic acid (the active form of aspirin) from the former was studied *in vitro* and from the latter was studied *in vivo* (Erdmann and Uhrich, 2000; Erdmann *et al.*, 2000). Similar polymers that release 5-amino salicylic acid, and *p*-nitro salicylic acid have been prepared by the same group for the treatment of Crohn's disease and tuberculosis, respectively (Anastasiou and Uhrich, 2000b; Krogh-Jespersen et al., 2000).

Jiang and Zhu (2001) reported on the synthesis of poly(p-carboxyphenoxy succinic monoester anhydride) and poly(p-carboxyphenoxy adipic monoester anhydride) (PCPSM and PCPAM), and the copolymer P(CPAM–CPSM) as polymeric antimicrobial prodrugs for diseases such as malaria and hepatitis B. They also reported that PCPSM exhibits strong fluorescence, the intensity of which increases linearly with its molecular weight (Jiang et al., 2001a,b). They showed that when co-polymerized the fluorescence is maintained, though diminished approximately in proportion to the copolymer composition.

7. Poly(anhydride-co-amide)s

The synthesis of poly(anhydride-co-amide)s (Table VII) of various chemistries was pursued by Hartmann and Schulz (1989) as a means of improving biocompatibility and extending the degradation times of polyanhydrides. This work also contains calorimetry data on the thermal transitions and spectroscopic characterization.

Jiang and Zhu (2001) became interested in synthesizing additional polyanhydrides with fluorescence after their discovery of the fluorescent properties of PCPS. They synthesized the series of poly(anhydride-co-amide)s poly{p-[carboxyphenoxy(ethyl/propyl/butyl)formamido]benzoic anhydride} (PCEFB, PCPFB, and PCBFB) (Jiang et al., 2001c). Only the ethyl polymer emitted strong fluorescence, which was consistent with their previous study of the poly(anhydride-co-ester)s of similar chemistry

TABLE VII
POLY(ANHYDRIDE-co-AMIDE)S

Structure	Name	
	$x=2$ poly{p-[carboxyphenoxy (ethyl)formamido]benzoic acid}	PCEFB
	$x=3$ poly{p-[carboxyphenoxy (propyl)formamido]benzoic acid}	PCPFB
	$x=4$ poly{p-[carboxyphenoxy (butyl)formamido]benzoic acid}	PCBFB
	Poly[o-acetyl-p(carboxyethylformamido) benzoic acid]	PACEFB

(Jiang and Zhu, 2001). PCEFB can be modified with an acetyl *ortho* to the anhydride bond to form poly[*o*-acetyl-*p*(carboxyethylformamido)benzoic acid] (PACEFB), which also fluoresces and may have potential as a polymeric prodrug for the treatment of tuberculosis (Jiang et al., 2001b). The copolymers of P(CEFB–SA) and P(CACEFB–SA) were also synthesized and shown to exhibit decreased fluorescence in proportion to the decrease in mole fraction of the fluorescent monomer (Jiang et al., 2001b). These polymers may prove to be very valuable for combining *in vivo* controlled release and drug targeting studies with non-invasive imaging techniques. The dependence of fluorescence on molecular weight may offer a powerful mechanism to conduct *in situ* analysis of *in vivo* degradation profiles (Jiang and Zhu, 2002).

8. Other Novel Anhydride Chemistries

The chemistry of polyanhydrides is by no means limited to the categories discussed in the preceding sections. A brief review of some of the additional chemistries that have recently been synthesized follows with a mention of their potential for application in drug delivery.

a. Branched polyanhydrides. Branched PSA was synthesized by Maniar et al. (1990) by reacting sebacic acid in the presence of 1,3,5-benzenetricarboxylic acid and polyacrylic acid to improve the processability and mechanical properties of PSA. Weight average molecular weights above 200,000 were obtained in four of the eight compositions tested and all of the branched polymers had weight average molecular weights above 140,000, though very little difference in the polymer properties from the properties of PSA other than molecular weight were observed (Maniar et al., 1990). Degradation profiles of the branched polymers were also similar to that for PSA (Maniar et al., 1990). Drug release profiles for these polymers are discussed in Section IV.A.

b. Poly(anhydride-co-alkylene carbonate)s. Xiao and Zhu (2000) suggested accelerating the degradation of polycarbonates by incorporating anhydrides into the polymer backbone. This was accomplished by melt polycondensation of acetylated bis-α,ω-(hydrodxy)alkalene carbonate oligomers. The polymers synthesized were poly(tetramethylene carbonate succinic half-ester anhydride) (PTMCSA) and poly(hexamethylene carbonate succinic half-ester anhydride) (PHMCSA). They observed an initially fast loss of molecular weight followed by much slower degradation in *in vitro* degradation studies and attributed this to initial hydrolysis of the more labile anhydride bond, followed by slower hydrolysis of the carbonate bonds.

c. Fluorinated polyanhydrides. Kaur et al. (2002) synthesized poly[4,4'-(hexafluoroisopropylidine)bis benzoic acid] (PHFB) as an alternative to aromatic polyanhydrides with relatively low solubilities. Acetylated prepolymer did not polymerize readily by melt polycondensation, so trifluoroacetylated prepolymer was used instead and weight average molecular weight of up to 14,000 was obtained with some unreacted monomer (Kaur et al., 2002). The authors suspected cyclization in the case of the acetylated prepolymer. The stability and degradation kinetics of PHFB were reported in the same study (Kaur et al., 2002).

d. Poly(lithocholic acid). Gouin et al. (2000) reported the synthesis of poly(lithocholic acid) (PLCA) and its copolymer with sebacic acid (P(LCA-co-SA)) via both melt polycondensation and dehydrative coupling. The material was characterized thermally, and drug release kinetics and biocompatibility studies were also reported. Modulation of the release kinetics was shown via changes in the copolymer composition (Gouin et al., 2000).

e. Poly(anhydride-co-urethane)s. In their investigation of polyanhydrides with novel chemistries, Hartmann et al. (1993) synthesized several poly(anhydride-co-urethane)s and compared their degradation kinetics to the poly(anhydride-co-ester)s and poly(anhydride-co-amide)s with similar structures. Poly(anhydride-co-amide)s, and poly(anhydride-co-urethane)s degraded by hydrolysis of the anhydride bond only, but poly(anhydride-co-ester)s degraded at both the ester and the anhydride bond.

III. Polyanhydride Characterization

A. CHEMICAL CHARACTERIZATION OF POLYANHYDRIDES

1. Chemistry of Polyanhydrides Assessed by FTIR and ^1H NMR

Fourier transform infrared spectroscopy (FTIR) and proton nuclear magnetic resonance spectroscopy (^{1}H NMR) have become standards for verifying the chemistry of polyanhydrides. The reader is referred to the synthesis literature in the previous section for spectra of specific polymers. The FTIR spectrum for PSA is shown in Fig. 2. In FTIR the absorption

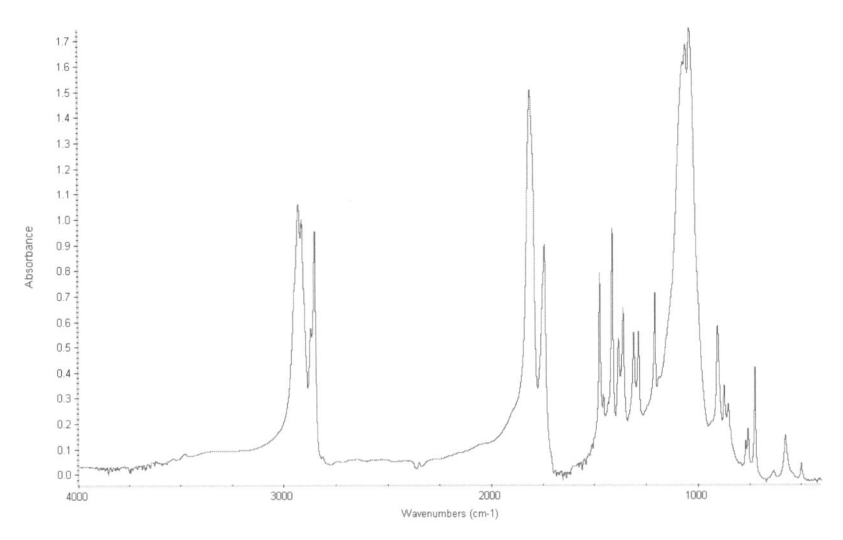

FIG. 2. FTIR spectra for PSA showing characteristic anhydride peaks between 1750 and 1900 cm^{-1}.

characteristic of the anhydride doublets are typically found around 1740 and 1810 cm^{-1} for the aliphatic residues and 1720 and 1780 cm^{-1} for the aromatic residues (Domb et al., 1993). Excitation of the anhydride bond also absorbs at 1050 cm^{-1} (Leong et al., 1985). The acidic O–H bond absorbs between 3300 and 2500 cm^{-1} (Rosen et al., 1983). The combination of these absorbances can be used to assess hydrolytic degradation, and the relative intensities of the anhydride bonds can be used to verify copolymer composition.

The analysis of ^{1}H NMR spectra of aliphatic and aromatic polyanhydrides has been reported by Ron et al. (1991), and McCann et al. (1999) and Shen et al. (2002), and ^{13}C NMR has been reported by Heatley et al. (1998). In ^{1}H NMR, the aliphatic protons have chemical shifts between 1 and 2 ppm, unless they are adjacent to electron withdrawing groups. Aliphatic protons appear at about 2.45 ppm when α to an anhydride bond and can be shifted even further when adjacent to ether oxygens. Aromatic protons typically appear with chemical shifts between 6.5 and 8.5 ppm and are also shifted up by association with anhydride bonds. The sequence distribution of copolymers can be assessed, for example in P(CPH–SA), by discerning the difference between protons adjacent to CPH–CPH bonds, CPH–SA bonds, and SA–SA bonds (Shen et al., 2002). FTIR and ^{1}H NMR spectra for many of the polymers mentioned in Section II can be found in their respective references.

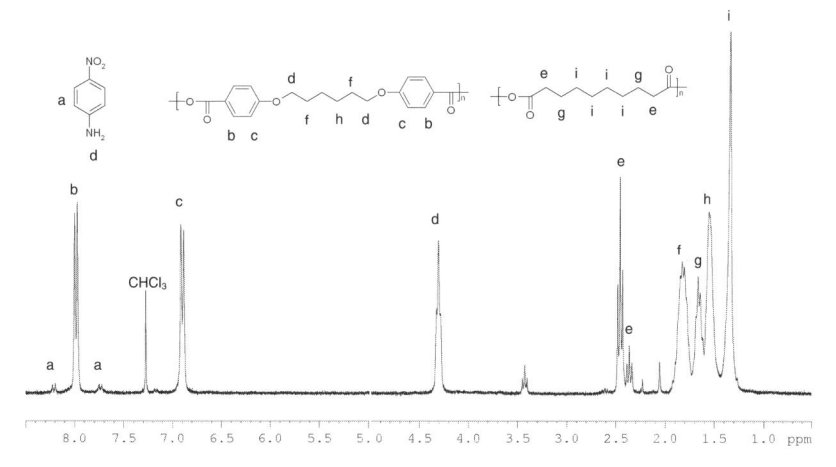

FIG. 3. ^{1}H NMR of P(CPH-SA) 50:50 loaded with *p*-nitroaniline.

Spectroscopy can also be used to assess drug-loading in these systems. Figure 3 is a ^{1}H NMR spectrum for *p*-nitroaniline-loaded P(CPH–SA) (50:50). The combination of these two techniques provides a standard for verifying the chemistry of polyanhydrides. UV spectroscopy has also been reported for determining the chemistry of copolymers (Leong *et al.*, 1985).

2. Solubility of Polyanhydrides

When Bucher and Slade first synthesized PTA and PIPA, they reported insolubility in low pH, aqueous media, and solubility of PTA in alkaline solutions. Most polyanhydrides synthesized in the century that has passed since then show similar behavior. Many polyanhydrides also exhibit extremely limited solubility in organic solvents. This can cause problems in both characterization and processing as many characterization techniques are conducted in solution, and co-dissolution is a common method of fabricating both polymer/polymer blends and polymer/drug systems. A careful survey of the literature reveals that chlorinated solvents (chloroform and dichloromethane (DCM)) are almost universal solvents (and in some cases the only solvents) for polyanhydrides. Leong *et al.* (1985) reported that PCPP and PCPH were soluble in tetrahydrofuran (THF) and *N,N'*-dimethylformamide (DMF) only immediately following polymerization, making characterization by GPC on these polymers rather inconvenient. Domb and Langer (1987, 1988b; Domb *et al.*, 1989) report the use of chloroform as a solvent for P(CPP–SA), PSA, PCPH, PPDP, PDDA, PCPV, and PCPO, but that PCPP, and PCPA are both insoluble in chloroform (Domb and Langer, 1988b; Domb et al., 1989). PDDA, PAA, and are also reported to be soluble in chloroform (Albertsson and Lundmark, 1990b). Domb (1992) also studied the solubilities of PTA, PCPP, PIPA, and PFA in DCM, chloroform, and carbon tetrachloride and reported that all of them had less than 0.1% solubility (w/v). However, altering copolymer composition proved to be an effective method of improving the solubility of aliphatic polyanhydrides. Domb (1992) indicated slightly increased solublities of the 70:30 copolymers P(TA–SA), P(CPP–SA), P(IPA–SA), and P(FA–SA), and increasing solubility as the PSA fraction was increased. More surprisingly, the copolymers made exclusively of the aromatic moieties (the homopolymers of which were insoluble) showed solubilities of greater than 1% (w/v) for some compositions (Domb, 1992).

Several of the synthetic efforts outlined in Section II were motivated partially by the necessity of increasing the processability of polyanhydrides. Solubilities of the 20:80 copolymers of P(CPP–SA) and P(FAD–SA) are compared by Domb and Maniar (1993). They reported improved solubility of the later over former in several organic solvents including (in order of decreasing solubility) THF, 2-butanone, 4-methyl-2-pentanone, acetone, and ethyl acetate.

Altering the linearity of aromatic polyanhydrides has proven to be a successful strategy for increasing solubility. Campo et al. (1999) reported the solubility of Po-CPP and Po-CPH in THF to be 124 mg/ml and 130 mg/ml, respectively. Anastasiou and Uhrich (2000a) reported that the *ortho*-isomers Po-o-CPX, Pm-o-CPX, Pp-o-CPX, and Po-p-CPX also had improved solubilities in DMF, and all but the Pp-o-CPX had improved solubility in THF, whereas the Pp-p-CPX could not be synthesized because its corresponding methyl ester monomer was not even soluble due to the rigidity of the three *para*-aromatic moieties in sequence. Other chemistries also demonstrated improved solubilities. The poly(anhydride-*co*-ester)s and poly(anhydride-*co*-imide)s synthesized by Jiang and Zhu (2001; Jiang et al., 2001c) demonstrated solubility in THF and the esters were also soluble in DMSO in addition to DCM.

B. CHARACTERIZATION OF THERMAL PROPERTIES, CRYSTALLINITY, AND PHASE BEHAVIOR OF POLYANHYDRIDES

1. Thermal Transitions

It is important to characterize the thermal properties of polyanhydrides that are proposed for drug delivery applications, as changes in crystallinity can affect degradation profiles and drug release kinetics. The anticipated dependences of chain structure on glass transition temperature (T_g) are evident in most of the polyanhydrides studied. The most rigid polymer, PTA, has a glass transition temperature of 245°C and a melting point reported alternatively at 372°C (Leong *et al.*, 1985) and 400°C (Yoda, 1963). As methylene groups are added to the *p*-aromatic polyanhydrides, the T_g and T_m generally exhibit systematic reductions. PCPM has a T_g reported at 86 and 92°C and a T_m reported at 196°C. PCPP has a T_g that has been reported to be between 92 and 96°C and T_m of between 230 and 266°C, while PCPH has a T_g that is difficult to detect, but found at 47–48°C and T_m between 123 and 147°C (Campo *et al.*, 1999; Domb and Langer, 1988b; Domb, 1992; Leong *et al.*, 1985, 1987; Mathiowitz *et al.*, 1990b; Rosen *et al.*, 1983).

The branched aromatic polyanhydrides synthesized by Sanders *et al.* (1999; Mathiowitz *et al.*, 1990b) demonstrated lower T_gs than the corresponding P(PCPP–SA) copolymers. The *para*-xylyl polymers synthesized by Anastasiou and Uhrich (2000a) (P*p-o*-CPX and P*p-m*-CPX) had systematically higher T_gs than the *ortho*-isomers (P*o-o*-CPX, P*m-o*-CPX, P*p-o*-CPX).

For the aliphatic polyanhydrides, Albertsson and Lundmark (1990a) report that the melting point increases as the number of methylenes between the anhydride bonds increases. For the series PAA, PSA, and PDDA, the melting points are 73, 80, and 107°C, respectively (Albertsson and Lundmark, 1990a). Also, altering PSA by addition of fatty acid terminals lowers the melting point by as much as 12°C from 82°C to as low as 70°C, depending on the specific fatty acid used (Teomim and Domb, 1999, 2001). And PFAD is completely amorphous (Tabata and Langer, 1993).

Staubli *et al.* (1991) offer an in depth analysis of the effects of sequence distribution on the T_g of poly(anhydride-*co*-imide)s and discuss the experimental results with respect to several applicable theoretical models of T_g.

The change in melting point and glass transition of the copolymers as a function of copolymer composition are also of particular interest because this reveals information about the copolymer microstructure. This is discussed along with the crystallinity characterization in the following section.

2. Crystalline Morphology of Polyanhydrides

Most of the commonly used polyanhydrides, including the copolymers, are semicrystalline. Crystallinity is characterized by a variety of techniques including differential scanning calorimetry (DSC) small-angle X-ray scattering (SAXS) and X-ray diffraction (XRD). Optical microscopy of films can also be used to investigate the crystallinity of polyanhydrides. Because most polyanhydrides have T_ms near or above room temperature, the crystallinity is a strong function of the thermal history. Therefore, the weight percents of crystallinity ($W_c\%$) reported here are primarily for neat polymer purified and precipitated from the synthesis reaction and dried under vacuum.

Most of the polyanhydride homopolymers discussed here have $W_c\%$ in the range of 50–60. For the aromatic polyanhydrides PTA and PCPP $W_c\%$ is around 60 (Domb, 1992; Mathiowitz et al., 1990b). As chain flexibility is increased, a corresponding decrease in the crystallinity is observed. PIPA and PCPH have $W_c\%$ of 50 and 20, respectively (Domb, 1992; Mathiowitz et al., 1990b). PFA, PSA, and PDDA all have a $W_c\%$ between 55 and 66 (Domb, 1992; Mathiowitz et al., 1988, 1990b). Mathiowitz et al. (1990b) provide an excellent summary of the crystallinity of homopolymers and copolymers of PSA, PCPP, PCPH, PFA, P(SA–FA), P(SA–CPP) and P(SA–CPH) (Fig. 4). Of the copolymers studied, only the copolymers P(FA–SA) in the composition range from 20:80 to 70:30 exhibited two melting temperatures, indicating two separate types of crystals (Mathiowitz et al., 1990b). Data on thermal transitions, $W_c\%$, and heats of fusion (ΔH_f) are presented for an extensive range of copolymer ratios. Plots of the copolymer crystallinities as a function of the composition are reproduced in Fig. 4. Crystallinity and heat of fusion data are summarized

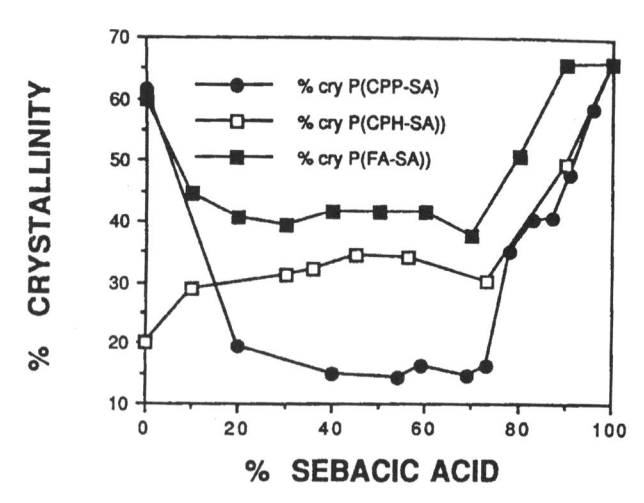

FIG. 4. Crystallinity of several polyanhydride copolymers as a function of composition. From Mathiowitz et al. (1990b). Reprinted with permission.

in Table VIII. X-ray diffraction spectra can be found in the work by Subramanyam and Pinkus (1985), Leong et al. (1985), Mathiowitz et al. (1990b), and Jiang et al. (2001c).

When drugs are incorporated into semicrystalline polymers, the crystallinity may be altered, depending on the interactions between the polymer and the drug (Shen et al., 2001b). The effects of drug loading on polymer crystallinity may offer some insights into release kinetics as will be discussed in Section IV.A. Mathiowitz et al. (1990a) reported the changes in melting point and degree of crystallinity for PSA and P(CPP–SA) 50:50 loaded with various model drugs at different loading levels. The effects on polymer crystallinity and melting point for different drugs provides information on the solubility of the drugs in the polymer matrix, which may be used to predict how drug loading will modify the polymer erosion kinetics and thus the drug release kinetics. Shen et al. (2001a) used wide-angle X-ray diffraction (WAXD) and DSC to characterize the changes in crystallinity of PSA as a function of the loading of a compatible drug, p-nitroaniline (PNA), and an incompatible drug, brilliant blue (BB) (Shen et al., 2001a). The compatible drug reduces the crystallinity, while the incompatible drug has no effect on the polymer crystallinity (Fig. 5).

3. Amorphous Phase Behavior and Microstructure of Polyanhydrides

Blending of polymers is a strategy commonly used to design materials with desirable properties for many applications. Few studies have investigated the amorphous phase behavior of polyanhydrides. Domb (1993) developed two techniques for qualitatively assessing polymer miscibility and reported the results for a variety of binary polyanhydride blends as well as blends of polyanhydrides with other biodegradable polymers. Shakesheff et al. (1995) studied the phase behavior of PSA blends with poly(DL-lactic acid) (PLA) and the effects of the phase behavior on erosion kinetics by novel techniques allowing *in situ* atomic force microscopy (AFM) and surface plasmon resonance (SPR). Surface enrichment in PSA/PLA blends has also been assessed by AFM (Chen et al., 1998). Chan and Chu (2002) used calorimetry and IR to characterize the phase behavior of PSA/poly(ethylene glycol) blends. Rigorous analysis of the phase behavior of polyanhydrides based on theoretical predictions is not found in the published literature.

When describing erosion of and drug release from surface erodible polymers, it is often implicitly assumed that the matrix erodes uniformly, thus resulting in a uniform release profile for a homogenously dispersed drug. While this may be a valid assumption for some homopolymer systems, neglecting the effects of crystallinity, some multicomponent

TABLE VIII
CRYSTALLINITY AND THERMAL PROPERTIES FOR A VARIETY OF POLYANHYDRIDES

Polymer	T_g (°C)	T_m (°C)	ΔH_f (J/g)	W_c%	References
Aliphatic polyanhydrides					
PAA		70–79	37–78		Albertsson and Lundmark, 1988, 1990b; Domb and Nudelman, 1995
PPA		71.5			Domb and Nudelman, 1995
PSU		77.9			Domb and Nudelman, 1995
PAZ		71.8			Domb and Nudelman, 1995
PSA	60	80–89	126–153	57–66	Albertsson and Lundmark, 1990b; Domb and Langer, 1987; Domb and Nudelman, 1995; Mathiowitz et al., 1990b, 1988
PDDA		88–95	107–123	56	Albertsson and Lundmark, 1990b; Domb and Langer, 1987; Domb and Nudelman, 1995; Mathiowitz et al., 1988
PDX		94.4			Domb and Nudelman, 1995
Aromatic polyanhydrides					
PTA	245	372–400		60	Leong et al., 1985; Yoda, 1963
PIA		259		50	Domb, 1992
PDP	[a]	100–113			Domb and Langer, 1987; Leong et al., 1987
PCPM	86–92	196			Leong et al., 1987; Rosen et al., 1983
PCPP	92–96	230–266	96.3–111	53–61.4	Campo et al., 1999; Domb and Langer, 1988b; Domb, 1992; Leong et al., 1985; Mathiowitz et al., 1990b, 1988

PCPH	47–48[b]	123–143	7.1	Campo et al., 1999; Domb and Langer, 1987; Leong et al., 1985, 1987; Mathiowitz et al., 1990b
PCPA	12	185–205		Domb et al., 1989
PCPV		50–74[c]		Domb et al., 1989; Mathiowitz et al., 1992
CPO		48–54		Domb et al., 1989
Po-CPP	50			Campo et al., 1999
Po-CPH	34			Campo et al., 1999
Po-o-CPX	82	[d]		Anastasiou and Uhrich, 2000a
Pm-o-CPX	71	[d]		Anastasiou and Uhrich, 2000a
Pp-o-CPX	84	114		Anastasiou and Uhrich, 2000a
Po-p-CPX	101	[d]		Anastasiou and Uhrich, 2000a
Pm-p-CPX	89			Anastasiou and Uhrich, 2000a
Other polyanhydrides				
PFA	41	246	60	Domb, 1992; Mathiowitz et al., 1990b
PFAD		25–30	0	Domb and Maniar, 1993
PCPAM	35.8			Jiang and Zhu, 2001
PCPSM	36.4			Jiang and Zhu, 2001
CEFB	81			Jiang et al., 2001c
CPFB	73			Jiang et al., 2001c
CBFB	60			Jiang et al., 2001c

[a] Leong et al. (1987) reported that no T_g was observed above room temperature.
[b] Leong et al. (1987) reported that no T_g was observed above −20°C.
[c] Mathiowitz et al. (1992) reported to be amorphous.
[d] No melting point observed (Anastasiou and Uhrich, 2000a).

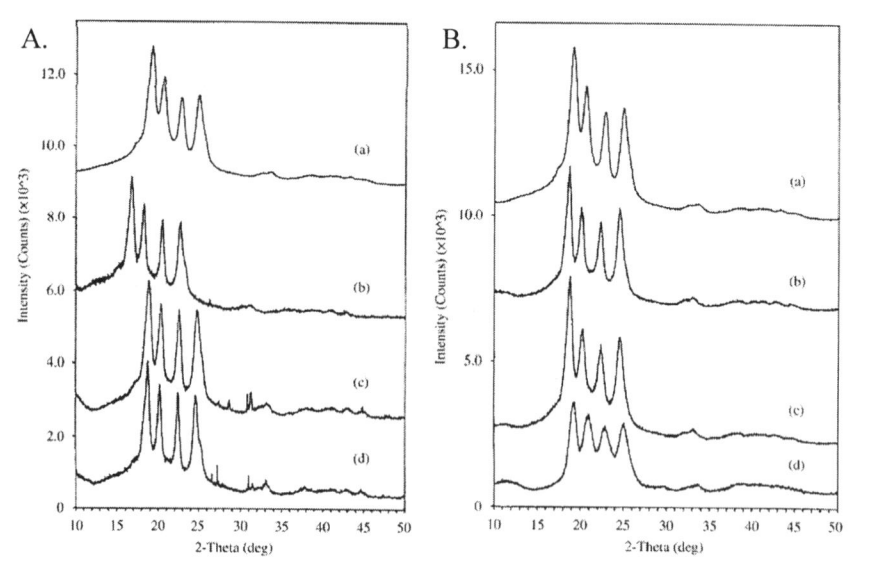

FIG. 5. WAXD spectra for: (A) BB-loaded PSA, and (B) PNA-loaded PSA. (A) BB loading is (a) 0, (b) 15, (c) 30, and (d) 45. Note that as loading increases, the spectrum shows no change for the PSA crystallinity, but crystals of BB appear, indicating that the solute and polymer are immiscible. (B) PNA loading is (a) 0, (b) 5, (c) 10, and (d) 15. Note that there are no peaks corresponding to PNA as the loading increases, however, the polymer crystallinity decreases with increased loading, indicating polymer/solute compatibility. From Shen et al. (2001a). Reprinted with permission.

polymer matrices may exhibit microphase separation, even when the copolymers are random (Shen et al., 2001b). In such phase-separated systems, a drug will thermodynamically partition.

The erosion of copolymers requires the hydrolytic cleavage of three bond types: the A–A bond, the A–B bond, and the B–B bond. If the degradation rates of these three bonds are unequal, as is likely the case, then the erosion will be inhomogeneous. And, if drugs are inhomogeneously distributed in the polymer matrix, the drug release profile will not follow overall device erosion (Shen et al., 2002). Therefore, it is necessary to accurately describe the microstructure of microphase-separated systems.

The length scale on which this microphase separation occurs can be obtained by considering the sequence distribution of monomers in the copolymers. For instance, number-average sequence lengths can be determined from ^{1}H NMR (Mathiowitz et al., 1990b; Ron et al., 1991; Shen et al., 2002; Tamada and Langer, 1992). One may estimate that the length scale of the phase-separated domains is likely to be less than < 10 nm. The characterization proves to be challenging as there are few microscopy or spectroscopy techniques that can resolve such small length scales. However, the effects on drug release kinetics are apparent (see Section IV.A).

C. BIOCOMPATIBILITY OF POLYANHYDRIDES

Biocompatibility is an essential property of new biomaterials for drug delivery. Biocompatibility is always assessed with respect to specific applications and may be assessed with respect to cytotoxicity, allergic responses, irritation, inflammation, mutagenicity, teratogenicity, and carcinogenicity (Katti et al., 2002). The reviews by Katti et al. (2002) and Domb et al. (1997) provide good discussions on the biocompatibility studies that have been conducted with polyanhydrides over the past two decades.

Leong et al. (1986) conducted experiments with the degradation products of P(CPP–SA) to determine mutagenicity and teratogenicity. In the same study, PCPP and PTA were implanted in rat corneas and PCPP was implanted subcutaneously in rat abdomens for histology. Endothelial and smooth muscle cell cultures on P(CPP–SA), P(SA–TA), and PTA were also conducted to assess cytotoxicity. Mutagenicity and teratogenicity tests were both negative, and the *in vivo* experiments revealed no inflammation. Cell cultures exhibited normal proliferation and no abnormal morphologies (Leong et al., 1986).

The biocompatibility of P(CPP–SA) implants in the brain was assessed by Brem et al. (1989) and Tamargo et al. (1989). In the former study the 50:50 copolymer was implanted in rabbit brains and compared to a gelatin based implant used in neurological surgery (Gelfoam) and induced similar mild reactions (Brem et al., 1989). In the latter study the 20:80 copolymer was implanted in rat brains and was compared to Gelfoam® and a cellulose-derived product (Surgicel®). Inflammatory response was similar to that induced by the Surgicel®, but more severe than the Gelfoam®. No local or systemic toxicity was observed (Tamargo et al., 1989). The brain biocompatibility of P(FAD–SA) was investigated by Brem et al. (1992) and found to be comparable to that of P(CPP-SA).

Laurencin et al. (1990) conducted extensive local and systemic toxicity studies with P(CPP–SA), which also showed excellent biocompatibility and toxicology. Domb (1992) studied the biocompatibility of P(CPP–IPA), P(CPP–IPA–SA), and P(CPP–SA) by subcutaneous and intramuscular implants in rabbits. Inflammation occurred at week one and was more pronounced for the intramuscular implants, but subsided in all cases by week 4 (Domb, 1992). Domb and Nudelman (1995) conducted subcutaneous biocompatibility studies in rats with poly(pimelic acid) (PPA), poly(azelaic acid) (PAZ), PSA, and PDDA resulting in mild inflammation but no encapsulation or other pathologies. The systemic and local biocompatibility of the ricinoleic acid-based polymers was investigated and confirmed by Teomim *et al.* (1999) by subcutaneous implantation in rats. Jiang *et al.* (2001a) assessed the biocompatibility of the poly(anhydride-*co*-ester)s PCPA, PCPS, and P(CPA-*co*-CPS) by subcutaneous implants in rats. Mutagenicity and toxicity were not observed, though mild inflammatory responses were observed.

IV. Degradation, Erosion, and Drug Release Kinetics

A. EXPERIMENTS

1. Polymer Stability

The degradation kinetics of several polyanhydrides have been assessed under different storage conditions, to determine the useful shelf life. Rate constants and activation energies for degradation of a variety of polyanhydrides in solution have been reported (Domb and Langer, 1989). In solution, degradation rate is an increasing function of temperature. Aromatic polymers such as PCPM, PCPP, and PCPH, and PDP all maintain their molecular weights both in the solid state and in organic solution for up to a year, but aliphatic polymers show a first order decrease in molecular weight with time (Chasin *et al.*, 1990; Domb and Langer, 1989). Domb *et al.* (1989) reported that the PCPV and PCPO were stable for six months when stored *in vacuo* at room temperature. However, when stored in concentrated chloroform solution, the molecular weights of both polymers were reduced by 50% in only about 3 h. The degradation products could be repolymerized, proving that the degradation occurred primarily via the anhydride interchange and could be reversed (Domb *et al.*, 1989). Chan and Chu (2003) showed that in humid environments, depolymerization results primarily in the formation of diacid products, and therefore occurs by hydrolysis. Domb (1992) also demonstrated the stability of aromatic copolymers stored both under dry argon and in DCM solution, and under exposure to γ-irradiation. The *ortho*-substituted aromatic polyanhydrides, salicylic acid-based poly(anhydride-*co*-ester)s, and ricinoleic acid based poly(anhydride-*co*-ester)s also demonstrate stability to γ-irradiation (Bedell *et al.*, 2001; Erdmann *et al.*, 2000; Krasko *et al.*, 2003). From a study of these results and the studies of other polyanhydrides, storage in a dry atmosphere below −20°C is recommended if polymers are not going to be used within a few days of synthesis (Tamada and Langer, 1992).

2. In vitro Degradation, Erosion, and Drug Release Kinetics

In vitro kinetics experiments are usually conducted on compression molded monolithic polymer tablets, slabs, or cylinders with well-defined surface areas. Compression molding is done above the glass transition and near the melting point. Drugs are incorporated by co-dissolution with the polymer or mechanical mixing in the melt. If erosion profiles are desired, the polymer samples can be removed from the dissolution media at the specified times, dried, and massed. Degradation and drug release requires an assay for the monomer or drug content of the dissolution media. UV Spectrophotometry or HPLC are common techniques. Monitoring the appearance of a single component in the dissolution media is not a reliable method for characterizing the overall erosion rate of a multicomponent system, even when that system is surface-erodible. Such generalizations should be carefully avoided, particularly when the system contains hydrophilic and hydrophobic moieties. For example, Shieh *et al.* (1994) demonstrate that different drugs release from the same matrix with different kinetics. In this study, the model hydrophilic drug acid orange (AO) released faster than the PSA monomer from P(FAD–SA) (50:50) systems, diffusing out of the polymer matrix, while rhodamine b base (RhoB) released more slowly than the PSA monomer from the same system (Shieh *et al.*, 1994). For other compositions, the AO release profile more closely matched the PSA degradation profile (Shieh *et al.*, 1994).

The *in vitro* degradation and drug release of polyanhydride formulations is not necessarily equivalent to the *in vivo* kinetics. For information on the *in vivo* kinetics, the interested reader is referred to the recent review by Katti *et al.* (2002) and the review by Domb *et al.* (1997).

a. Modulating erosion rates and drug release rates. The erosion rate constants reported in the literature or estimated from degradation or erosion data for many of the polyanhydrides discussed in this review are summarized in Table IX. Many of the homopolymers exhibit zero-order degradation over the majority of the release time. As polymer hydrophobicity is increased, the erosion rates generally decrease, presumably due to the decrease in reactivity of the anhydride bond. However, increase in polymer hydrophobicity corresponds to increase in monomer hydrophobicity as well. The corresponding decrease in erosion may therefore be

TABLE IX
EROSION RATE CONSTANTS FOR MANY COMMON POLYANHYDRIDES

Polymer	Erosion rate constant (mol cm^{-2} day^{-1})	Weight-average molecular weight	Reference
PSA	2.7×10^{-5}	23,900	Leong et al., 1987
PDDA	5.4×10^{-5a}	32,700	Albertsson and Lundmark, 1990a
PCDA	9.3×10^{-5}		Zhang et al., 2001
PCPA	3.1×10^{-5}		Domb et al., 1989
PCPV	1.3×10^{-5}	44,600	Domb et al., 1989
PCPO	2.5×10^{-6}	33,300	Domb et al., 1989
PTA	3.2×10^{-5}		Leong et al., 1985
PCPM	3.4×10^{-5b}	11,800	Rosen et al., 1983
PCPP	1.1×10^{-7}	15,000	Leong et al., 1985
Po-CPP	6.3×10^{-7}		Bedell et al., 2001
PCPH	1.4×10^{-8}	9530	Leong et al., 1985
Po-CPH	1.2×10^{-5}		Bedell et al., 2001
PCPS	1.2×10^{-5}		Jiang et al., 2001a
PCPA	5.3×10^{-5}	21,000	Jiang et al., 2001a
PXDA	3.1×10^{-5}	7920	Leong et al., 1987
PFAD			Tabata and Langer, 1993
PHFB	1.6×10^{-6}	15,700	Kaur et al., 2002

CopolymerP (CPP–SA)	Erosion rate constant (μg cm^{-2} day^{-1})	Weight-average molecular weight	Reference
100:0	1.4	15,000	Leong et al., 1985
85:15	6.0	9,840	Leong et al., 1985
45:55	80.0	6,140	Leong et al., 1985
21:79	160.0	12,030	Leong et al., 1985
0:100	210	23,900	Leong et al., 1987

Polyanhydrides with other functional groups	Erosion rate constant (μg cm^{-2} day^{-1})	Number-average molecular weight	Reference
P(A-co-U)	8400	5900	Hartmann et al., 1993
	3600	9100	
	2160	13,700	
P(A-co-A)	9120	6800	Hartmann et al., 1993
	5280	10,800	
P(A-co-E)	2880	6,390	Hartmann et al., 1993
	480	10,900	

[a] Erosion experiment conducted at pH 7.2.
[b] Estimated from linear portion of sigmoidal profile.

due to both degradation kinetics and/or monomer dissolution kinetics (Hanes *et al.*, 1998). Evidence has also been presented (see, for example, Shakesheff *et al.*, 1994) that crystalline domains erode much more slowly than amorphous domains. Thus, careful control of crystallinity may be necessary to accurately modulate erosion and drug release kinetics.

Erosion rates of copolymers can also be modulated by changing the copolymer composition. As an example, erosion rates for three compositions of P(CPP–SA) are reported in Table IX. Similar results were reported by Domb and Maniar (1993) for the copolymers of P(FAD–SA). This study also showed that the copolymers degrade in a heterogeneous fashion, that is, at later times, the composition is richer in the more slowly degrading monomer. Note that erosion rates are varied over two orders of magnitude (Table IX). The same phenomenon was demonstrated by Shakesheff *et al.* (1995) for PSA/PLA blends by a novel technique allowing *in situ* AFM and SPR measurements. Further characterization of these blends revealed surface segregation of the PLA phase, which slowed erosion for high PLA content blends (Davies *et al.*, 1996).

Whether in copolymers or blends, inhomogeneous erosion has a nontrivial effect on drug release kinetics as will be shown later. Leong *et al.* (1985) demonstrated that the pH of the degradation media also has a dramatic effect on the erosion rate, which increases with increasing pH. The acceleration of degradation of polyanhydrides with increase in pH is widely reported and has been used to speed up experiments (Shakesheff *et al.*, 1994).

Molecular weight may also affect the erosion rate. Table IX shows the degradation rate of a representative poly(anhydride-*co*-urethane), a poly(anhydride-*co*-amide), and a poly(anhydride-*co*-ester) of different molecular weights (Hartmann *et al.*, 1993). For all of these polymers reported, the erosion rate decreases as the molecular weight increases.

In their study of branched PSA, Maniar *et al.* (1990) found that the molecular architecture of branched polymers affects the release kinetics in a variety of ways. They found that the branched polymers degraded faster than linear PSA of comparable molecular weight (Maniar *et al.*, 1990). They also noted that drug (morphine) release profiles were more characteristic of bulk erosion than surface erosion: An initial lag time during which very little drug was released was associated with the time required for water to swell the polymer. This was followed by a period of relatively fast release, which tapered off as the device disintegrated. The polymer matrix lost its mechanical integrity before the release experiment was complete (Maniar *et al.*, 1990). Despite the increase in degradation rate, release rates from the polymer randomly branched with 1,3,5-benzene tricarboxylic acid were much lower than release rates from PSA (Maniar et al., 1990). The release from the graft type polymer branched with poly(acrylic acid) approached that of PSA (Maniar et al., 1990).

Evidence that drug loading modifies the erosion rate can be found in many drug release studies. Particularly at higher loadings, hydrophilic drugs tend to increase the overall erosion rate of the polymer (Park et al., 1996; Shen et al., 2002). This phenomenon is attributed to the contribution that the drug makes to the overall chemistry of the system, as well as porosity and voids that may form as hydrophilic drug crystals rapidly dissolve from the exposed surface (Sandor et al., 2002). One study of drug release from bioerodible polyanhydrides found a change in the drug release kinetics from zero-order to first order by simply changing the pH of the media or by changing the hydrophobicity of the drug (Park et al., 1997).

Finally, drug release profiles can be altered by altering the distribution of the drug in the polymer matrix. For purely surface eroding systems, it is theoretically possible to obtain any desired drug release profile by fabricating a device with the corresponding drug distribution profile. Design and fabrication of devices with non-uniform drug distribution is discussed in Section V.

b. Surface changes during erosion. Albertsson and Lundmark (1990a) reported that during the degradation of PDDA, the surface showed a lower C/O ratio (from electron spectroscopy for chemical analysis (ESCA) studies) than in the neat polymer, indicating partial oxidation. Mathiowitz et al. (1993) discussed the effects of crystallinity and liquid crystallinity on the degradation kinetics in P(CPH–SA) and P(CPP–SA) copolymers. Evidence that crystalline domains degrade more slowly than amorphous domains is also reported in several studies (Shakesheff et al., 1994).

The monomer solubility has a crucial effect on the surface characteristics of eroding polymer systems. Undissolved monomer deposited on the surface complicates erosion and release kinetics by presenting a diffusional barrier for drug release as well as water ingress. The compounding effect slows not only the release of monomer and drug, but also the prerequisite hydrolysis of the polymer backbone that results in release (Goepferich et al., 1996). The solubilities of the class of aliphatic polyanhydride monomers from adipic acid (six carbons) to dodecandicarboxylic acid (14 carbons) vary from 50 mg/ml to <0.01 mg/ml, generally decreasing as the length of the methylene chain increases (Domb and Nudelman, 1995).

c. Chemical changes during erosion. Because the degradation products of polyanhydrides are acidic (see pKa's reported in Goepferich and Langer, 1993a), and the degradation is a strong function of pH, it has been hypothesized that during erosion the pH of the microenvironment very near the surface of a device may not be the same as that of the dissolution media. Dissolved drugs may also affect the local pH. This local pH is difficult to measure or estimate (Goepferich and Langer, 1993a), but may have profound effects on the erosion and drug release profiles. Mäder *et al.* (1997) employed spectral spatial paramagnetic resonance imaging and measured pH values inside eroding samples of P(CPP–SA) as low as 4.5, though the dissolution media was buffered at 7.4.

The composition of copolymers usually changes during erosion due to the disparity between the degradation kinetics of the two corresponding homopolymers. Actually, in binary copolymers there are three types of bonds that may all have different degradation kinetics: the A–A bond, the A–B bond, and the B–B bond. Spectroscopic techniques such as IR and NMR can be used to follow the kinetics of specific bond cleavage in copolymers (Heatley *et al.*, 1998; McCann *et al.*, 1999; Uhrich *et al.*, 1998). Changes in molecular weight during degradation are frequently reported. The formation of relatively stable oligomers in copolymer erosion studies has been shown (Santos *et al.*, 1999). The changes in molecular weight may also result in drastic shifts in thermal transitions during erosion (Bedell *et al.*, 2001).

Figure 6 summarizes some of the important effects contributing to drug release kinetics discussed in this section. Drug release from a simple, homogeneous surface eroding system is shown schematically in Fig. 6a and graphically in Fig. 6c. Zero order release is obtained when the drug (represented by the circles) is uniformly distributed and the system erodes uniformly from the surface. Drug release from a phase-separated surface eroding system is shown schematically in Fig. 6b. In this system, two polymer phases are present, one which erodes quickly (light gray), and one which erodes slowly (dark gray). Drug release accelerates initially because the inhomogeneous erosion and bursting of drug from the slow eroding phase lead to increase in surface area. At later times, the fast eroding phase is completely gone, and the degradation products from the slow eroding phase (triangles) form an insoluble barrier to transport, retarding the release. The result is a sigmoidal release profile shown in Fig. 6d. Additional effects, such as partitioning of the drug are not represented.

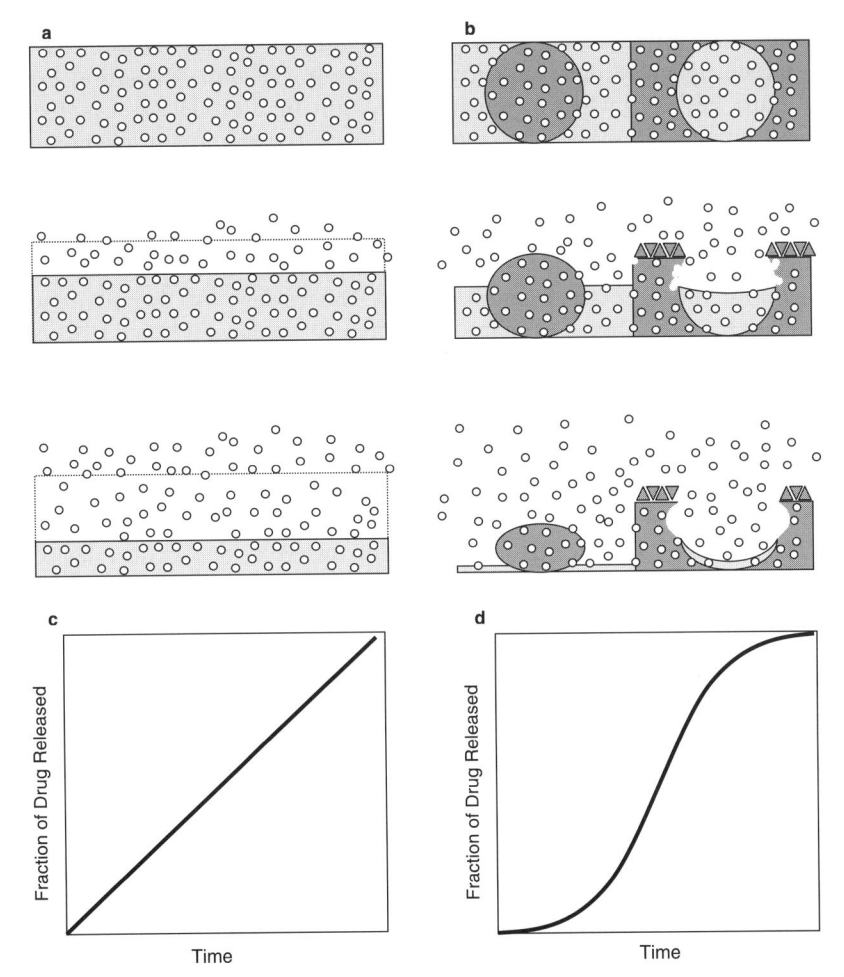

FIG. 6. Mechanism of drug release from (a) homogenous, surface-eroding system, and (b) phase-separated surface-eroding system demonstrating some of the key factors affecting release as discussed in Section IV.A. The corresponding drug release profiles are represented in (c) and (d). Length scale of phase separation is enlarged for emphasis.

B. Modeling Degradation, Erosion, and Drug Release Kinetics

Modeling the behavior of bioerodible polyanhydrides is complicated by the many phenomena contributing to release profiles described in the previous section. The degradation kinetics may be coupled to other processes, such as diffusion and dissolution, and the overall erosion kinetics represent the sum of all of these multiple processes (Goepferich, 1996a).

The phenomena that contribute to erosion kinetics may be difficult or impossible to study independently (Goepferich, 1996b). Therefore, great care must be taken when formulating or applying a model to ensure that the phenomena described by the model are the dominant phenomena controlling the kinetics. A variety of models have been developed that account for different aspects of polymer microstructure, degradation kinetics, and drug loading. The recent review by Goepferich and Tessmar (2002) discusses degradation and erosion of polyanhydrides with an eye to developing more accurate models. And the review by Siepmann and Goepferich (2001) discusses many of the recent models and could be used to aid in selection of the appropriate model for a given system.

Burkersroda et al. (2002) provide a model that can be used to estimate whether a polymer is more accurately characterized as surface eroding or bulk eroding. In this model, the ratio of a characteristic time scale for diffusion to a characteristic time scale for degradation (comparable to a Deborah number) determines the "erosion number," ε (Burkersroda et al., 2002). For $\varepsilon \gg 1$, a device is surface eroding, whereas for $\varepsilon \ll 1$, a device is bulk eroding (Burkersroda et al., 2002). A key component of this model is the device dimensions. Theoretically, even very hydrophobic polymers can be bulk eroding, provided the device is sufficiently small. If the polymer matrix itself is hydrophobic, the polymer degradation rate can be decreased by several orders of magnitude.

The simplest model for pure erosion control with kinetics dominated by a single rate constant and uniformly distributed drugs was described by Hopfenberg (1976). This model says nothing about the various physical phenomena that contribute to erosion, and therefore fails to describe drug release profiles from many polyanhydride systems. Below we classify some of the models that can be found in the literature.

1. Phenomenological Models

The broadest class of models, phenomenological models, account explicitly for individual phenomena such as swelling, diffusion, and degradation by incorporation of the requisite transport, continuity, and reaction equations. This class of models is useful only if it can be accurately parameterized. As phenomena are added to the model, the number of parameters increases, hopefully improving the model's accuracy, but also requiring additional experiments to determine the additional parameters. These models are also typically characterized by implicit mean-field approximations in most cases, and model equations are usually formulated such that explicit solutions may be obtained. Examples from the literature are briefly outlined below.

The transport and continuity equations for surface eroding polymers with two moving boundaries (defining a diffusion zone for drugs inside the polymer matrix) were solved by Thombre and Himmelstein (1984). No account was made for inhomogeneities either in polymer matrix or the drug distribution, but the model was extended to account for the presence of a membraneous diffusive barrier at the surface. A later extension of the model accounted for an external mass transfer coefficient and changes in degradation rate and drug diffusivity with pH and the progress of degradation (Thombre and Himmelstein, 1985). This model was solved numerically.

Batycky *et al.* (1997) developed a model applicable for bulk eroding systems. An interesting component of this model is the explicit accounting of the changes in the molecular weight distribution with time via both end chain scission and random chain scission. Larobina *et al.* (2002) developed a model for release from copolymers that accounts for microphase separation in copolymers and partitioning of drugs into the phase separated microdomains. Two moving erosion fronts are assumed, leading to three regimes of release. Analytical solutions are obtained.

2. Discretized Models

Zygourakis (1990; Zygourakis and Markenscoff, 1996) developed a discretized model in which cells are assigned a degradation time, upon exposure to solvent, based on their identity as either drug, polymer, solvent, or void. The initial distribution of cells can be modeled after the microstructure of the polymer matrix and multiple phases are explicitly accounted for. The solution is found numerically.

Goepferich and Langer (1993b) developed a similar model, except that finite probabilities are assigned for the erosion of each cell type rather than predetermined erosion times. No account of drug release was made in this model, but the model was applied to materials with two types of polymer cells, designed to signify crystalline and amorphous phases. In a second publication, Goepferich and Langer (1995) also accounted for monomer diffusion through the eroding zone. The solution to this model is also obtained numerically.

V. Design of Polyanhydride Carriers for Controlled Release

Many model formulations of polyanhydrides have been tested both *in vitro* and *in vivo*. The delivery schemes that polyanhydrides have been used for can be broadly grouped into three classifications—implantable systems for localized drug release, injectable systems, and aerosols for mucosal delivery. Each of these delivery routes presents a unique set of challenges and these are discussed below.

A. IMPLANTABLE SYSTEMS

1. BCNU-Loaded Polyanhydride Discs for Treatment of Glioblastoma Multiforma

The encapsulation and release of 1,3-bis(2-chloroethyl)nitrosourea (BCNU) in P(CPP-SA) 20:80 wafers was the first implantable controlled release device based on polyanhydrides that was FDA-approved and marketed (Gliadel®) (Chasin et al., 1988). BCNU was encapsulated by two techniques, trituration and co-dissolution, resulting in different release profiles (Chasin et al., 1990, 1991). The triturated samples released faster than those prepared by co-dissolution, presumably due to more homogeneous loading in the samples prepared by co-dissolution.

2. Laminated Devices for Pulsatile Release

Jiang and Zhu (2000) and Qiu and Zhu (2001) have reported the fabrication of multilayered devices composed of stacks of compression-molded disks of alternating compositions. One type of disk is either P(SA–EG) or P[SA-co-TMAgly)-b-EG] and the other is a pH-sensitive, protein-loaded blend of, for example, poly(methacrylic acid) and polyethoxazoline. The release of model proteins, myoglobin, bovine serum albumin, and FITC-dextran, and compounds such as brilliant blue have been studied and pulsatile release profiles have been demonstrated (Jiang and Zhu, 2000; Qiu and Zhu, 2001).

3. Other Devices

Erdmann et al. (2000) report the fabrication of devices for the localized delivery of salicylic acid from the poly(anhydride-co-ester)s mentioned in Section II.C. A unique feature of this drug delivery system is that the drug compound is part of the polymer backbone. Devices were implanted intraorally and histopathology was reported (Erdmann et al., 2000). Chasin et al. (1990) review fabrication and testing of implantable formulations for other drugs including angiogenesis inhibitors for treatment of carcinomas and bethanechol for the treatment of Alzheimer's disease.

B. INJECTABLE SYSTEMS

Injectable polyanhydride systems for drug delivery usually consist of polymer microspheres suspended in an injection media. Langer and co-workers reported on three techniques for the fabrication of drug loaded polyanhydride microspheres: hot-melt, solvent removal, and spray drying (Bindschaedler *et al.*, 1988; Mathiowitz and Langer, 1987; Mathiowitz *et al.*, 1988, 1990a, 1992). The hot-melt technique used by Mathiowitz and Langer (1987) is performed by heating the polymer and drug in a nonsolvent to a temperature above the melting point of the polymer and stirring to disperse the molten droplets. Subsequent cooling freezes polymer microspheres loaded with dissolved drug. This technique is only useful for polymers with melting points sufficiently low that the activity of the drugs is not affected by the heating. In the spray drying technique, polymer and drug are dissolved in a suitable solvent and a spray dryer is used to disperse small droplets into air where precipitation occurs (Mathiowitz *et al.*, 1992). The third and most common technique found in the literature is solvent removal. In this technique, a polymer solution (containing drug) is dispersed in a non-solvent (Mathiowitz *et al.*, 1988). An emulsion is formed. The solvent is extracted out of the droplets by the non-solvent, precipitating the microspheres. Variations on the solvent removal technique have been optimized for several polymer/drug systems. Double emulsion or phase inversion techniques are used when the drug and polymer are not soluble in the same solvent (Chiba *et al.*, 1997; Chickering *et al.*, 1997; Thomas *et al.*, 1997). Double walled microspheres have been produced by precipitating a second polymer solution onto previously fabricated microspheres (Goepferich *et al.*, 1994), and by allowing thermodynamic partitioning of two polymer solutions during the solvent removal process (Leach *et al.*, 1999; Pekarek *et al.*, 1994). *In vitro* and *in vivo* degradation studies showed that the inner layer of P(CPP–SA) degraded before an outer layer of PLA in double walled systems (Leach and Mathiowitz, 1998; Leach *et al.*, 1998).

Microspheres with precisely controlled sizes have been produced by a novel apparatus that uses acoustic excitation and a non-solvent carrier stream to form each droplet in the emulsion separately (Berkland *et al.*, 2003). The morphology and hence the drug release kinetics of the microspheres are affected by the fabrication technique. The size of the microspheres can be modulated by changing the stirring rate in the hot melt and solvent removal techniques, however both of these techniques produce highly polydisperse size distributions (Mathiowitz and Langer, 1987; Mathiowitz *et al.*, 1988). The surface and internal morphology of microspheres produced by various techniques have also been characterized, as these will affect the drug release kinetics. The hot-melt technique produces non-porous microspheres with crenellated surfaces (Mathiowitz and Langer, 1987). Solvent removal techniques can produce smooth microspheres, though porosity is difficult to control and crystalline polymers tend to have greater surface roughness (Mathiowitz et al., 1988, 1990a). Spray dried microspheres also have polydisperse size distributions and can have very porous structures. Mathiowitz et al. (1992) had difficulty preventing the microspheres made from some polymers from fusing into aggregates with this technique. Drug loading efficiencies and uniformity can vary depending on the compatibility of the drug with the polymer matrix and other characteristics of the fabrication technique. These morphological variations will also have a significant impact on the drug release kinetics, which are discussed in the next subsection.

An advantage of this type of delivery system is that microspheres displaying different release profiles (e.g., being composed of different polymers or different sizes) can be combined in cocktails to obtain release profiles that are the sum of the various release profiles from the individual formulations (Kipper et al., 2002). Multiple drugs could also be delivered this way in a single injection.

Berkland et al. (2003) showed that for systems made by solvent removal, the precipitation kinetics play a crucial role in determining drug distribution within the microspheres, and thus the release profiles. For drugs that are incompatible with the polymer matrix, slow precipitation may result in surface segregation of the drug (Berkland et al., 2003). One way of controlling the precipitation kinetics is to carefully control the microsphere size. *Smaller* microspheres precipitate more quickly and therefore exhibit the most *extended* release profiles when the polymer/drug compatibility is low (Berkland et al., 2003). In a study comparing release profiles from tablets and injectable granules (Tabata et al., 1994), it was shown that inhomogeneously distributed drug has little or no detectable effect on release profiles from tablets, while the release profiles from granules exhibit drug bursts at the beginning of the experiment.

Proteins may be stabilized by encapsulation in polyanhydride microspheres. Stability of proteins with respect to water-induced aggregation has been demonstrated to be a function of polymer hydrophobicity for insulin and bovine somatotropin as model proteins (Ron et al., 1993). Encapsulation and enzymatic activity of a variety of other proteins encapsulated in P(SA–FAD) was studied by Tabata et al. (1993).

C. Aerosols and Systems Designed for Mucosal Delivery

Many therapeutic proteins must be delivered by injection as alternative delivery routes (e.g., oral) result in low bioavailability. This can be difficult, inconvenient, and painful, particularly for long-term treatments, for example, in the case of insulin administration for diabetes patients. Mucosal delivery offers an attractive alternative to injection, but poses some unique challenges. The formulation must stabilize the drug, target delivery to the mucosa, remain at the delivery site for extended periods, and facilitate trans-mucosal transport of the drug (Harris and Robinson, 1990). The characteristics of the various mucosa (buccal, nasal, gastrointestinal, and ocular) that can be quantified for design of controlled release devices are summarized by Harris and Robinson (1990). Theories of bioadhesion are briefly outlined by Chickering *et al.* (1995).

Chickering and Mathiowitz (1995) developed a technique for investigating the bioadhesive properties of polymers and showed that p(FA–SA) demonstrated good bioadhesion. Two mechanisms of bioadhesion were proposed: surface free energy effects and hydrogen bonds between carboxylic acid residues in degradation products and mucin or epithelia (Chickering and Mathiowitz, 1995). The same authors showed that encapsulation of a model drug (ducimerol) in P(FA–SA) improved bioavailability in oral delivery experiments (Chickering *et al.*, 1996).

Fu *et al.* (2002) report the optimization of a fabrication procedure for microspheres based on the poly(anhydride-*co*-ether) P(SA–EG). The microspheres are fabricated by solvent removal process that produces a porous structure with densities in the range of 0.344 and 0.077 g cm^{-3} and sizes that are optimized for delivery to the deep lung by inhalation (Fu *et al.*, 2002). An appropriate *in vitro* cell culture model for characterization of the particle–epithelia system was also developed (Fiegel *et al.*, 2003).

VI. Conclusions and Future Opportunities

The past two decades have produced a revival of interest in the synthesis of polyanhydrides for biomedical applications. These materials offer a unique combination of properties that includes hydrolytically labile backbone, hydrophobic bulk, and very flexible chemistry that can be combined with other functional groups to develop polymers with novel physical and chemical properties. This combination of properties leads to erosion kinetics that is primarily surface eroding and offers the potential to stabilize macromolecular drugs and extend release profiles from days to years. The microstructural characteristics and inhomogeneities of multi-component systems offer an additional dimension of drug release kinetics that can be exploited to tailor drug release profiles.

The development of new polyanhydrides has sparked researchers to developed new device fabrication and characterization techniques, instrumentation, and experimental and mathematical models that can be extended to the study of other systems. The growing interest in developing new chemistries and drug release systems based on polyanhydrides promises a rich harvest of new applications and drug release technologies, as well as new characterization techniques that can be extended to other materials. Future endeavors will likely focus on multicomponent polyanhydride systems, combining new chemical functionalities to tailor polyanhydrides for specific applications.

The release characteristics of polyanhydride systems could be used not only to develop clinical treatments, but also to induce chronic disease states as models for studying immune function. Many current models of chronic diseases are based on induction of acute effects, which do not exhibit the same long-term behavior as the disease being modeled.

REFERENCES

Albertsson, A. C., and Lundmark, S. *J. Macromol. Sci. Pure. Appl. Chem.* **A25**, 247 (1988).
Albertsson, A.-C., and Lundmark, S. *Brit. Polym. J.* **23**, 205 (1990a).
Albertsson, A.-C., and Lundmark, S. *J. Macromol. Sci. Chem.* **A27**, 397 (1990b).
Albertsson, A.-C. *J. Appl. Polym. Sci.* **57**, 87 (1995).
Anastasiou, T. J., and Uhrich, K. E. *Macromolecules* **33**, 6217 (2000a).
Anastasiou, T. J., and Uhrich, K. E. *Polym. Prepr.* **42**, 1366 (2000b).
Batycky, R. P., Hanes, J., Langer, R., and Edwards, D. *J. Pharm. Sci.* **86**, 1464 (1997).
Bedell, C., Deng, M., Anastasiou, T. J., and Uhrich, K. E. *J. Appl. Polym. Sci.* **80**, 32 (2001).
Berkland, C., Kipper, M. J., Kim, K. K., Narasimhan, B., and Pack, D. W., *J. Controlled Rel.* **94**, 129 (2004).
Bindschaedler, C., Leong, K., Mathiowitz, E., and Langer, R. *J. Pharm. Sci.* **77**, 696 (1988).
Brem, H., Domb, A., Lenartz, D., Dureza, C., Olivi, A., and Epstein, J. I. *J. Control. Rel.* **19**, 325 (1992).
Brem, H., Kader, A., Epstein, J. I., Tamargo, R. J., Domb, A., Langer, R., and Leong, K. W. *Sel. Canc. Ther.* **5**, 55 (1989).
Bucher, J. E., and Slade, W. C. *J. Am. Chem. Soc.* **31**, 1319 (1909).
Burkersroda, F. V., Schedl, L., and Goepferich, A. *Biomaterials* **23**, 4221 (2002).
Cabré-Castellví, J., Palomo-Coll, A., and Palomo-Coll, A. L., Synthesis 616 (1981).
Campo, C. J., Anastasiou, T., and Uhrich, K. E. *Polym. Bull.* **42**, 61 (1999).
Chan, C.-K., and Chu, I.-M. *Biomaterials* **23**, 2353 (2002).
Chan, C.-K., and Chu, I.-M. *J. Appl. Polym. Sci.* **89**, 1423 (2003).
Chasin, M., Domb, A., Ron, E., Mathiowitz, E., Langer, R., Leong, K., Laurencin, C., Brem, H., and Grossman, S. *Drugs Pharm. Sci.* **45**, 43 (1990).
Chasin, M., Hollenbeck, G., Brem, H., Grossman, S., Colvin, M., and Langer, R. *Drug Dev. Ind. Pharm.* **16**, 2579 (1991).
Chasin, M., Lewis, D., and Langer, R. *Biopharm. Manuf.* **1**, 33 (1988).

Chen, X., McGurk, S. L., Davies, M. C., Roberts, C. J., Shakesheff, K. M., Tendler, S. J. B., Williams, J. R., Davies, J., Dawkes, A. C., and Domb, A. *Macromolecules* **31**, 2278 (1998).
Chiba, M., Hanes, J., and Langer, R. *Biomaterials* **18**, 893 (1997).
Chickering, D. E., and Mathiowitz, E. *J. Control. Rel.* **34**, 251 (1995).
Chickering, D. E. I., Jacob, J. S., Desai, T. A., Harrison, M., Harris, W. P., Morrell, C. N., Chaturvedi, P., and Mathiowitz, E. *J. Control. Rel.* **48**, 35 (1997).
Chickering, D. E. I., Jacob, J. S., and Mathiowitz, E. *React. Polym.* **25**, 189 (1995).
Chickering, D., Jacob, J., and Mathiowitz, E. *Biotechnol. Bioeng.* **52**, 96 (1996).
Conix, A. *Makromol. Chem.* **24**, 76 (1957).
Conix, A. *J. Polym. Sci.* **29**, 343 (1958).
Conix, A. *Macromol. Synthesis* **2**, 95 (1966).
Davies, M. C., Shakesheff, K. M., Shard, A. G., Domb, A., Roberts, C. J., Tendler, S. J. B., and Williams, J. R. *Macromolecules* **29**, 2205 (1996).
De Abajo, J., Babé, S. G., and Fontán, J. *Angew. Makromol. Chem.* **19**, 121 (1971).
Deng, X., Li, Z., Yuan, M., and Hao, J. *J. Appl. Polym. Sci.* **88**, 2194 (2003).
Domb, A. *J. Polym. Sci. A.* **31**, 1993 (1973).
Domb, A. J. *Macromolecules* **25**, 12 (1992).
Domb, A., and Langer, R. *J. Polym. Sci. A.* **25**, 3373 (1987).
Domb, A. J., and Langer, R. S. US Patent 4,789,724 (1988a).
Domb, A. J., and Langer, R. *Macromolecules* **21**, 1925 (1988b).
Domb, A. J., and Langer, R. *Macromolecules* **22**, 2117 (1989).
Domb, A. J., and Maniar, M. *J. Polym. Sci. A.* **31**, 1275 (1993).
Domb, A. J., and Nudelman, R. *Biomaterials* **16**, 319 (1995).
Domb, A., Amselem, S., Shah, J., and Manoj, M. *Adv. Polym. Sci.* **107**, 93 (1993).
Domb, A. J., Elmalak, O., Shastri, V. R., Ta-shma, Z., Masters, D. M., Ringel, I., Teomim, D., and Langer, R. *Drug Target. Deliv.* **7**, 135 (1997).
Domb, A., Gallardo, C., and Langer, R. *Macromolecules* **22**, 3200 (1989).
Domb, A. J., Mathiowitz, E., Ron, E., Giannos, S., and Langer, R. *J. Polym. Sci. A* **29**, 571 (1991).
Edlund, U., and Albertsson, A.-C. *J. Appl. Polym. Sci.* **72**, 227 (1999).
Erdmann, L., and Uhrich, K. E. *Biomaterials* **21**, 1941 (2000).
Erdmann, L., Macedo, B., and Uhrich, K. E. *Biomaterials* **21**, 2507 (2000).
Fiegel, J., Ehrhardt, C., Schaefer, U. F., Lehr, C.-M., and Hanes, J. *Pharm. Res.* **20**, 788 (2003).
Fu, J., Fiegel, J., Krauland, E., and Hanes, J. *Biomaterials* **23**, 4425 (2002).
Goepferich, A. *Biomaterials* **17**, 103 (1996a).
Goepferich, A. *Eur. J. Pharm. Biopharm.* **42**, 1 (1996b).
Goepferich, A., and Langer, R. *J. Polym. Sci. A* **31**, 2445 (1993a).
Goepferich, A., and Langer, R. *Macromolecules* **26**, 4105 (1993b).
Goepferich, A., and Langer, R. *J. Control. Rel.* **33**, 55 (1995).
Goepferich, A., and Tessmar, J. *Adv. Drug Deliv. Rev.* **54**, 911 (2002).
Goepferich, A., Alonso, M. J., and Langer, R. *Pharm. Res.* **11**, 1568 (1994).
Goepferich, A., Schedl, L., and Langer, R. *Polymer* **37**, 3861 (1996).
González, J. I., De Abajo, J., González-Bebé, S., and Fontán, J. *Angew. Makromol. Chem.* **55**, 85 (1976).
Gouin, S., Shu, X. X., and Lehnert, S. *Macromolecules* **33**, 5379 (2000).
Gupta, B., US Patent 4,868,265 (1989).
Hanes, J., Chiba, M., and Langer, R. *Macromolecules* **29**, 5279 (1996).
Hanes, J., Chiba, M., and Langer, R. *Biomaterials* **19**, 163 (1998).
Harris, D., and Robinson, J. R. *Biomaterials* **11**, 652 (1990).

Hartmann, M., and Schulz, V. *Makromol. Chem.* **190,** 2141 (1989).
Hartmann, M., Geyer, A., Wermann, K., Schulz, V., Knips, C., and Pinther, P. *J. Macromol. Sci. Pure Appl. Chem.* **A30,** 91 (1993).
Heatley, F., Humadi, M., Law, R. V., and D'Emanuele, A. *Macromolecules* **31,** 3832 (1998).
Hill, J. W., and Carothers, W. H. *J. Am. Chem. Soc.* **54,** 1569 (1932).
Hill, J. W. *J. Am. Chem. Soc.* **52,** 4110 (1930).
Hopfenberg, H. B., *in* "Controlled Release Polymeric Formulations, ACS Symposium Series No. 33" (D. R. Paul and F. W. Harris, Eds.), p. 26. American Chemical Society, Washington DC (1976).
Jiang, H. L., and Zhu, K. *J. Polym. Int.* **48,** 47 (1999).
Jiang, H. L., and Zhu, K. *J. Int. J. Pharm.* **194,** 51 (2000).
Jiang, H. L., and Zhu, K. *J. Biomaterials* **22,** 211 (2001).
Jiang, H. L., and Zhu, K. *J. Biomaterials* **23,** 2345 (2002).
Jiang, H. L., Tang, G. P., Weng, L. H., and Zhu, K. *J. J. Biomater. Polym. Ed.* **12,** 1281 (2001a).
Jiang, H. L., Zhu, K. J., and Dai, L. *J. Macromol. Rapid. Commun.* **22,** 414 (2001b).
Jiang, H. L., Zhu, K. J., and Dai, L. *J. Polym. Int.* **50,** 722 (2001c).
Katti, D. S., Lakshmi, S., Langer, R., and Laurencin, C. T. *Adv. Drug Deliv. Rev.* **54,** 933 (2002).
Kaur, S., Doerr, A., Thompson, A., and Dalby, C. *J. Polym. Sci. A* **40,** 3027 (2002).
Kipper, M. J., Shen, E., Determan, A., and Narasimhan, B. *Biomaterials* **23,** 4405 (2002).
Krasko, M. Y., Shikanov, A., Kumar, N., and Domb, A. *J. Polym. Adv. Technol.* **13,** 960 (2002).
Krasko, M. Y., Shikanov, A., Ezra, A., and Domb, A. *J. J. Polym. Sci. A* **41,** 1059 (2003).
Kricheldorf, H. R., and Jürgens, C. *Eur. Polym. J.* **30,** 281 (1994).
Krogh-Jespersen, E., Anastasiou, T. J., and Uhrich, K. E. *Polym. Prepr.* **41,** 1048 (2000).
Larobina, D., Kipper, M. J., Mensitieri, G., and Narasimhan, B. *AIChE J.* **48,** 2960 (2002).
Laurencin, C., Domb, A., Morris, C., Brown, V., Chasin, M., McConnell, R., Lange, N., and Langer, R. *J. Biomed. Mater. Res.* **24,** 1463 (1990).
Leach, K. J. P., and Mathiowitz, E. *Biomaterials* **19,** 1973 (1998).
Leach, K. J. P., Takahashi, S., and Mathiowitz, E. *Biomaterials* **19,** 1981 (1998).
Leach, K., Noh, K., and Mathiowitz, E. *J. Microencap.* **16,** 153 (1999).
Leong, K. W., Brott, B. C., and Langer, R. *J. Biomed. Mat. Res.* **19,** 941 (1985).
Leong, K. W., D'Amore, P., Marletta, M., and Langer, R. *J. Biomed. Mater. Res.* **20,** 51 (1986).
Leong, K., Simonte, V., and Langer, R. *Macromolecules* **20,** 705 (1987).
Li, Z., Hao, Z., Yuan, M., and Deng, M. *Eur. J. Phys.* **39,** 313 (2003).
Mäder, K., Nitschke, S., Stosser, R., Borchert, H.-H., and Domb, A. *Polymer* **38,** 4785 (1997).
Maniar, M., Xie, X., and Domb, A. J. *Biomaterials* **11,** 690 (1990).
Mathiowitz, E., and Langer, R. *J. Control. Rel.* **5,** 13 (1987).
Mathiowitz, E., Saltzman, W. M., Domb, A., Dor, P., and Langer, R. *J. Appl. Polym. Sci.* **35,** 755 (1988).
Mathiowitz, E., Amato, C., Dor, P., and Langer, R. *Polymer* **31,** 547 (1990a).
Mathiowitz, E., Ron, E., Mathiowitz, G., Amato, C., and Langer, R. *Macromolecules* **23,** 3212 (1990b).
Mathiowitz, E., Bernstein, H., Giannos, S., Dor, P., Turek, T., and Langer, R. *J. Appl. Polym. Sci.* **45,** 125 (1992).
Mathiowitz, E., Jacob, J., Pekarek, K., and Chickering, D. I. *Macromolecules* **26,** 6756 (1993).
McCann, D. L., Heatley, F., and D'Emanuele, A. *Polymer* **40,** 2151 (1999).
Mestres, R. *Synthesis* 218 (1981).
Park, E.-S., Maniar, M., and Shah, J. *J. Controlled Rel.* **40,** 111 (1996).
Park, E.-S., Maniar, M., and Shah, J. C. *J. Controlled Rel.* **48,** 67 (1997).

Pekarek, K., Jacob, J. S., and Mathiowitz, E. *Nature* **367**, 258 (1994).
Pierre, T. S., and Chiellini, J. *Bioactive Compatible Polym.* **1**, 467 (1986).
Pinther, P., and Hartmann, M. *Makromol. Chem. Rapid Commun.* **11**, 403 (1990).
Qiu, L. Y. *Polym. Int.* **51**, 481 (2002).
Qiu, L. Y., and Zhu, K. J. *Polym. Int.* **49**, 1283 (2000).
Qiu, L. Y., and Zhu, K. J. *Int. J. Pharm.* **219**, 151 (2001).
Ron, E., Mathiowitz, E., Mathiowitz, G., Domb, A., and Langer, R. *Macromolecules* **24**, 2278 (1991).
Ron, E., Turek, T., Mathiowitz, E., Chasin, M., Hageman, M., and Langer, R. *Proc. Nat. Acad. Sci. USA.* **90**, 4176 (1993).
Ropson, N., Dubois, P., Jérôme, R., and Teyssié, P. *J. Polym. Sci. A* **35**, 183 (1997).
Rosen, H. B., Chang, J., Wnek, G. E., Linhardt, R. J., and Langer, R. *Biomaterials* **4**, 131 (1983).
Sanders, A. J., Li, B., Bieniarz, C., and Harris, F. W. *Polym. Prepr.* **40**, 888 (1999).
Sandor, M., Bailey, N. A., and Mathiowitz, E. *Polymer* **43**, 278 (2002).
Santos, C. A., Freedman, B. D., Leach, K. J., Press, D. L., Scarpulla, M., and Mathiowitz, E. *J. Control. Rel.* **60**, 11 (1999).
Shakesheff, K. M., Chen, X., Davies, M. C., Domb, A., Roberts, C. J., Tendler, S. J. B., and Williams, P. M. *Langmuir* **11**, 3921 (1995).
Shakesheff, K. M., Davies, M. C., Roberts, C. J., Tendler, S. J. B., Shard, A. G., and Domb, A. *Langmuir* **10**, 4417 (1994).
Shen, E. E., Chen, H.-L. and Narasimhan, B. *Proc. Mat. Res. Soc.* 662 (2001a).
Shen, E., Pizsczek, R., Dziadul, B., and Narasimhan, B. *Biomaterials* **22**, 201 (2001b).
Shen, E., Kipper, M. J., Dziadul, B., Lim, M.-K., and Narasimhan, B. *J. Control. Rel.* **82**, 115 (2002).
Shieh, L., Tamada, J., Tabata, Y., Domb, A., and Langer, R. *J. Control. Rel.* **29**, 73 (1994).
Siepmann, J., and Goepferich, A. *Adv. Drug Deliv. Rev.* **48**, 229 (2001).
Slivniak, R., and Domb, A. *Biomacromolecules* **3**, 754 (2002).
Staubli, A., Mathiowitz, E., and Langer, R. *Macromolecules* **24**, 2224 (1991).
Staubli, A., Ron, E., and Langer, R. *J. Am. Chem. Soc.* **112**, 4419 (1990).
Subramanyam, R., and Pinkus, A. V. *J. Macromol. Sci. Chem.* **A22**, 23 (1985).
Tabata, Y., and Langer, R. *Pharm. Res.* **10**, 391 (1993).
Tabata, Y., Domb, A., and Langer, R. *J. Pharm. Sci.* **83**, 5 (1994).
Tabata, Y., Gutta, S., and Langer, R. *Pharm. Res.* **10**, 487 (1993).
Tamada, J., and Langer, R. *Biomater. Sci. Polym. Ed.* **3**, 315 (1992).
Tamada, J. A., and Langer, R. *Proc. Nat. Acad. Sci. USA* **90**, 552 (1993).
Tamargo, R. J., Epstein, J. I., Reinhard, C. S., Chasin, M., and Brem, H. *J. Biomed. Mater. Res.* **23**, 253 (1989).
Teomim, D., and Domb, A. J. *J. Polym. Sci. A.* **37**, 3337 (1999).
Teomim, D., and Domb, A. J. *Biomacromolecules* **2**, 37 (2001).
Teomim, D., Nyska, A., and Domb, A. J. *J. Biomed. Mater. Res.* **45**, 258 (1999).
Thomas, P. A., Padmaja, T., and Kulkarni, M. G. *J. Control. Rel.* **43**, 273 (1997).
Thombre, A. G., and Himmelstein, K. J. *Biomaterials* **5**, 249 (1984).
Thombre, A. G., and Himmelstein, K. J. *AIChE J.* **31**, 759 (1985).
Uhrich, K. E., Gupta, A., Thomas, T. T., Laurencin, C. T., and Langer, R. *Macromolecules* **28**, 2184 (1995).
Uhrich, K. E., Ibim, S. E. M., Larrier, D. R., Langer, R., and Laurencin, C. T. *Biomaterials* **19**, 2045 (1998).
Weinberg, J. M., Gitto, S. P., and Wooley, K. L. *Macromolecules* **31**, 15 (1998).
Windholz, T. B., US Patent 3,082,191 (1965).

Wu, C., Fu, J., and Zhao, Y. *Macromolecules* **33,** 9040 (2000).
Xiao, C., and Zhu, K. J. *Macromol. Rapid Commun.* **21,** 1113 (2000).
Xu, H.-B., Zhou, Z.-B., Huang, K.-X., Lei, T., Zhang, T., and Liu, Z.-L. *Polym. Bull.* **46,** 435 (2001).
Yoda, N. *Makromol. Chem.* **32,** 1 (1959).
Yoda, N. *Makromol. Chem.* **55,** 179 (1962a).
Yoda, N. *Makromol. Chem.* **56,** 10 (1962b).
Yoda, N. *Makromol. Chem.* **56,** 36 (1962c).
Yoda, N. *J. Polym. Sci. Pt. A.* **1,** 1323 (1963).
Yoda, N., and Akihisa, M. *Bull. Chem. Jpn.* **32,** 1120 (1959).
Zhang, T., Gu, M., and Yu, X. *Polym. Bull.* **45,** 223 (2000).
Zhang, T., Gu, M., and Yu, X. *J. Biomater. Polym. Ed.* **12,** 491 (2001).
Zygourakis, K. *Chem. Eng. Sci.* **45,** 3259 (1990).
Zygourakis, K., and Markenscoff, P. A. *Biomaterials* **17,** 125 (1996).

INDEX

A

Acrylamides, 118
Actin cytoskeleton, 17–18
Adenosine deaminase deficiency, 131
Adhesive peptide sequences within ECM proteins, 12
Adhesive peptides, 37
Adsorbed proteins, conformation of, 22
Aliphatic polyanhydrides, 177
  copolymers, 182
Allografts, 47
Alpha, 1-glycoprotein (alpha 1-GP) 65
Alzheimer's disease, 64, 67, 210
Amine-modified surfaces, 29
Amyotrophic lateral sclerosis (ALS), 67
Angiogenesis inhibitors, 210
Angiogenic biomaterials, 3
Anhydride interchange mechanism, 175
Anti-adhesive matrix molecules, 17–18
Anti-PECAM, 120
Apoptosis, 23–24
  adhesion-dependent control, 23
Appropriate host response, 3
Arg–Gly–Asp peptides (RGD), 11, 37–38, 63, 104
Asialoglycoprotein, 40
Astrocytes, 48
Atomic force microscopy (AFM), 195
ATR–FTIR spectroscopy, 111
Autografts, 47
Axonal growth
  control of, 55
  electrically mediated guidance, 60
  longitudinally directed, 61
Azo-compounds, 121

B

Baby hamster fibroblast cell line (BHK), 67–68
Basic fibroblast growth factor (b-FGF), 65
BCECF–am, 122

BCNU, 210
Bethanechol, 210
Bioactive agents, 2
Bioactive factor delivery, 159–160
Biocompatibility, 1–5
  concept of, 3
  host response central to, 5
Biodegradable conduits, comparative studies, 59
Biodegradable materials, 50
Biodegradable polymer scaffolds, 61
Bioerodible polymers, 169
  functional groups found in, 171
Biohybrid nerve guide, 56
Biological response, 5
Biologically active materials vs. drugs, 4
Biomaterials
  as agonists of biological response, 3
  inert, 1–2
  overview, 1–6
  synthesis, 15
  three-dimensional polymeric networks as, 76–105
Blood compatibility, 3
Bone and GAMs
  larger animals, 160–161
  small animals, 160
  summary, 161
Bone morphogenetic proteins (BMPs), 159
Bone regeneration, 158–159
Bone tissue engineering, 159–161
Bovine serum albumin (BSA), 65
Bulk erosion, 172

C

^{13}C-NMR studies, 96
Carbohydrates, 13, 15
Carcinomas, 210
Cationic lipids, 136–138
Cationic polymers, 138–141
CD36, 17
CD44, 16–17

CD44–ligand interaction, 16
CD44 receptors, 16
Cell adhesion, 7–8, 11, 21–25, 28–29, 32–33, 40
Cell-adhesion ligands, 36–41
Cell attachment to quaternary amine surfaces, 29
Cell contractility, 25
Cell-derived matrix, 21
Cell differentiation, 21–23
Cell encapsulation *see* Cell encapsulation
Cell integrity, 28
Cell–material interactions, 7–46
  controlled, 33–41
  nonspecific, 25–33
Cell migration, 24–25
Cell motility, 24–25
Cell placement and growth, 55–56
Cell-recognition processes, 14
Cell–substrate contacts, 22
Cell–substrate interactions, 8, 18–19, 24
Cell–surface glycosaminoglycan, 29
Cell surface receptors
  activation, 13
  and their ligands, 8–18
  recognition, 34
Cellular differentiation, 32
Central nervous systems, polymers for regeneration, 60–64
Cetyltrimethylammonium bromide (CTAB), 153
Charge transfer complexes, 92
Charged surfaces, 28
  cell response to, 29
Chemical cues, 50–51
Chemical potential change due to elastic retractive forces, 79
Chemotherapeutic agents delivery using hydrogels, 121
Chinese hamster ovary (CHO) cells, 28
Chitosan, 112, 142, 153, 155
Chitosan–DNA microspheres, 156
Chitosan–DNA nanoparticles, 155
Chitosan–DNA nanospheres, 155
Chloroquine, 155
Chondroitin sulfate, 29
Chondroitinase ABC, 29
Ciliary neurotrophic factor (CNTF), 67–68
Collagen, 16, 20–21, 36, 50–51, 55, 57, 60
Collagen GAMs, 161

Collagen nerve guide, 56
Collagen–NGF mixtures, 51
Combinatorial chemistry, 75
Complementary DNA, 122
Complexation in polymers, 92–98
  effect of PEG chain length, 92–96
  interpolymer, 92–96
  overview, 92
Complexation of poly(ethylene glycols), 92
Compound muscle action potential (CMAP), 59
Compression molding, 201
Concanavalin-A (Con-A), 118
Conduit materials, comparative studies, 57–60
Configurational biomimetic imprinted networks, 78
Controlled cell–material interactions, 33–41
Controlled delivery, polymers for, 141
Controlled DNA delivery, polymeric scaffolds for, 157–162
Controlled DNA release, polymer based particles for, 141–157
Controlled release, polyanhydride carriers for, 209–213
Controlled-release device, 86
Controlled-release polymers, 64–66
Corticospinal tract (CST), 60
Covalently immobilized adhesive peptide sequences, 36–37
Cystic fibrosis, 131
Cytoplasmic alkalinization, 19
Cytoskeletal organization, 30

D

DDAB, 151–153
Degradation, use of term, 170
Degradation half-lives, 170
Dehydrative coupling, 175–176
Dehydrochlorination, 173, 175
Dendrimers, 121
Dextran, 139
Dichloromethane (DCM), 191–192, 200
Differential scanning calorimetry (DSC), 194
Diffusion, fundamentals of, 84–87
Diffusion coefficients, 85–86
Diffusion equations, 83
Dimethylformamide (DMF), 191

Directed growth methods, 52
DMAEMA, 114
DMSO, 192
DNA
  degradation, 147
  delivery, 136–137, 141
  denaturation, 146
  release from scaffolds, 161–162
  release in vaccination applications, 153–157
  sequences, 122
  synthesis, 21
  vaccinations, 142, 162
  see also Plasmid DNA
DNA/DDAB complexes, 151
DNA–gelatin microspheres, 154
DOTAP, 153
Double-emulsion solvent-evaporation technique, 146
Drug delivery, 2
  surface-erodible biomaterials for, 169–218
Drug release
  chemically-controlled, 84
  control mechanisms, 170
  diffusion-controlled, 84
  swelling-controlled, 84
Drugs vs. biologically active materials, 4

E

E–selectin, 15, 40
ECM, 9–10, 17, 104
  coatings, 22
  components, 16, 20, 24, 48–49, 104
  environment, 20
  geometry, 22
  layers, 31
  ligands, 19
  molecules, 15–16, 22
  orientation, 31–32
  production, 33, 39
  properties, 31
  proteins, 11, 34, 36, 41
    adhesive peptide sequences within, 12
  synthesis, 39
ECM–integrin interactions, 21
EILDV, 37
Electrical cues, 51

Encapsulation, 66–68
  advantages over injection, 143
  plasmid DNA, 143–150, 152, 154
Endothelial cells, 21, 33, 104
Entubulization, 48
  degradable polymers for, 52–57
  nondegradable polymers for, 50–52
Equilibrium swelling theory, 79–81
Erosion
  characterization, 170
  use of term, 170
Ethyl cellulose, 113
Eucaryotic cells, 13
Eudragit 100 gels, 119
Extracellular matrix *see* ECM

F

Fabrication methods for porous conduits, 56–57
Factor XII, 3
FAD, 178
FDA, 2
Fibrillar adhesions, 20
Fibroblast growth factor (FGF), 51
Fibroblasts, 20–21, 33, 50
Fibronectin, 16, 20, 22, 27, 36, 50, 55, 64
Fickian diffusion theory, 85
Fick's law of diffusion, 84
Flory–Rehner theory, 79–80
Fluorinated polyanhydrides, 189
Focal adhesions, 19, 25
Foreign body response, 101–102
FT-IR spectroscopy, 94

G

Galactose, 15
Gelatin, 142, 153–154
Gene activated matrices (GAMs), 157–158
  and bone
    larger animals, 160–161
    small animals, 160
    summary, 161
Gene delivery
  advantages, 133
  methods, 133–136

Gene therapy, 131–168
 and protein delivery, 132–133
 concept of, 162
 ex vivo, 133
 in vivo, 133–134
 nonviral, 136
  biomaterials for, 136–141
 overview, 131–132
 viral, 135
Genetic immunization, 142–143
Gibbs free energy, 79
Glial cell line-derived neurotrophic factor (GDNF), 65
Glial growth factor (GGF), 53
Glioblastoma multiforma, polyanhydride discs for treatment of, 210
Glucose response following infusion of human insulin, 107
Glucose-sensitive systems, 117–119
Glycocalyx, 14, 29
Glycopeptides, 39
Glycoproteins, 14
Glycosaminoglycann (GAG), 15
GPC, 191
GRGDY, 37
Growth factor administration, 64

H

^{1}H-NMR spectroscopy, 96, 198
Hemocompatibility testing, 5
Hemophilia, 131–132
Heparin immobilization, 1
Hepatocytes, 39
Host response central to biocompatibility, 5
Human insulin concentration, 107
Human nerve growth factor gene (hNGF), 67
Huntington's disease, 68
Hyaluronic acid (HA), 16–17
Hydrogel tubes, 64
Hydrogels, 60, 76
 applications, 76, 105–122
 chemotherapeutic agents delivery using, 121
 classification, 77
 complexing, 91, 115–117
 drug delivery applications, 121
 environmentally responsive, 88–91
 glucose-sensitive systems, 117–119
 macroporous, 82
 microporous, 82
 network structure, 77–83
 neutral, 105–110
 nonporous, 82
 pH-sensitive, 89–90, 110–112, 114–115
 poly(glyceryl methacrylate) p(GMA)–collagen, 63
 protein-based, 120
 solute permeability properties, 77
 solute transport in, 83–87
 swollen temperature, 89
 synthetic, 63
 temperature-sensitive, 90–91, 112–115
Hydrogen-bonding complexes, 92
Hydrogen bonds, 97–98
 inter-associating, 97
 self-associating, 97
Hydrophilic polymer networks, 76
Hydrophilicity/hydrophobicity, 30, 76, 104
Hydrophobic monomers, 100
Hydrophobicity/hydrophobicity, 30, 76, 104
2-Hydroxyethyl methacrylate (HEMA), 96, 99
Hydroxypropyl cellulose (HPC), 113

I

ICAM-1, 11
ICAMs, 16
Ideal surfaces, 34–35
Immunoglobulins, 9, 16–17
Inert biomaterials, 1–2
Inflammatory response, 102
Infrared spectroscopy, 96–97
 and polymer complexation, 97–98
Inside-out signaling, 12–13
Insulin delivery systems, 119–120
Insulin-like growth factor (IGF), 159
Integrin–ligand binding, 18–25
Integrin–ligand interactions, 12
Integrins, 9–13, 17, 19, 36–39
Intracellular domain, 9

K

Ketene, polymerization with, 176
KRSR, 38

INDEX

L

L-selectin, 15
Lactose, 15
Laminin, 16, 48, 50, 55, 58, 60
Lectin–carbohydrate interactions, 40
Lectins, 15, 40
Leukocyte adhesion, 28
Leukocyte binding, 40
Lower critical solution temperature (LCST), 91, 112–114

M

Macrophages, 103
Matrix-based systems, solute transport in, 87
Medical devices, 2
Melt polycondensation, 174–175
Membrane proteins, 13
Methacrylic acid (MAA), 96
Methyl methacrylate, 100
Mitogen-activated protein kinases (MAPK), 21
Molecular design, 75
Monocyte activation, 3
Monosaccharide asialoglycoprotein ligands, 40
Monosaccharides, 15
Mucosal delivery, aerosols and systems designed for, 212–213
Multigrooved substrates, 32

N

N-acetyllactosamine, 40
N-methyl pyrrolidinone (NMP), 98
Naked plasmid DNA (pDNA), 142
  limitations, 134–135
NCAM, 16
Neomembranes, 56
Nerve growth factor (NGF), 48, 51, 64–65
  silicone tubes prefilled with, 59
Nerve growth factor (NGF)-treated nitrocellulose implants, 60
Nerve guide conduit, 58
Nerve regeneration, polymeric biomaterials for, 47–74

Neural glial cell adhesion molecule (NgCAM), 16
Neural stem cells, 61
Neurotrophic factors, 64, 66
Neurotrophin-3 (NT-3), 64
Neutral networks, tissue engineering, 98–105
Nitrocellulose implants, 60
Nonviral gene therapy, 136
  biomaterials for, 136–141
Nonviral plasmid DNA, 160
Nucleic acids, 131–132

O

Office of Combination Products, 2
Oligosaccharides, 14
Osteoblasts, 33
Osteopontin, 16
Outside-in signaling, 13, 20

P

p-nitroaniline (PNA), 191, 195
  encapulation, 154
P–selectin, 15, 40–41
PAA, 93, 111, 118, 175, 192–193
PAA/PEG complexes, 93–94
Parkinson's disease, 64, 66
PBA, 118
PCDA, 177
PCPA, 179, 191, 200
PCPAM, 187
PCPH, 174, 179, 191, 193–194, 200
P(CPH–CPS), 186
PCPM, 173, 179, 193, 200
PCPO, 179, 191, 200
PCPP, 174–175, 179, 191–194, 199–200
P(CPP–DDA), 174
P(CPP–SA), 174
PCPS, 186, 200
PCPSM, 187
PCPV, 179, 191, 200
PDDA, 174–175, 177, 191–194, 200, 205
PDEAEMA, 110
P(DEAEMA-*co*-HEMA), 111
PDLA, 56–58
PDLLA, 62
PDMAEMA, 110, 118

P(DMAEMA-co-HEMA), 111
pDNA see Plasmid DNA
PDX, 177
PEG, 34–35, 38, 95, 105, 109–110, 115, 119–120, 139, 152, 156
PEG 400, 66
PEG chain length, 92–96
PEG-dimethacrylates, 110
PEG-monomethacrylates, 110
PEG–PLA, 151–152
PEI, 139
PEI/DNA complexes, 139–140
PELA, 62
PEO, 2, 105, 109–110, 112, 121
Peptide-modified surfaces, 36–37
Peripheral nerve damage, 47
Peripheral nervous system, polymers for regeneration, 48–60
PEVAc, 105, 161
PFA, 177, 192, 194
PFAD, 178, 193
PFG-NMR technique, 95
PGA, 59
pH effect on polymer mesh size, 116
pH-sensitive hydrogels, 89–90, 110–112
Phagocytosis, 102
Pharmacotectonics concept, 66
PHB, 54, 64
PHEMA, 34, 63–64, 77, 97–101, 104–106, 115, 118–119
PHEMA-co-AA, 111
PHEMA-co-MAA, 111
p(HEMA-co-MMA), 64
PHFB, 189
PHMCSA, 188
Photolithographic methods, 22
PHPMA, 63, 139
PHSRN, 37
PIPA, 179, 191–192, 194
P(IPA–SA), 174
PLA, 121, 211
PLA/PLGA, 144
Plasmid DNA, 133, 136, 138, 141, 157–158, 161–162
   encapsulation, 143–150, 152, 154
   entrapment and release, 157
   interaction with cationic lipids, 137
   nonviral, 160
PLC, 54, 59–60
PLCA, 189

PLGA, 53, 55, 57, 65–66, 142–157, 161
PLGA–CTAB microspheres, 153
PLGA–CTAB nanospheres, 153
PLL, 139, 147–148
PLLA, 53, 56–57, 59
PMAA, 93, 110, 115–117, 122
PMAA hydrogels, 95
P(MAA-g-EG), 118–119
PMAA/PEG complexes, 93–94
PNA, 198
PNIPAAm, 112–113, 115, 118
PNVP, 105
Polylactic acid, 57
Polyacrylamide, 34
Polyacrylamide (PAAm), 110
Poly(acrylic acid) (PAA), 110
Poly(adipic acid) (PAA), 177
Poly(alpha-hydroxy acid), 61
Poly(amidoamine) dendrimers, 139
Poly(amidoamine) (PAMAM) dendrimers, 140
Polyanhydride carriers for controlled release, 209–213
Polyanhydride discs for treatment of glioblastoma multiforma, 210
Poly(anhydride-co-alkylene carbonate)s, 188
Poly(anhydride-co-amide)s, 187–188
Poly(anhydride-co-ester)s, 183–187
Poly(anhydride-co-ether)s, 183–187
Poly(anhydride-co-imide)s, 183
Poly(anhydride-co-urethane)s, 189
Polyanhydrides
   additional chemistries, 188–189
   aliphatic, 193
   amorphous phase behavior, 195–199
   aromatic, 179–182, 194
   as surface erodible biomaterials, 171
   biocompatibility, 199–200
   branched, 188
   characterization, 189–200
   chemical changes during erosion, 206
   chemical characterization, 189–192
   chemistry and synthesis, 172–189
   crystalline morphology, 193–195
   crystallinity, 196–197
   degradation kinetics, 200–208
   discretized models, 209
   drug release kinetics, 201, 207–209
   drug release rates, 201–205
   early synthesis, 172–173

erosion, 201, 207–209
erosion number, 208
erosion rate constants, 202–203
experiments, 200–206
from unsaturated and fatty acid-derived monomers, 177–179
FTIR, 189–191
future opportunities, 213–214
^{1}H NMR, 189–191
implantable systems, 210
in vitro degradation, 201
injectable systems, 211–212
laminated devices for pulsatile release, 210
microstructure, 195–199
model formulations testing *in vitro* and *in vivo*, 209
modeling, 207–209
modulating erosion rates, 201–205
phenomenological models, 208–209
solubility, 191–192
surface changes during erosion, 205–206
synthesis for drug delivery, 173–176
thermal properties, 196–197
thermal transitions, 192–193
Poly[α, ω(p-carboxyphenoxy)alkanes], 173
Poly(azelaic acid) (PAZ), 200
Poly(bis(hydroxyethyl)terephthalate-ethyl ortho-phosphate/terephthaloyl chloride), 58
Polydimethylsiloxane, 48
Polyelectrolyte complexes, 92
Polyesters, 169
Polyethers, 169
Poly(glyceryl methacrylate) p(GMA)–collagen hydrogels, 63
Poly(glycolic acid), 50
Poly(lactic acid) (PLA), 50, 186, 195
Polylactic-*co*-glycolic acid, 57
Poly(lactide)-*co*-glycolide, 65–66
Poly(lithocholic acid), 189
Polymer-based particles for controlled DNA release, 141–157
Polymer complexation and infrared spectroscopy, 97–98
Polymeric biomaterials for nerve regeneration, 47–74
Poly(phosphoester) conduits, 57
Poly(vinylidene fluoride), 51
Porogens, 101

Porous materials, tissue response to, 102–103
PPA, 200
PPDP, 174, 179, 191
Protein adsorption, 26–28, 34, 39
Protein-based hydrogels, 120
Protein conformation, 26–27
Protein delivery
  and gene therapy, 132–133
  limitations, 132–133
Protein diffusion coefficient, 27
Protein diffusivity, 27
Protein–surface interactions, 28
Proteoglycans, 13–15, 39–41
PSA, 175, 177–178, 191–195, 198, 200–201, 204–205
  FTIR spectrum, 189
P(SA-*alt*-TA), 179
PSA–fatty acid-based copolymers, 179
PTA, 173, 175, 179, 191–192, 194, 199
PTFE, 104
PTMCSA, 188
PTPA, 179
PVA, 34, 103–105, 107–109, 111, 118, 145, 148, 152, 161
PVP, 145, 152
PXDA, 179

R

Receptor affinity, 11
Receptor binding to ligands, 10
Receptor diffusivity, 10
Receptor–ligand binding, 9
REDV (Arginine–Glutamine–Aspartic acid–Valine), 11, 38
Responsive networks, 110–119
RGD (Arginine–Glycine–Aspartic acid), 11, 37–38, 63, 104
Ricinoleic acid, 179
Ricinoleic half-esters, 179
Ring opening polymerization, 176
Rubber elasticity theory, 81–82

S

Saccharides, 14
Salicylic acid, 210

Scaffolds
  biodegradable polymer, 61
  DNA release from, 161–162
  for controlled DNA delivery, 157–162
  tissue engineering, 162
Schwann cells, 48, 50, 52, 58, 61
Secreted protein acidic and rich in cysteine (SPARC), 17
Selectins, 9, 13–15, 39–41
Severe combined immunodeficiency (SCID), 131
Sialyl-Lewis^x (sLe^x), 41
Signal transduction, 18–25
Silicone, 60
Silicone chambers, 49–50
Silicone conduits, comparative studies, 59
Silicone rubber, 48
Silicone tubes, 50
  electrical circuit within, 61
  prefilled with NGF, 59
Small-angle X-ray scattering (SAXS), 194
Sodium chloride, 66
Solute transport
  in hydrogels, 83–87
  in matrix-based systems, 87
Specificity, 5
Spinal cord injuries, 47
Spinal cord regeneration, 61–62
Spinal cord tissue, 60–61
Spray-drying technique, 149–150
Star polymers, 121
Stereocomplexes, 92
Styrene, 119
Surface chemistry, 28–30
Surface-erodible biomaterials for drug delivery, 169–218
Surface erosion, 172
Surface plasmon resonance (SPR), 195
Surface receptors, 11, 24
Surface topography, 31–33
Syndecans, 17

T

Teflon, 60
Tenascins, 17
Tetrahydrofuran (THF), 191–192
Three-dimensional polymeric networks
  as biomaterials, 76–105
  structural characteristics, 82–83

Thrombogenicity, 3
Thrombospondins (TSPs), 17
Tissue attachment, chemical and physical determinants, 103–105
Tissue culture polystyrene (TCPS) vs. laminin-coated surfaces, 8
Tissue engineering
  neutral networks, 98–105
  scaffolds, 162
Tissue–implant interactions, 101–105
Tissue regeneration, 162
Tissue response to porous materials, 102–103
Transforming growth factor β (TGF-β), 159
Transmembranous domain, 9
Trifluoroethanol (TFE), 151
Trophic factors, 48, 50
Tyrosine-phosphorylated proteins, 20

U

Ulex europaeus I (UEA I), 40
Unsintered hydroxyapatite/poly-L-lactide (u-HA/PLLA), 62

V

Vaccination applications, DNA release in, 153–157
VCAMs, 16
Viral gene therapy, 135
VP/AAm matrix, 95

W

Weibel-Palade bodies, 15
Wide-angle X-ray diffraction (WAXD), 195, 198
Wound healing, 158–159

X

X-ray diffraction (XRD), 194

Y

YISGR, 104

CONTENTS OF VOLUMES IN THIS SERIAL

Volume 1

J. W. Westwater, *Boiling of Liquids*
A. B. Metzner, *Non-Newtonian Technology: Fluid Mechanics, Mixing, and Heat Transfer*
R. Byron Bird, *Theory of Diffusion*
J. B. Opfell and B. H. Sage, *Turbulence in Thermal and Material Transport*
Robert E. Treybal, *Mechanically Aided Liquid Extraction*
Robert W. Schrage, *The Automatic Computer in the Control and Planning of Manufacturing Operations*
Ernest J. Henley and Nathaniel F. Barr, *Ionizing Radiation Applied to Chemical Processes and to Food and Drug Processing*

Volume 2

J. W. Westwater, *Boiling of Liquids*
Ernest F. Johnson, *Automatic Process Control*
Bernard Manowitz, *Treatment and Disposal of Wastes in Nuclear Chemical Technology*
George A. Sofer and Harold C. Weingartner, *High Vacuum Technology*
Theodore Vermeulen, *Separation by Adsorption Methods*
Sherman S. Weidenbaum, *Mixing of Solids*

Volume 3

C. S. Grove, Jr., Robert V. Jelinek, and Herbert M. Schoen, *Crystallization from Solution*
F. Alan Ferguson and Russell C. Phillips, *High Temperature Technology*
Daniel Hyman, *Mixing and Agitation*
John Beck, *Design of Packed Catalytic Reactors*
Douglass J. Wilde, *Optimization Methods*

Volume 4

J. T. Davies, *Mass-Transfer and Interfacial Phenomena*
R. C. Kintner, *Drop Phenomena Affecting Liquid Extraction*
Octave Levenspiel and Kenneth B. Bischoff, *Patterns of Flow in Chemical Process Vessels*
Donald S. Scott, *Properties of Concurrent Gas-Liquid Flow*
D. N. Hanson and G. F. Somerville, *A General Program for Computing Multistage Vapor-Liquid Processes*

Volume 5

J. F. Wehner, *Flame Processes–Theoretical and Experimental*
J. H. Sinfelt, *Bifunctional Catalysts*
S. G. Bankoff, *Heat Conduction or Diffusion with Change of Phase*
George D. Fulford, *The Flow of Liquids in Thin Films*
K. Rietema, *Segregation in Liquid–Liquid Dispersions and Its Effects on Chemical Reactions*

Volume 6

S. G. Bankoff, *Diffusion-Controlled Bubble Growth*
John C. Berg, Andreas Acrivos, and Michel Boudart, *Evaporation Convection*
H. M. Tsuchiya, A. G. Fredrickson, and R. Aris, *Dynamics of Microbial Cell Populations*
Samuel Sideman, *Direct Contact Heat Transfer between Immiscible Liquids*
Howard Brenner, *Hydrodynamic Resistance of Particles at Small Reynolds Numbers*

Volume 7

Robert S. Brown, Ralph Anderson, and Larry J. Shannon, *Ignition and Combustion of Solid Rocket Propellants*
Knud Østergaard, *Gas–Liquid–Particle Operations in Chemical Reaction Engineering*
J. M. Prausnitz, *Thermodynamics of Fluid–Phase Equilibria at High Pressures*
Robert V. Macbeth, *The Burn-Out Phenomenon in Forced-Convection Boiling*
William Resnick and Benjamin Gal-Or, *Gas–Liquid Dispersions*

Volume 8

C. E. Lapple, *Electrostatic Phenomena with Particulates*
J. R. Kittrell, *Mathematical Modeling of Chemical Reactions*
W. P. Ledet and D. M. Himmelblau, *Decomposition Procedures for the Solving of Large Scale Systems*
R. Kumar and N. R. Kuloor, *The Formation of Bubbles and Drops*

Volume 9

Renato G. Bautista, *Hydrometallurgy*
Kishan B. Mathur and Norman Epstein, *Dynamics of Spouted Beds*
W. C. Reynolds, *Recent Advances in the Computation of Turbulent Flows*
R. E. Peck and D. T. Wasan, *Drying of Solid Particles and Sheets*

Volume 10

G. E. O'Connor and T. W. F. Russell, *Heat Transfer in Tubular Fluid–Fluid Systems*
P. C. Kapur, *Balling and Granulation*

Richard S. H. Mah and Mordechai Shacham, *Pipeline Network Design and Synthesis*
J. Robert Selman and Charles W. Tobias, *Mass-Transfer Measurements by the Limiting-Current Technique*

Volume 11

Jean-Claude Charpentier, *Mass-Transfer Rates in Gas–Liquid Absorbers and Reactors*
Dee H. Barker and C. R. Mitra, *The Indian Chemical Industry—Its Development and Needs*
Lawrence L. Tavlarides and Michael Stamatoudis, *The Analysis of Interphase Reactions and Mass Transfer in Liquid–Liquid Dispersions*
Terukatsu Miyauchi, Shintaro Furusaki, Shigeharu Morooka, and Yoneichi Ikeda, *Transport Phenomena and Reaction in Fluidized Catalyst Beds*

Volume 12

C. D. Prater, J. Wei, V. W. Weekman, Jr., and B. Gross, *A Reaction Engineering Case History: Coke Burning in Thermofor Catalytic Cracking Regenerators*
Costel D. Denson, *Stripping Operations in Polymer Processing*
Robert C. Reid, *Rapid Phase Transitions from Liquid to Vapor*
John H. Seinfeld, *Atmospheric Diffusion Theory*

Volume 13

Edward G. Jefferson, *Future Opportunities in Chemical Engineering*
Eli Ruckenstein, *Analysis of Transport Phenomena Using Scaling and Physical Models*
Rohit Khanna and John H. Seinfeld, *Mathematical Modeling of Packed Bed Reactors: Numerical Solutions and Control Model Development*
Michael P. Ramage, Kenneth R. Graziano, Paul H. Schipper, Frederick J. Krambeck, and Byung C. Choi, *KINPTR (Mobil's Kinetic Reforming Model): A Review of Mobil's Industrial Process Modeling Philosophy*

Volume 14

Richard D. Colberg and Manfred Morari, *Analysis and Synthesis of Resilient Heat Exchange Networks*
Richard J. Quann, Robert A. Ware, Chi-Wen Hung, and James Wei, *Catalytic Hydrometallation of Petroleum*
Kent David, *The Safety Matrix: People Applying Technology to Yield Safe Chemical Plants and Products*

Volume 15

Pierre M. Adler, Ali Nadim, and Howard Brenner, *Rheological Models of Suspensions*
Stanley M. Englund, *Opportunities in the Design of Inherently Safer Chemical Plants*
H. J. Ploehn and W. B. Russel, *Interations between Colloidal Particles and Soluble Polymers*

Volume 16

Perspectives in Chemical Engineering: Research and Education
Clark K. Colton, *Editor*

Historical Perspective and Overview

L. E. Scriven, *On the Emergence and Evolution of Chemical Engineering*
Ralph Landau, *Academic–Industrial Interaction in the Early Development of Chemical Engineering*
James Wei, *Future Directions of Chemical Engineering*

Fluid Mechanics and Transport

L. G. Leal, *Challenges and Opportunities in Fluid Mechanics and Transport Phenomena*
William B. Russel, *Fluid Mechanics and Transport Research in Chemical Engineering*
J. R. A. Pearson, *Fluid Mechanics and Transport Phenomena*

Thermodynamics

Keith E. Gubbins, *Thermodynamics*
J. M. Prausnitz, *Chemical Engineering Thermodynamics: Continuity and Expanding Frontiers*
H. Ted Davis, *Future Opportunities in Thermodynamics*

Kinetics, Catalysis, and Reactor Engineering

Alexis T. Bell, *Reflections on the Current Status and Future Directions of Chemical Reaction Engineering*
James R. Katzer and S. S. Wong, *Frontiers in Chemical Reaction Enginerring*
L. Louis Hegedus, *Catalyst Design*

Environmental Protection and Energy

John H. Seinfeld, *Environmental Chemical Engineering*
T. W. F. Russell, *Energy and Environmental Concerns*
Janos M. Beer, Jack B. Howard, John P. Longwell, and Adel F. Sarofim, *The Role of Chemical Engineering in Fuel Manufacture and Use of Fuels*

Polymers

Matthew Tirrell, *Polymer Science in Chemical Engineering*
Richard A. Register and Stuart L. Cooper, *Chemical Engineers in Polymer Science: The Need for an Interdisciplinary Approach*

Microelectronic and Optical Material

Larry F. Thompson, *Chemical Engineering Research Opportunities in Electronic and Optical Materials Research*
Klavs F. Jensen, *Chemical Engineering in the Processing of Electronic and Optical Materials: A Discussion*

Bioengineering

James E. Bailey, *Bioprocess Engineering*
Arthur E. Humphrey, *Some Unsolved Problems of Biotechnology*

Channing Robertson, *Chemical Engineering: Its Role in the Medical and Health Sciences*

Process Engineering

Arthur W. Westerberg, *Process Engineering*
Manfred Morari, *Process Control Theory: Reflections on the Past Decade and Goals for the Next*
James M. Douglas, *The Paradigm After Next*
George Stephanopoulos, *Symbolic Computing and Artificial Intelligence in Chemical Engineering: A New Challenge*

The Identity of Our Profession

Morton M. Denn, *The Identity of Our Profession*

Volume 17

Y. T. Shah, *Design Parameters for Mechanically Agitated Reactors*
Mooson Kwauk, *Particulate Fluidization: An Overview*

Volume 18

E. James Davis, *Microchemical Engineering: The Physics and Chemistry of the Microparticle*
Selim M. Senkan, *Detailed Chemical Kinetic Modeling: Chemical Reaction Engineering of the Future*
Lorenz T. Biegler, *Optimization Strategies for Complex Process Models*

Volume 19

Robert Langer, *Polymer Systems for Controlled Release of Macromolecules, Immobilized Enzyme Medical Bioreactors, and Tissue Engineering*
J. J. Linderman, P. A. Mahama, K. E. Forsten, and D. A. Lauffenburger, *Diffusion and Probability in Receptor Binding and Signaling*
Rakesh K. Jain, *Transport Phenomena in Tumors*
R. Krishna, *A Systems Approach to Multiphase Reactor Selection*
David T. Allen, *Pollution Prevention: Engineering Design at Macro-, Meso-, and Microscales*
John H. Seinfeld, Jean M. Andino, Frank M. Bowman, Hali J. L. Forstner, and Spyros Pandis, *Tropospheric Chemistry*

Volume 20

Arthur M. Squires, *Origins of the Fast Fluid Bed*
Yu Zhiqing, *Application Collocation*
Youchu Li, *Hydrodynamics*
Li Jinghai, *Modeling*
Yu Zhiqing and Jin Yong, *Heat and Mass Transfer*
Mooson Kwauk, *Powder Assessment*

Li Hongzhong, *Hardware Development*
Youchu Li and Xuyi Zhang, *Circulating Fluidized Bed Combustion*
Chen Junwu, Cao Hanchang, and Liu Taiji, *Catalyst Regeneration in Fluid Catalytic Cracking*

Volume 21

Christopher J. Nagel, Chonghun Han, and George Stephanopoulos, *Modeling Languages: Declarative and Imperative Descriptions of Chemical Reactions and Processing Systems*
Chonghun Han, George Stephanopoulos, and James M. Douglas, *Automation in Design: The Conceptual Synthesis of Chemical Processing Schemes*
Michael L. Mavrovouniotis, *Symbolic and Quantitative Reasoning: Design of Reaction Pathways through Recursive Satisfaction of Constraints*
Christopher Nagel and George Stephanopoulos, *Inductive and Deductive Reasoning: The Case of Identifying Potential Hazards in Chemical Processes*
Keven G. Joback and George Stephanopoulos, *Searching Spaces of Discrete Soloutions: The Design of Molecules Processing Desired Physical Properties*

Volume 22

Chonghun Han, Ramachandran Lakshmanan, Bhavik Bakshi, and George Stephanopoulos, *Nonmonotonic Reasoning: The Synthesis of Operating Procedures in Chemical Plants*
Pedro M. Saraiva, *Inductive and Analogical Learning: Data-Driven Improvement of Process Operations*
Alexandros Koulouris, Bhavik R. Bakshi and George Stephanopoulos, *Empirical Learning through Neural Networks: The Wave-Net Solution*
Bhavik R. Bakshi and George Stephanopoulos, *Reasoning in Time: Modeling, Analysis, and Pattern Recognition of Temporal Process Trends*
Matthew J. Realff, *Intelligence in Numerical Computing: Improving Batch Scheduling Algorithms through Explanation-Based Learning*

Volume 23

Jeffrey J. Siirola, *Industrial Applications of Chemical Process Synthesis*
Arthur W. Westerberg and Oliver Wahnschafft, *The Synthesis of Distillation-Based Separation Systems*
Ignacio E. Grossmann, *Mixed-Integer Optimization Techniques for Algorithmic Process Synthesis*
Subash Balakrishna and Lorenz T. Biegler, *Chemical Reactor Network Targeting and Integration: An Optimization Approach*
Steve Walsh and John Perkins, *Operability and Control inn Process Synthesis and Design*

Volume 24

Raffaella Ocone and Gianni Astarita, *Kinetics and Thermodynamics in Multicomponent Mixtures*

Arvind Varma, Alexander S. Rogachev, Alexandra S. Mukasyan, and Stephen Hwang, *Combustion Synthesis of Advanced Materials: Principles and Applications*
J. A. M. Kuipers and W. P. M. van Swaaij, *Computational Fluid Dynamics Applied to Chemical Reaction Engineering*
Ronald E. Schmitt, Howard Klee, Debora M. Sparks, and Mahesh K. Podar, *Using Relative Risk Analysis to Set Priorities for Pollution Prevention at a Petroleum Refinery*

Volume 25

J. F. Davis, M. J. Piovoso, K. A. Hoo, and B. R. Bakshi, *Process Data Analysis and Interpretation*
J. M. Ottino, P. DeRoussel, S. Hansen, and D. V. Khakhar, *Mixing and Dispersion of Viscous Liquids and Powdered Solids*
Peter L. Silverston, Li Chengyue, Yuan Wei-Kang, *Application of Periodic Operation to Sulfur Dioxide Oxidation*

Volume 26

J. B. Joshi, N. S. Deshpande, M. Dinkar, and D. V. Phanikumar, *Hydrodynamic Stability of Multiphase Reactors*
Michael Nikolaou, *Model Predictive Controllers: A Critical Synthesis of Theory and Industrial Needs*

Volume 27

William R. Moser, Josef Find, Sean C. Emerson, and Ivo M. Krausz, *Engineered Synthesis of Nanostructure Materials and Catalysts*
Bruce C. Gates, *Supported Nanostructured Catalysts: Metal Complexes and Metal Clusters*
Ralph T. Yang, *Nanostructured Absorbents*
Thomas J. Webster, *Nanophase Ceramics: The Future Orthopedic and Dental Implant Material*
Yu-Ming Lin, Mildred S. Dresselhaus, and Jackie Y. Ying, *Fabrication, Structure, and Transport Properties if Nanowires*

Volume 28

Qiliang Yan and Juan J. DePablo, *Hyper-Parallel Tempering Monte Carlo and Its Applications*
Pablo G. Debenedetti, Frank H. Stillinger, Thomas M. Truskett, and Catherine P. Lewis, *Theory of Supercooled Liquids and Glasses: Energy Landscape and Statistical Geometry Perspectives*
Michael W. Deem, *A Statistical Mechanical Approach to Combinatorial Chemistry*
Venkat Ganesan and Glenn H. Fredrickson, *Fluctuation Effects in Microemulsion Reaction Media*
David B. Graves and Cameron F. Abrams, *Molecular Dynamics Simulations if Ion–Surface Interactions with Applications to Plasma Processing*
Christian M. Lastoskie and Keith E. Gubbins, *Characterization of Porous Materials Using Molecular Theory and Simulation*

Dimitrios Maroudas, *Modeling of Radical-Surface Interactions in the Plasma-Enhanced Chemical Vapor Deposition of Silicon Thin Films*
Sanat Kumar, M. Antonio Floriano, and Athanassiors Z. Panagiotopoulos, *Nanostructured Formation and Phase Separation in Surfactant Solutions*
Stanley I. Sandler, Amadeu K. Sum, and Shiang-Tai Lin, *Some Chemical Engineering Applications of Quantum Chemical Calculations*
Bernhardt L. Trout, *Car-Parrinello Methods in Chemical Engineering: Their Scope and Potential*
R. A. van Santeen and X. Rozanska, *Theory of Zeolite Catalysis*
Zhen-Gang Wang, *Morphology, Fluctuation, Metastability and Kinetics in Ordered Block Copolymers*

Volume 29

Michael V. Sefton, *The New New Biomaterials*
Kristi S. Anseth and Kristyn S. Masters, *Cell–Material Interactions*
Surya K. Mallapragada and Jennifer B. Recknor, *Polymeric Biomaterials for Nerve Regeneration*
Anthony M. Lowman, Thomas D. Dziubla, Petr Bures, and Nicholas A. Peppas, *Structural and Dynamic Response of Neutral and Intelligent Networks in Biomedical Environments*
F. Kurtis Kasper and Antonios G. Mikos, *Biomaterials and Gene Therapy*
Balaji Narasimhan and Matt J. Kipper, *Surface-Erodible Biomaterials for Drug Delivery*

ISBN 0-12-008529-1

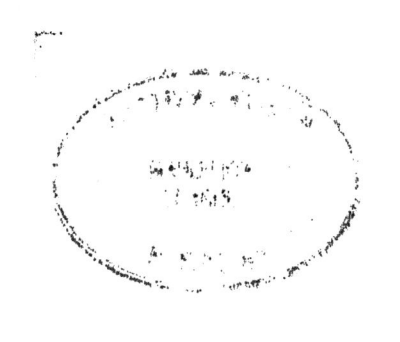